Digital Mammography

Peter Hogg • Judith Kelly
Claire Mercer
Editors

Digital Mammography

A Holistic Approach

Springer

Editors
Peter Hogg
University of Salford
Salford
UK

Judith Kelly
Breast Care Unit
Countess of Chester Hospital
NHS Foundation Trust
Chester
UK

Claire Mercer
The Nightingale Centre and
Genesis Prevention Centre
Wythenshawe Hospital
University Hospital of South Manchester
Manchester
UK

ISBN 978-3-319-38071-1 ISBN 978-3-319-04831-4 (eBook)
DOI 10.1007/978-3-319-04831-4

Springer Cham Heidelberg New York Dordrecht London

Softcover reprint of the hardcover 1st edition 2015

Printed on acid-free paper

Springer is part of Springer Science+Business Media (www.springer.com)

Foreword

This book is aimed at all those involved in breast imaging. It provides an in-depth analysis of current imaging techniques which will provide the basis of learning for those new to breast imaging; particularly those taking up this speciality for the first time. For those already experienced in the field, the breadth of subject areas covered will make this an excellent reference text.

Technology has changed significantly over recent years in all aspects of breast imaging but particularly as digital mammography has replaced traditional analogue film. The techniques involved for the processes of both image acquisition and image reporting are, whilst fundamentally similar, also profoundly different, and this book is timely in addressing these issues.

The inclusion of a patient's story is both innovative and extremely moving. Understanding the patient's perspective will assist all breast professionals in their work, and Sue and her husband provide great insight into many areas of practice often neglected. Of particular note is the requirement for everything that happens to patients to be explained in full, together with the benefit of human contact and conversation at times of stress. Social media impacts on almost all aspects of the modern world, and it is refreshing to see the impact of this on breast imaging services analysed here.

There has been significant recent controversy concerning the benefits and harms of screening programmes for breast cancer. The chapter which explores this provides a balanced overview of the current debate with a further section devoted to describing these services in Europe. At a time of increasing interest in personalised healthcare, a separate chapter on breast density, its evolution and significance makes important reading. This topic will undoubtedly become more important following the American adoption of processes to inform all women of their mammographic breast density assessment. Explaining these findings to women may become part of routine UK and European practice in years to come.

This book is likely to become a standard text for breast imaging professionals and, if read by many, will improve the service we provide.

Norwich, UK — Erika Denton

Preface

Extensive implementation of full field digital mammography in recent years, coupled with an increasing desirability within healthcare to continue delivering patient-centred care, provided the impetus for writing this text. It is hoped it will supplement the imperative within professional practice to adopt a continuing reflective approach in providing such care. Historically, much of the evidence underpinning mammographic practice was intended for analogue systems, hence the need for a comprehensive and new evidence base to underpin the principles of digital mammography and optimise the potential of this technology.

In addition, significant gaps in the guidance informing aspects of mammographic practice have been identified, and recent research attempts to address some of these deficits. A notable example is the variation in compression force applied by practitioners on serial mammograms and the important question of how much compression force is necessary to produce a diagnostic mammogram [1]. Conventional wisdom suggested that applying as much compression force as tolerable contributed to the best possible image quality. However, a recent study demonstrated that continuing to apply compression force does not reduce breast thickness in a linear fashion. In fact, too high a compression force may not achieve the desired impact on image quality and might be counterproductive to the patient/client experience [2]. Significantly, evidence also suggests that some women are deterred from attending for a mammogram due to the discomfort or pain that may be experienced and therefore, *ipso facto*, a minimum amount of compression force is desirable, provided image quality and radiation dose reduction are not compromised [3]. This issue is extremely important particularly within breast screening since the success of any screening programme depends on uptake [4].

Rapid technological advances enabling easy access to web-based information have resulted in the public becoming increasingly well-informed and empowered regarding their healthcare. Expectations of healthcare are high. These expectations include listening to the patient and taking account of their perspectives. Attention to such detail – moving towards the holistic approach, illustrated and evidence-based in this text – should assist in gaining the trust and confidence of the patient/client and result in an optimal experience for both practitioner and patient/client. For this reason a chapter has been included in this book from a patient who has experienced breast cancer. Her detailed description, recalling the diagnostic and treatment pathways, is greatly appreciated.

It is now widely recognised that healthcare should be holistic, an approach which takes account of the physical, mental, emotional and social factors of patients/clients. In a mammographic context this implies delivering tailored care to the 'whole person' (who is not simply an accessory to the breast being imaged), whilst being acutely aware that such a procedure can be a significant ordeal for many people. Again, this is the rationale for including comprehensive information relating to the care component of this book, which is highly patient-centred. The challenge for practitioners today is how to choreograph their delivered care – balancing art and science in their approaches to patients. The current healthcare culture of quantification-at-all-costs and scientific management can, on occasion, overestimate the science and impoverish the art [5]. Perhaps most novel of all in this book is the chapter covering tissue viability which can sometimes be a significant issue when mammography results in skin tearing or damage particularly around the infra-mammary angle regions.

Though there is a heavy use of UK practice and policy, this book has a multinational authorship and it is intended to appeal to an international readership. Whilst it is recognised that aspects of mammographic practice vary considerably across different regions and countries, many issues and principles within healthcare remain generic and are transferable across populations.

An important issue to address for a wide readership is the terminology used in clinical practice. For example, the individual performing the mammogram is described variously as radiographer, mammographer, mammography practitioner, and radiologic technologist – all performing similar roles. In this book we describe the person performing the imaging as the practitioner. Similar differences exist in naming the subject of the mammography procedure as woman, client, patient and man, and this may also vary according to whether the individual is undergoing a screening or symptomatic mammogram. Within this book the term 'client' is often used for screening purposes; similarly patient is often used for symptomatic purposes.

Our intention has been to produce a comprehensive text which is informative, based on the latest published evidence, having direct relevance for a range of healthcare professional groups who work in the delivery of mammography services, not necessarily exclusively those performing clinical mammography. It may also provide valuable reference material for those who work within other breast imaging modalities, such as ultrasound or MRI. Whatever the role or professional background, it is hoped that healthcare workers will approach this text with an enquiring mind and be willing to challenge established practices and identify further, as yet unaddressed, gaps in the research base. Whilst we attempted to include all the main subjects necessary in the delivery of a state-of-the-art mammographic service, inevitably it is impossible to cover every topic in depth in a single text. An extensive range of references is included to facilitate further reading and literature searches. In addition, readers are encouraged to avail themselves of up-to-date texts or journal articles specific to their particular area of interest.

The editors would like to express their sincere gratitude to all the authors of this book, without which none of this would have been possible.

The editors would like to express their sincere gratitude to the following people for their assistance in reviewing some of the chapters

William Mairs, Consultant Physicist, The Christie Hospital, Manchester UK
Raed Ali, PhD Student, University of Salford; Assistant Lecturer, University of Kufa, Iraq

Salford, UK — Peter Hogg
Chester, UK — Judith Kelly
Manchester, UK — Claire E. Mercer

References

1. Mercer C.E, Szczepura K, Kelly J, Millington SR, Denton ERE, Borgen R, Hilton B, Hogg P. A 6-year study of mammographic compression force: practitioner variation within and between screening sites. Radiography. 2014. http://dx.doi.org/10.1016/j.radi.2014.07.004.
2. Hogg, P, Taylor, M, Szczepura, K, Mercer, C and Denton, E 2013, Pressure and breast thickness in mammography an exploratory calibration study', British journal of Radiology, 86, 2, 1–7. http://usir.salford.ac.uk/29530/.
3. Whelehan P, Evans A, Wells M, Macgillivray S. The effect of mammography pain on repeat participation in breast cancer screening: a systematic review. Breast. 2013; 22(4):389–94.
4. Marmot M, Altman DG, Cameron DA, Dewer JA, Thompson SG, Wilcox M. The benefits and harms of breast cancer screening: an independent review. Lancet. 2012; 380(9855):1778–86.
5. Zigmond D. Five executive follies. How commodification imperils compassion in person healthcare. J Holist Healthc. 2011;9:7–10.

Contents

Part I Introduction and Background

1 **Anatomy of the Breast** 3
Alison J. Darlington

2 **Breast Density and Influencing Factors** 11
Dawn M. McDonald

3 **Aetiology and Epidemiology of Breast Cancer** 17
Lisa Hackney

4 **Other Breast Diseases** 27
Lisa Hackney and Susan Williams

5 **Signs and Symptoms of Breast Cancer with Management Pathways** 49
Zebby Rees and Susan E. Garnett

6 **Disease Progression: Local and Distal Spread (Mechanisms)** 53
Susan Williams

7 **Mammography Screening: Philosophy – Evidence for and against** 59
John A. Dewar

8 **Screening Programmes for Breast Cancer in Europe** 67
Solveig S.H. Hofvind and Chris J.M. de Wolf

Part II Caring for Patients and Clients

9 **Sue's Story: The Big Journey** 77
Susan Cliffe and Colin Cliffe

10 **Psychological Considerations in Attending for Mammography Screening** 83
Anne Pearson and Ashley Weinberg

11 **Emotional Intelligence** 89
Stuart J. Mackay

12 **Client-Practitioner Interactions within Breast Care Services** 97
Julie M. Nightingale, Fred J. Murphy, and Rita M. Borgen

13 **The Use of Digital Health Technology and Social Media to Support Breast Screening** 105
Leslie Robinson, Marie Griffiths, Julie Wray, Cathy Ure, Julie R. Stein-Hodgins, and Geraldine Shires

14 **Pain in Mammography** 113
Patsy Whelehan

15 **Tissue Viability and Skin Tearing in Mammography** 119
Melanie Stephens

Part III Equipment

16 **Mammography Equipment** 125
C. John Kotre and Cláudia Sá dos Reis

17 **Equipment Quality Control** 143
Cláudia Sá dos Reis

18 **Radiation Dose in Mammography** 153
Ingrid Helen Ryste Hauge

19 **Mammographic Density** 163
Solveig S.H. Hofvind, Gunvor Gipling Waade, and Sue Astley

Part IV Imaging Techniques

20 **Recording Clinical and Client Information Prior to Imaging** 171
Bernadette Bickley

21 **Practical Mammography** 175
Claire E. Mercer, Catherine A. Hill, Allison Kelly, and Helen L. Smith

22 **Mammographic Compression: A Need for Mechanical Standardisation** 189
Jerry E. de Groot, Woutjan Branderhorst, Ralph Highnam, Ariane Chan, Marcela Böhm-Vélez, M.J.M. Broeders, C.A. Grimbergen, and G.J. den Heeten

23 **Repetitive Strain Injury – RSI** 195
Claire D. Borrelli

24 **Supplementary Mammographic Projections** 203
Judith Kelly

25 **Magnification and Compression Views** 211
Victoria L. Hipperson

26 **Specimen Imaging** 219
Amanda Coates

27 **Imaging the Augmented Breast** 223
Claire D. Borrelli

28 Imaging Bariatric, Post Surgical and Limited Mobility Clients 231
Lisa Bisset

29 Male Mammography 239
Susan E. Garnett

30 Digital Breast Tomosynthesis 241
Yit Y. Lim and Anthony J. Maxwell

31 Reflection on the Oslo Tomosynthesis Screening Trial 247
Robin Lee Hammond, Randi Gullien, and Per Skaane

32 Purpose of Interventional Procedures 251
Susan E. Garnett

33 Stereotactic Image Guided Interventional Techniques 255
Rita M. Borgen

34 Contrast Enhanced Investigations 263
Eva M. Fallenberg

Part V Service Quality Assurance

35 Radiographic Service Quality 273
Caroline J. Dobson and Clare S. Alison

36 Observer Studies in Mammography 291
Peter Hogg, Sara Millington, David Manning, and Hussien Mraity

Index 303

Contributors

Clare S. Alison, Clinical Instructor, Breast Imaging, Thirlestaine Breast Centre, Cheltenham, UK

Sue Astley, Centre for Imaging Sciences, Institute of Population Health, Manchester Academic Health Science Centre, The University of Manchester, Manchester, UK

Bernadette Bickley, Consultant Practitioner in Breast Imaging, South Staffs Breast Screening, Stafford, UK

Lisa Bisset, Consultant Radiographer, Dorset Breast Screening Unit, Poole General Hospital, Poole, UK

Marcela Bohm-Velez, Weinstein Imaging Associates, Pittsburgh, PA, USA

Rita M. Borgen, Consultant Radiographer, Breast Screening Service, East Lancashire Hospitals NHS Trust, Burnley, UK

Claire D. Borrelli, Head of Education and Clinical Training, Lead Radiographer for the UK - Cancer Screening and Prevention, St George's National Breast Education Centre, The Rose Centre, St George's Healthcare NHS Trust, London, UK

Woutjan Branderhorst, Post-doctoral researcher, Biomedical Engineering and Physics, Academic Medical Center, Amsterdam, The Netherlands

M.J.M. Broeders, LRCB Dutch Reference Center for Screening, Nijmegen, The Netherlands

Ariane Chan, Volpara Solutions, Wellington, New Zealand

Amanda Coates, Consultant Radiographer, Breast Imaging, Mid Yorkshire Hospitals Trust, Pinderfields Hospital, Wakefield, UK

Alison J. Darlington, Consultant Radiographer Breast Imaging, The Victoria Breast Unit, The Royal Oldham Hospital, Pennine Acute NHS Trust, Oldham, UK

Jerry E. de Groot, PhD candidate Biomedical Engineering and Physics, Academic Medical Center, Amsterdam, The Netherlands

Chris J.M. de Wolf, MD, Consultant Quality Assurance Breast Screening, Swiss Cancer Screening, Bern, Switzerland

G.J. den Heeten, Department of Radiology, Academic Medical Center, Amsterdam, The Netherlands

LRCB Dutch Reference Center for Screening, Nijmegen, The Netherlands

John A. Dewar, Honorary Professor of Clinical Oncology, Department of Surgery and Molecular Oncology, University of Dundee, Chipping Norton, UK

Caroline J. Dobson, Superintendent Radiographer, Breast Imaging, Thirlestaine Breast Centre, Cheltenham, UK

Cláudia Sá dos Reis, Department of Radiography, Associate Professor, Escola Superior de Tecnologia da Saúde de Lisboa (ESTeSL), Lisbon School of Health Technology, Lisbon, Portugal

Eva Fallenberg, Clinic of Radiology, Charite-Universitätsmedizin Berlin, Berlin, Germany

Susan E. Garnett, Consultant Radiographer, Breast Unit, Ground Floor West Wing University Hospital, Coventry, UK

Marie Griffiths, Reader, Salford Business School, University of Salford, Salford, UK

C.A. Grimbergen, Biomedical Engineering and Physics, Academic Medical Center, Amsterdam, The Netherlands

Randi Gullien, Senior Radiographer, Department of Radiology and Nuclear Medicine, Breast Imaging Centre, Oslo University Hospital, Oslo, Norway

Lisa Hackney, Consultant Radiographer, Breast Care Unit, University Hospital of North Staffordshire, Stoke-on-Trent, UK

Robin Lee Hammond, Lead Mammographer, Mammography Screening, Department of Radiology and Nuclear Medicine, Breast Imaging Centre, Oslo University Hospital, Oslo, Norway

Ingrid Helen Ryste Hauge, Researcher, Department of Monitoring and Research, Section for Radiation Research, Norwegian Radiation Protection Authority, Oesteraas, Norway

Ralph Highnam, Volpara Solutions, Wellington, New Zealand

Catherine A. Hill, Training and Education Lead, Breast Imaging, The Nightingale Centre & Genesis Prevention Centre, Wythenshawe Hospital, University Hospital South Manchester, Wythenshawe, Manchester, UK

Victoria L. Hipperson, Consultant Radiographer, Breast Imaging, Whipps Cross Hospital, Barts Health NHS Trust, London, UK

Solveig S.H. Hofvind, Head of the Norwegian Breast Cancer Screening Program, Cancer Registry of Norway and Oslo and Akershus University College of Applied Sciences, Oslo, Norway

Peter Hogg, Professor of Radiography, School of Health Sciences, University of Salford, Salford, UK

Allison Kelly, Senior Mammographer, Breast Imaging, The Nightingale Centre and Genesis Prevention Centre, Wythenshawe Hospital, University Hospital South Manchester, Wythenshawe, Manchester, UK

Judith Kelly, Breast Imaging Consultant, Breast Care Unit, The Countess of Chester Hospitals NHS Foundation Trust, Chester, UK

C. John Kotre, Consultant Clinical Scientist, Christie Medical Physics and Engineering, The Christie NHS Foundation Trust, Manchester, UK

Yit Y. Lim, Consultant Radiologist, The Nightingale Centre and Genesis Prevention Centre, University Hospital of South Manchester, Manchester, UK

Dawn M. McDonald, Consultant Mammographer, Breast Unit, Worthing Hospital, Worthing, West Sussex, UK

Stuart J. Mackay, Senior Lecturer and Head of Directorate, Medical Imaging and Radiotherapy Directorate, School of Health Sciences, University of Liverpool, Liverpool, UK

David Manning, Visiting Professor, Department of Radiography, University of Salford, Salford, UK

Lancaster Medical School, Faculty of Health & Medicine, Furness College, Lancaster University, Lancaster, UK

Anthony J. Maxwell, Consultant Academic Breast Radiologist, The Nightingale and Genesis Prevention Centre, University Hospital of South Manchester, Manchester, UK

Claire E. Mercer, Breast Imaging, The Nightingale Centre & Genesis Prevention Centre, Wythenshawe Hospital, University Hospital South Manchester, Wythenshawe, Manchester, UK

Sara Millington, Advanced Practitioner, Breast Care Unit, The Countess of Chester Hospitals NHS Foundation Trust, Chester, UK

Hussien Mraity, PhD student, Department of Physics, College of Science, University of Kufa, Kufa, Iraq

School of Health Sciences, Allerton Building, University of Salford, Salford, UK

Fred J. Murphy, Senior Lecturer, School of Health Sciences, University of Salford, Salford, UK

Julie M. Nightingale, Director of Radiography and Occupational Therapy, School of Health Sciences, University of Salford, Salford, UK

Anne Pearson, Psychology Lecturer, Department of Psychology, University of Salford, Salford, UK

Zebby Rees, Consultant Breast Radiographer, The Breast Centre, University Hospital Llandough, Cardiff, UK

Leslie Robinson, Senior Lecturer, Department of Radiography, University of Salford, Salford, UK

Geraldine Shires, Senior Radiographer, Nightingale Centre, University Hospital of South Manchester (Wythenshawe Hospital), Manchester, UK

Per Skaane, Professor, Department of Radiology and Nuclear Medicine, Breast Imaging Centre, Oslo University Hospital, Oslo, Norway

Helen L. Smith, Consultant Radiographer, Breast Care Unit, Royal Lancaster Infirmary, University Hospitals of Morecambe Bay NHS Foundation Trust, Lancaster, Lancashire, UK

Julie R. Stein-Hodgins, Mammographer, Breast Unit, Bolton Trust, Bolton, UK

Melanie Stephens, Senior Lecturer in Adult Nursing, School of Nursing, Midwifery, Social Work and Social Sciences, University of Salford, Salford, UK

Cathy Ure, Postgraduate Student, Department of Media Psychology, University of Salford, Salford, UK

Gunvor Gipling Waade, Department of Radiography, University of Salford, Student MSc Biomedicine, Oslo and Akershus University College, Oslo, Norway

College of Health & Social Care, University of Salford, Salford, UK

Ashley Weinberg, Senior Lecturer in Psychology, Department of Psychology, University of Salford, Salford, UK

Patsy Whelehan, Senior Research Radiographer, Medical Research Institute, Ninewells Hospital and Medical School, University of Dundee, Dundee, UK

Susan Williams, Consultant Radiographer, Breast Imaging Treatment Centre, Royal Shrewsbury Hospital, Shrewsbury, UK

Julie Wray, Senior Lecturer, School of Nursing, Midwifery, Social Work and Social Science, University of Salford, Salford, UK

Terminology and Abbreviations

Terminology

Client	The representative term used for women, men, patients and clients
Image receptor	Image platform table to which the breast is placed upon
Practitioner	This term is used to encompass assistant practitioners, mammographers, practitioners and advanced practitioners who specialise in mammography

Abbreviations

ACR	American College of Radiology
ADH	Atypical ductal hyperplasia
AEC	Automatic exposure control
AGR	Average glandular dose
ALARA	As low as reasonably achievable
ALH	Atypical lobular hyperplasia
ANDI	Aberrations in the normal development and involution of the breast
AP	Assistant practitioners
a-Se	Amorphous selenium
ATM	Ataxia telangiectasia mutated
BI-RADS	Breast Imaging-Reporting and Data System
BMI	Body mass index
BRCA1	Breast cancer gene 1
BRCA2	Breast cancer gene 2
BRIP1	BRCA1 interacting protein C-terminal helicase 1
C2DE	Social group: 'blue-collar'/'working class'
CC	Cranio-caudal view
CCD	Charge-coupled devices
CHEK2	Checkpoint kinase 2
CI	Confidence interval
cm	Centimetres
CNR	Contrast to noise ratio
CPD	Continued professional development
CR	Computerised radiography
CT	Computerised tomography
daN	decaNewtons
DBT	Digital breast tomosynthesis
DCIS	Ductal carcinoma in situ

DICOM	Digital imaging and communications in medicine
DoH	Department of Health
DR	Digital radiography
DSN	Digital social network
DVDs	Digital versatile disc
EAR	Excellent, acceptable, repeat
ECI-U	Emotional competence inventory-university version
EFOMP	European Federation of Organisations in Medical Physics
EFTA	European Free Trade Association
EI	Emotional intelligence
EP	European protocol
EPUAP	European Pressure Ulcer Advisory Panel
EU	European Union
EUREF	European Reference Organisation for Quality Assured Breast Screening and Diagnostic Services
FAQ	Frequently asked question
FDA	Food and Drug Administration
FFDM	Full field digital mammography
FN	False negative
FNA	Fine needle aspiration
FOM	Figure of merit
FP	False positive
GDU	Good, diagnostic, un-diagnostic
GP	General practitioner
GSDF	Greyscale standard display function
Gy	Gray
HRT	Hormone replacement therapy
HVL	Half value layer
IAEA	International Atomic Energy Agency
IASP	International Association for the Study of Pain
IMF	Infra-mammary fold
IPEM	Institute of Physics and Engineering in Medicine
IQ	Image quality
IR	Image receptor
IRMER	Ionising Radiation (Medical Exposure) Regulations
JND	Just noticeable difference
K	Kerma
KeV	Kiloelectronvolt
kPa	Kilopascal
KPI	Key performance indicator
kV	Kilovolts
kVp	Kilovolt peak
LCD	Liquid-crystal display
LCIS	Lobular carcinoma *in situ*
MD	Mammographic density
MDT	Multi-disciplinary team
MGD	Mean glandular dose
mGy	Milligray

MLO	Medio-lateral oblique view
mm	Millimetres
Mo/Mo	Molybdenum-molybdenum
Mo/Rh	Molybdenum/rhodium
MP	Megapixels
MQSA	Mammography Quality and Standards Act
MR	Magnetic resonance
MRI	Magnetic resonance imaging
MRMC	Multiple reader, multiple case
MSCEIT	Mayer, Salovey and Caruso Emotional Intelligence Test
MSKD	Musculoskeletal disorders
N	Newtons
NCI	National Cancer Institute
NHS	National Health Service
NHSBSP	National Health Service Breast Screening Programme
NL	Needle localisation
NPUAP	National Pressure Ulcer Advisory Panel
NRS	Numerical rating scale
PALB2	Partner and localizer of BRCA2
PASH	Pseudoangiomatous stromal hyperplasia
PERFORMS	Personal Performance in Mammographic Screening
PGMI	Perfect, good, moderate, inadequate
PMMA	Poly-methyl methacrylate
PNL	Posterior nipple line
PROCAS	Predicting risk of breast cancer at screening
QA	Quality assurance
QC	Quality control
Rh/Rh	Rhodium/rhodium
ROC	Receiver operating characteristics
ROI	Region of interest
RSI	Repetitive strain injury
s	Second
SCB	Stereotactic core biopsy
SCM	Screen-film mammography
SdNR	Signal difference to noise ratio
SDT	Signal detection theory
SEGs	Socio-economic groups
SFM	Screen film mammography
SMS	Short message service
SNR	Signal to noise ratio
STAR	Skin tear audit research
STF	Signal transfer function
STP	Signal transfer property
T/F	Target/filter
TC	Technical recall
TDLU	Terminal ductal lobular units
TEIQue	Trait emotional intelligence questionnaire
TN	True negative

TP	True positive
TP	Technical repeat
TP53	Tumour protein 53
TR	Technical recall
2AFC	Two-alternative forced choice
UK	United Kingdom
UKNHSBSS	United Kingdom National Health Service Breast Screening Service
USA	United States of America
VAB	Vacuum assisted biopsy
VAS	Visual analogue scale
VRS	Verbal rating scale
W/Ag	Tungsten/silver
W/Rh	Tungsten/rhodium
Wi-Fi	Local area wireless technology (Trademarked name)
θ	Projection angle
μGy	Microgray

Part I

Introduction and Background

1 Anatomy of the Breast

Alison J. Darlington

Introduction

This chapter aims to describe breast anatomy and relate it to mammographic appearances where appropriate. Breasts are made up of fat and glandular tissue, with nerves, arteries and veins, and connective tissue that provides the support structure. Breast anatomy is such that the internal and external support structures enable the breast to be mobile inferiorly and at the lateral border. The superior and medial aspects are relatively fixed. This allows the breast to be positioned for mammography.

The breast is a modified apocrine sweat gland. It develops at puberty and is sited on the anterior chest wall overlying the pectoralis major muscle between the 2nd to 6th ribs vertically and from the sternum medially to the mid axillary line laterally. Various physiological changes occur throughout life in response to hormonal stimulation, pregnancy and lactation and eventually a process of involution takes place. These changes are apparent on mammography and should be understood in order to appreciate the visual impact on mammograms.

A.J. Darlington
Consultant Radiographer Breast Imaging,
The Victoria Breast Unit, The Royal Oldham Hospital,
Pennine Acute NHS Trust, Rochdale Road,
Oldham OL1 2JH, UK
e-mail: Alison.darlington@pat.nhs.uk

Embryology and Development

The breast is composed of a collection of glands arising from the epidermis during foetal development. They are sited between the deep and superficial fascia of the anterior thorax which is derived from the dermis. The nipple is a local proliferation of the stratum spinosum of the epidermis.

Breast development begins during the second month of gestation, two lines of thickened ectoderm form on the ventral body wall of the foetus; these extend from the axilla to the groin as illustrated in Fig. 1.1 and are called the milk lines. Mammary glands can develop at any point along these. By the 9th week of foetal development this ridge regresses: usually leaving a single functional bud in the pectoral region, which persists and, at puberty, develops into an adult mammary gland, however, in 2–6 % of the population ectopic or accessory breast tissue may be present along the milk line. This may or may not have a visible nipple, but should be borne in mind during breast imaging as breast disease can develop wherever breast tissue is present.

The glandular component of the breast develops from the ectoderm. It arises from local thickening of the epidermis, 15–20 groups of ectodermal cells grow into the underlying mesoderm (dermis) during the 12th week of gestation. These groups of cells then develop spaces that

P. Hogg et al. (eds.), *Digital Mammography: A Holistic Approach*,
DOI 10.1007/978-3-319-04831-4_1, © Springer International Publishing Switzerland 2015

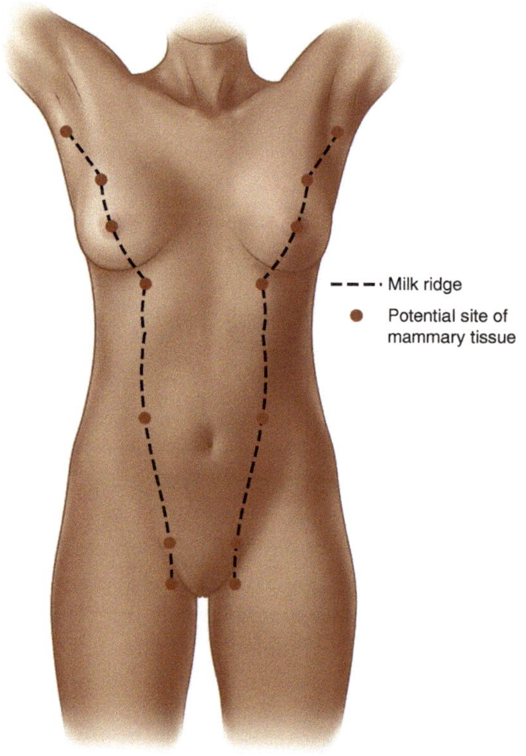

Fig. 1.1 Illustration of milk (ridge) line

will become the lactiferous ducts. The nipple initially develops as a shallow epidermal indentation which becomes everted near term.

The connective tissue stroma of the breast forms from the mesoderm, which also forms the dermis of the skin and the superficial fascia. Fibres forming the Cooper's suspensory ligaments develop from both layers. At birth males and females have the same breast anatomy. In the female, at puberty, hormonal stimuli cause the breast to develop, initially oestrogen causes fat to be deposited in the breast, and the lactiferous milk ducts to enlarge.

Following the onset of menstruation the ovaries begin to produce progesterone and this causes lobules and acini or milk glands to develop at the ends of the lactiferous ducts. The breasts develop from the buds sited bilaterally on the anterior chest wall overlying the pectoralis major muscle and once formed will lie between the 2nd to 6th ribs vertically and from the sternum medially to the mid axillary line laterally. The process of development usually takes about 3–5 years.

Male breast development, when present, is termed gynaecomastia. This condition arises as a response to hormonal imbalances which can occur at puberty or in later life as a result of disease, medication, recreational drug use or excessive alcohol consumption. The condition is investigated in the same way as female breast disease utilising mammography and ultrasound. Pseudogynaecomastia occurs when fat is deposited on the anterior chest wall under the nipple areolar complex and looks very similar outwardly to true gynaecomastia, however, in gynaecomastia proper breast tissue development is evident, in pseudogynaecomastia the enlargement is purely due to adipose tissue.

Macroscopic and Microscopic Anatomy

Once fully developed the breast is 'tear drop' shaped. The breast itself can be described in terms of both its external and internal composition and by its macroscopic and microscopic anatomy.

Externally the breast comprises of:

- The nipple
- The areolar
- Skin
- Inframammary Fold
- Montgomery's Glands (Tubercles)

Internally the breast comprises of:

- Glandular Tissue – 15–20 lobes
- Lactiferous Ducts
- Lactiferous Sinuses (Ampullae)
- Terminal Ductal Lobular Units (TDLU)
- Adipose Tissue
- Superficial Fascia
- Deep Fascia
- Retromammary Space
- Cooper's Ligaments
- Blood vessels

Figure 1.2 illustrates the gross anatomical structures of the breast

It is important to understand the external anatomy when positioning the breast for mammography and the internal anatomy when assessing the mammographic image. On mammography the fat

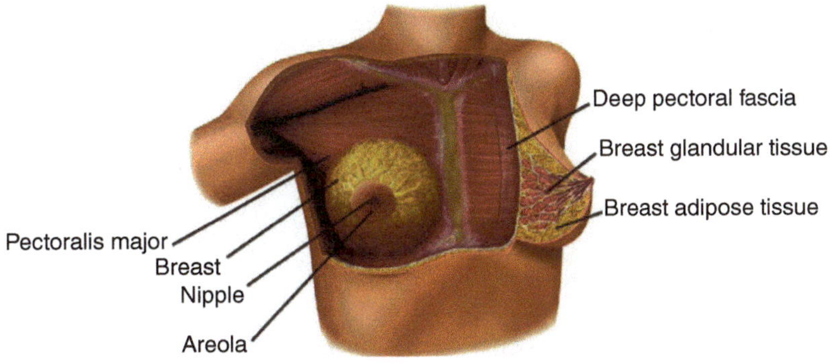

Fig. 1.2 Overview of external and internal breast anatomy (Reprinted with permission from: Shiffman MA, Di Giuseppe A. *Cosmetic Surgery*. Springer, 2013)

contained within the breast is radiolucent whilst the glandular component appears as areas of increased density.

Macroscopic Anatomy

The breast can be macroscopically divided into two main parts. The glandular component is the first of these and is concerned with milk production. The second part consists of all the other tissues that make up and support the breast. These include fat, fascia (connective tissue), and muscles.

Breast tissue extends into the low axilla as a triangular shaped projection – this portion of the breast is called the axillary tail or 'Tail of Spence'. The glandular component consists of 15–20 lobes which radiate out from the nipple. Each one of these is made up of 10–100 lobules which contain multiple acini - where milk is produced and stored during lactation.

These are drained by a network of small ducts (intralobular ducts) which come together to form a single duct draining each lobule (interlobular duct). The interlobular ducts in turn join to form intralobar ducts which jointly form a single lactiferous duct which drains that lobe. The purpose of the ducts is to transport milk; the lactiferous ducts dilate just under the nipple to form the lactiferous sinus or ampulla and then narrow and terminate at the surface of the nipple. The lobes are separated by fibrous septae and connective tissue stroma.

The skin overlying the breast is typically 0.5–2.0 mm in thickness. Beneath the skin is a superficial layer of fascia that divides into the superficial and deep layers as it reaches the breast. Between these layers the breast proper develops. The deep layer of fascia lies directly on the fascia of the pectoralis major muscle. This allows slight movement of the breast on the chest wall. The breast is supported by the Cooper's ligaments, and also by the skin, deep and superficial layers of the fascia and pectoralis major muscle. The superficial fascia is covered by a layer of adipose tissue 2–2.5 cm thick and is attached to the skin by the Cooper's Ligaments which pierce the fat. The retro mammary space lies between the deep fascia of the breast and the fascia of the pectoralis major muscle and is filled by loose connective tissue. The main internal components of the breast and the corresponding mammographic features are demonstrated in Fig. 1.3.

Externally the whole of the breast is covered by skin; the skin of the nipple areolar complex contains sweat glands, sebaceous glands and hair follicles. The nipple promontory is surrounded by a circular area of pigmented skin called the areolar. Montgomery's glands are sited around, but not on the nipple, and are transitional between sweat and lactiferous glands. They lubricate the nipple during lactation and are visible as small bumps on the areolar. The infra mammary fold is the lower border of the breast where the breast tissue meets the chest wall.

Most women have a degree of breast asymmetry; that is the size, shape and position on the chest wall differs slightly from right to left. Nipple characteristics also vary greatly.

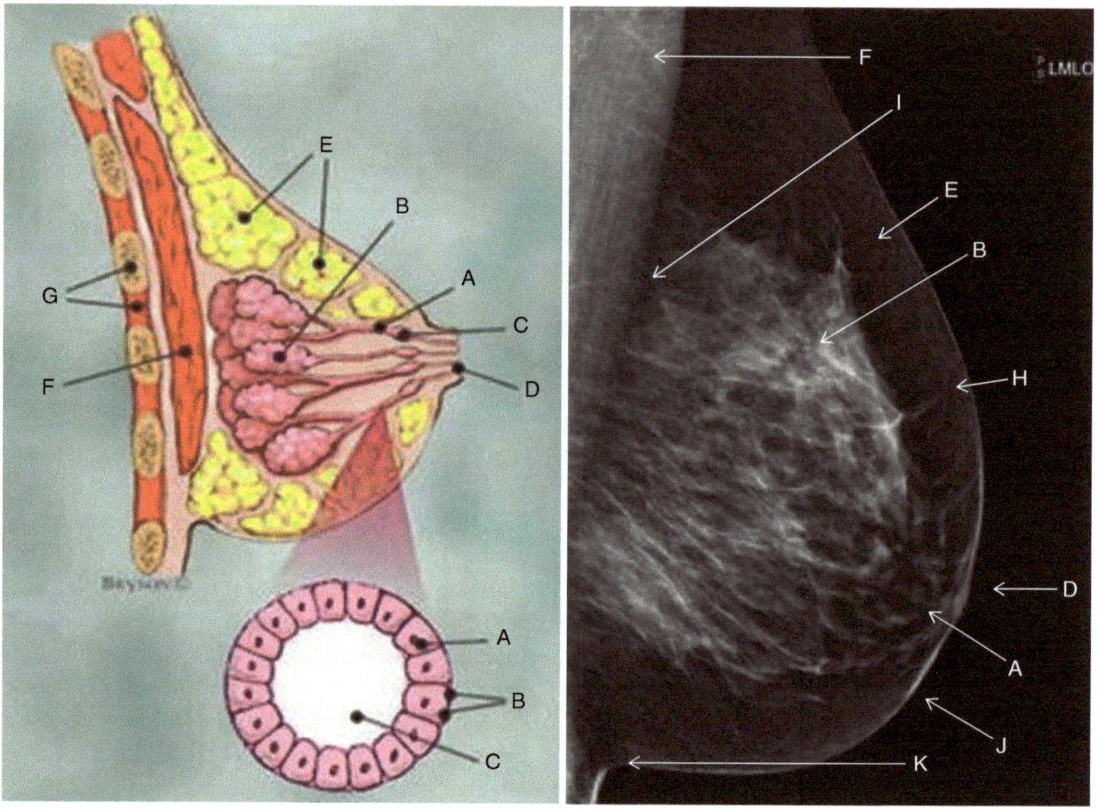

A Lactiferous duct
B Lobules
C Cross section of lactiferous duct
D Nipple
E Adipose tissue
F Pectoralis major muscle
G Chest wall / ribs
H Cooper's ligaments
I Retromammary space
J Skin
K Inframammary fold

Fig. 1.3 Internal anatomy of the breast: schematic and mammographic illustrations (Reprinted with permission from A new approach for breast skin-line estimation in mammograms, from Sun Y, Suri JS, Leo Desautels JE, Rangayyan RM. *Pattern Analysis and Applications.* Springer Verlag, London, 2009, Vol 9. Issue 1, 34–47)

Microscopic Anatomy

Microscopic description of the breast centres on the TDLU. This is the functional unit of the breast and is composed of acini, an intralobular terminal duct and an extralobular duct. Over 90 % of breast carcinomas originate in these units as do many benign breast diseases.

The acini and ducts are made up of three layers:

- Basement Membrane
- Myoepithelial Layer
- Epithelial Lining

The epithelial layer is usually only one cell thick but if this becomes two or three cells thick it is called hyperplasia. Further proliferation is categorised according to how many layers of cells are present and how atypical the cells appear; these conditions range from atypical ductal hyperplasia to ductal carcinoma in situ.

The basement membrane acts as a barrier to the spread of a cancer. A carcinoma is termed invasive if this is breached. Figure 1.4 shows a simplified diagram of the structure of a TDLU.

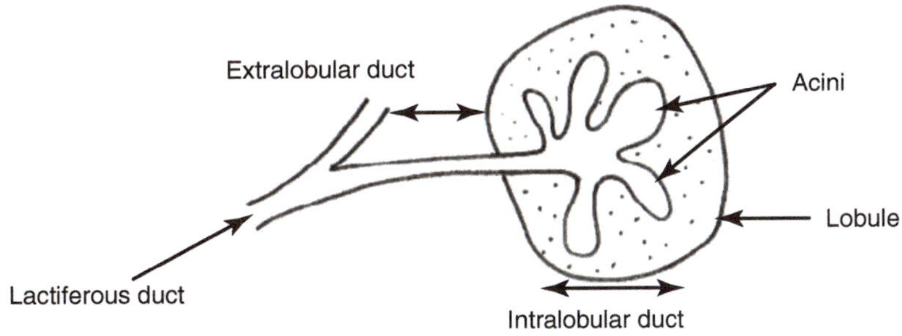

Fig. 1.4 Illustration of Terminal Ductal Lobular Unit (TDLU)

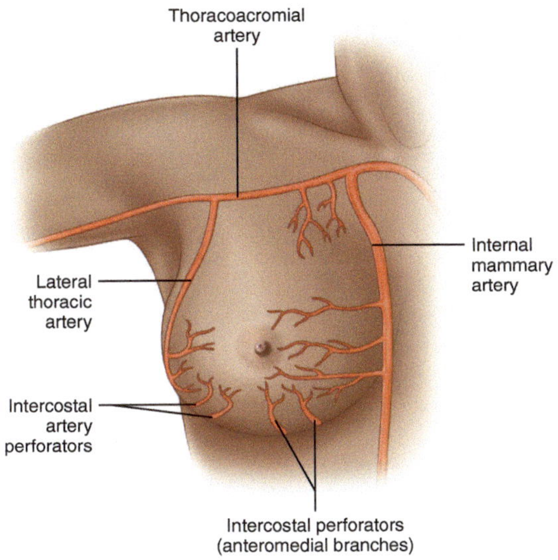

Fig. 1.5 Illustration of vascular supply to the breast

Vascular Supply

Arterial Supply

The blood supply to the breast skin comes from the subdermal plexus, which is in communication with deeper underlying vessels supplying the breast parenchyma. The main arterial supply is from perforating branches of the internal mammary artery (most notably the second to fifth perforators). The superomedial perforator supply, arising from the internal mammary artery, accounts for around 60 % of the total breast arterial blood supply. Additional arterial supply is derived from the thoracoacromial artery, the lateral thoracic artery and the intercostal arteries. Figure 1.5 gives a pictorial representation of the breast arterial vasculature.

Venous Drainage

Venous drainage of the breast is mainly through the axillary vein, with some through the internal mammary and thoracic veins. In general, the venous drainage system of the breast follows the arterial system. The superficial venous system of the breast drains into the internal thoracic vein. The deep venous system drains into the perforating branches of the internal thoracic vein, lateral thoracic, axillary vein, and upper intercostal veins. A circular venous plexus lies around the areola.

Innervation

The nerve supply to the breast is from the anterior and lateral branches of the second to sixth intercostal (T2–6) nerves. The nipple supply is complex but is mainly from the anterior branch of the lateral cutaneous ramus of T4. Nerve endings in the nipple are activated during suckling and initiate the 'let down' reflex via the central nervous system.

Lymphatic Drainage

Lymphatic drainage of the breast begins in a perilobular plexus sited in the connective tissue stroma of the breast, lymphatic fluid flows from here alongside the lactiferous ducts into a subareolar plexus; Sappey's Plexus. Internal mammary lymph nodes may be present along these channels. From this plexus the breast drains into the axillary, subscapular, central, pectoral and apical and clavicular node groups laterally and the parasternal (internal mammary) nodes medially.

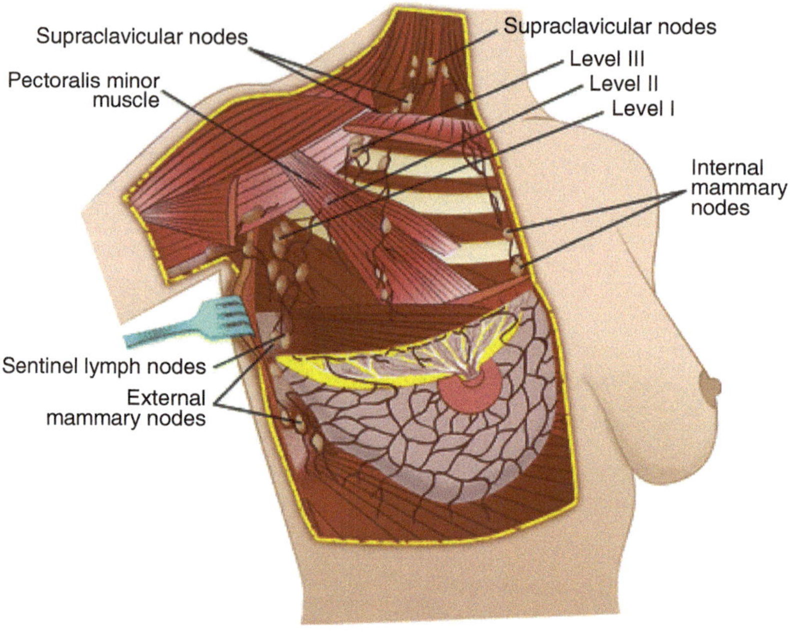

Fig. 1.6 Lymphatic drainage of the breast indicating position of the sentinel lymph node (Reprinted with permission from Urban C, Rietjens M, Kuroda F, Hurley J. *Oncoplastic and Reconstructive Anatomy of the Breast*. Springer, Italia, 2013)

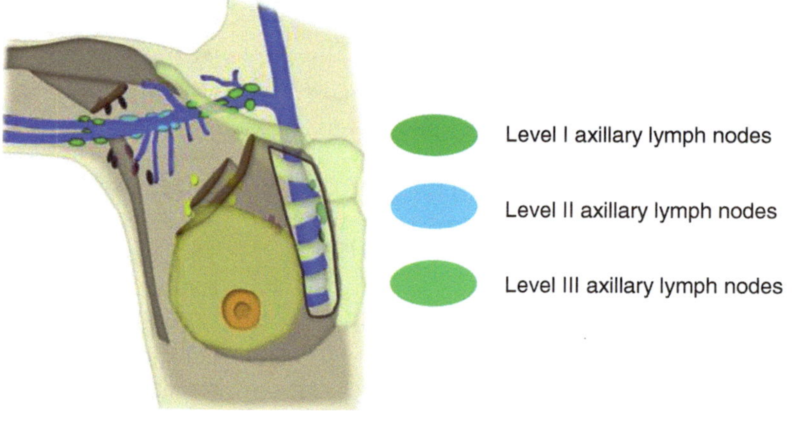

Fig. 1.7 Illustration of Level I, level II and Level III axillary lymph nodes (Reprinted from Harisinghani MG. *Chest Lymph Node Anatomy, Atlas of Lymph Node Anatomy*. Springer Science + Business Media, New York, 2013)

Drainage to the internal mammary nodes means that lymphatic fluid can cross to the contralateral breast. Communication between these groups frequently occurs. Lymphatic fluid may also reach the abdominal nodal groups from the inferomedial breast. Knowledge of these pathways is important in order to understand potential metastatic pathways in breast carcinoma. Seventy-five percent of the breast lymphatic drainage is to the axillary nodal groups. The sentinel lymph node is the first node to which cancer cells are most likely to spread from a primary tumour; in breast carcinoma this is most likely to lie low in the axilla and is the node removed at surgery in order to assess the spread of disease. This gives prognostic information regarding likelihood of local recurrence. Figure 1.6 illustrates the relative lymph node groups providing the breast lymphatic drainage.

Axillary lymph nodes are divided into three groups: Level I, Level II, and Level III as demonstrated below in Fig. 1.7. Level I nodes lie lateral to the lateral border of the pectoralis major muscle and can extend into the axillary tail, Level II nodes lie beneath the pectoralis minor muscle and Level III nodes lie medially and superiorly to the pectoralis minor muscle up to the clavicle. Level I nodes are often visible on mammogram, as are intramammary nodes when present.

Pregnancy and Lactation

During pregnancy, rises in oestrogen, progesterone and prolactin lead to growth of the acini, hyperplasia of the lactogenic (milk producing) epithelium and an increase in myoepithelial cells in preparation for milk production. The lobules enlarge until only thin fibrous septations separate them. Once breastfeeding ceases the breasts undergo a degree of involution and may appear less glandular than before pregnancy. This return to a new baseline takes around 3 months to complete.

Involution

The female breast undergoes gradual regression starting at the end of the fourth decade. This is called involution. The function of the ovaries declines which causes the supporting connective tissues in the breast to be replaced by adipose tissue. Changes are also seen in the TDLU, the epithelium shrinks to one layer, there is progressive lobular atrophy. There is a reduction in glandular component with an increase in fatty tissue. The regressive process continues until and after menopause.

The breasts of post-menopausal women may be entirely fatty on mammogram, however, most post-menopausal women produce enough endogenous oestrogen to maintain some glandular component. As the woman ages the support structures of the breast weaken causing corresponding 'sag' of the breast tissue – this is called ptosis. A mammographic image of an involuted breast is shown in Fig. 1.8b; note that the glandular component seen in Fig. 1.8a has been almost entirely replaced by fatty tissue.

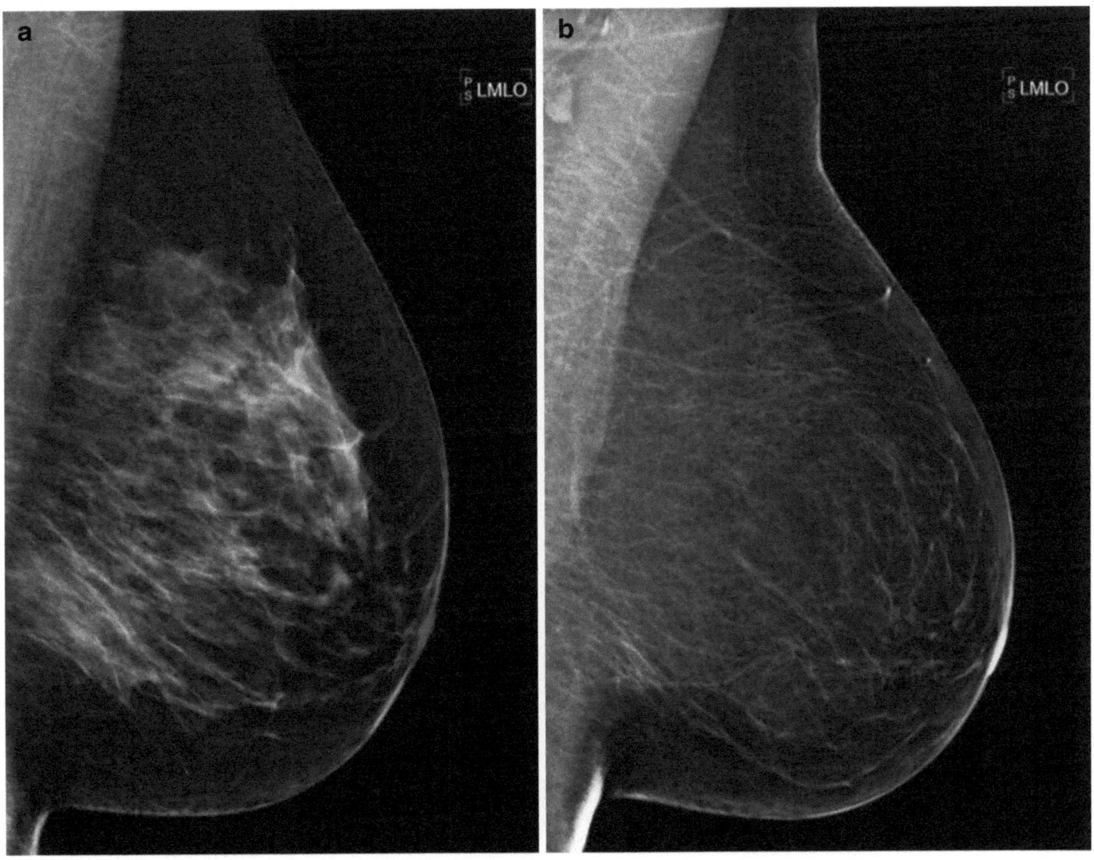

Fig. 1.8 Mammographic illustration of (**a**) Mature female breast, (**b**) Involuted breast

Bibliography and Further Reading

David J, Dabbs MD. Breast pathology. Philadelphia: Elsevier; 2012.

Drake R, et al. Gray's anatomy for students. 3rd ed. London: Churchill Livingstone; 2014.

Jaspers JJP, Posma AN, van Immerseel AAH, Gittenberger-de Groot AC. The cutaneous innervations of the female breast and nipple-areola complex: implications for surgery. Br J Plast Surg. 1997;50:249–59.

Kopans DB. Breast imaging. 3rd ed. Philadelphia: Lippincott, Williams & Wilkins; 2007.

Lee L, Strickland V, Wilson R, Roebuck E. Fundamentals of mammography. London: WB Saunders Comp. Ltd; 1995.

Moore KL, Agur MR. Essential clinical anatomy. Philadelphia: Lippincott, Williams & Wilkins; 1996.

Tabar L, Dean PB. Teaching atlas of mammography. New York: Thieme Verlag; 1985.

Wellings SR, Wolfe JN. Correlative studies of the histological and radiological appearance of the breast parenchyma. Radiology. 1978;129:299–306.

Breast Density and Influencing Factors

2

Dawn M. McDonald

Breast Structure

Breast parenchyma consists of three types of tissue – skin, subcutaneous adipose tissue and functional glandular tissue. The breast itself is divided into approximately 15–18 lobes. Lobes consist of branching ductal systems which lead from the collecting ducts to the terminal ductal lobular units (TDLU). Most breast diseases – with the exception of papillomas in major ducts – arise in the TDLU. The TDLU normally regresses at menopause [1].

The main duct within each lobe has an opening, draining 20–40 lobules. The acini, consisting of a number of lobules, are the site of milk production in the lactating breast [1]. The number of lobules per lobe varies according to age, lactation, parity, and hormonal status. Towards the end of the reproductive life there is an increase in the amount of adipose tissue, and a considerable loss of lobular units, although the main ductal system is preserved. This process, in which there is a reduction in the number, and size, of the acini per lobule, and replaced by fatty tissue, is known as age-related lobular involution, or physiologic atrophy of the breast [2–4].

The changes in breast composition can be demonstrated by variations in breast density on mammography. Usually, younger women tend to have more dense glandular tissue. In older women, the mammographic density tends to decrease with the replacement of glandular tissue by fatty tissue [5].

The images, below, illustrate this (Figs. 2.1 and 2.2).

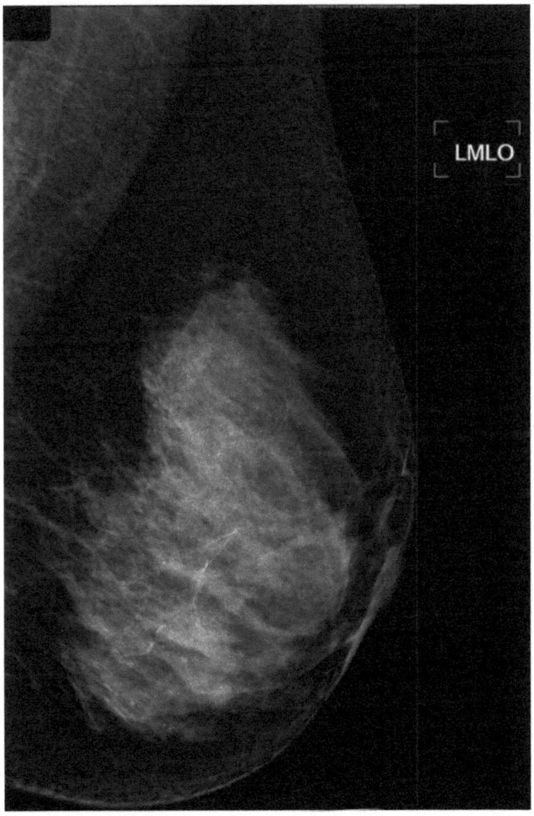

Fig. 2.1 Example of a 40 year old with dense breast tissue pattern

D.M. McDonald
Breast Unit, Worthing Hospital,
Lyndhurst Road, Worthing, West Sussex
BN11 2DH, UK
e-mail: dawn.mcdonald1@nhs.net

P. Hogg et al. (eds.), *Digital Mammography: A Holistic Approach*,
DOI 10.1007/978-3-319-04831-4_2, © Springer International Publishing Switzerland 2015

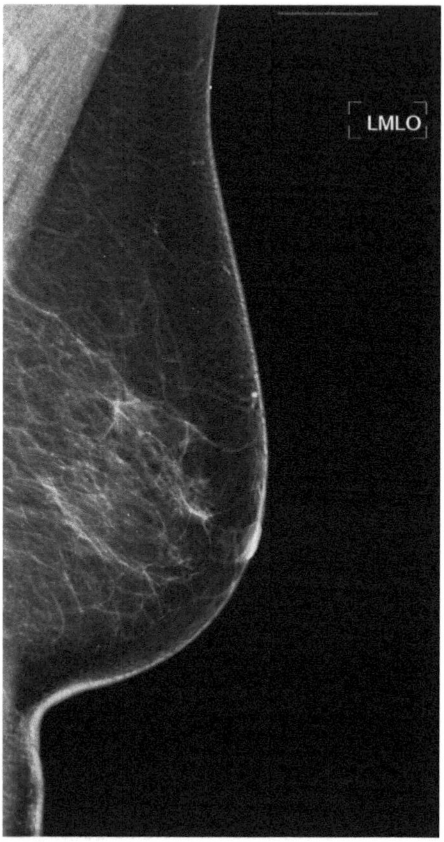

Fig. 2.2 Example of a 65 year old with fatty tissue pattern

Breast Density Classification (See Also Chap. 16)

Classification of breast composition by Wolfe [6], is such that in 'fatty breasts' almost all of the tissue appears to be fat, and less than 25 % will be fibro-glandular tissues. If a breast has scattered fibro-glandular tissue, 26–50 % volume of the breast is visible as fibro-glandular tissue. Heterogeneously dense tissue will have 51–75 % tissue. Extremely dense breasts will have more than 75 % of fibrous connective tissue [6]. Ten per cent of postmenopausal and 20 % of pre-menopausal women have a breast density of above 50 %. It is estimated that one in three women have a high mammographic density [7].

Further classifications of breast composition include Boyd's [8], in which mammographic density is divided into six categories:

- A : 0 %
- B : >0–10 %
- C : >10–25 %
- D : >25–50 %
- E : >50–75 %
- F : >75 %

and Tabar [9], which classifies the mammograms into five patterns:

- I: balanced proportion of all components of breast tissue with a slight predominance of fibrous tissue
- II: predominance of fat tissue (fatty breast)
- III: predominance of fat tissue with retro-areolar residual fibrous tissue
- IV: predominantly nodular densities
- V: predominantly fibrous tissue (dense breast)

The **BI-RADS** system, (Breast Imaging Reporting and Data System), an American system used to categorise breast density and mammographic abnormalities, has been updated in 2013 to reflect a more recent and relevant method for defining breast density, seen below:

(a) The breasts are almost entirely fatty
(b) There are scattered areas of fibroglandular density
(c) The breasts are heterogeneously dense
(d) The breasts are extremely dense.

It uses a sequential method to visually define the amount of fibro glandular tissue seen within the breast as opposed to numerical [10]. It is also a widely accepted risk assessment and quality assurance assessment tool used in the USA and parts or Europe.

Sensitivity

The sensitivity of mammography in the detection of breast cancer ('*... **the number of true positives as a proportion of all those with breast cancer present***') [11] is directly related to the density of the breast tissue. Generally, mammographic sensitivity is higher in older, post-menopausal

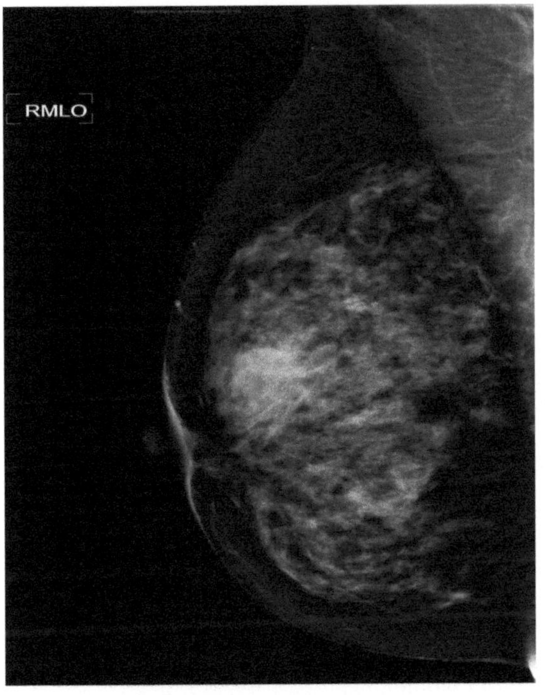

Fig. 2.3 Focal lesion in 'dense' breast

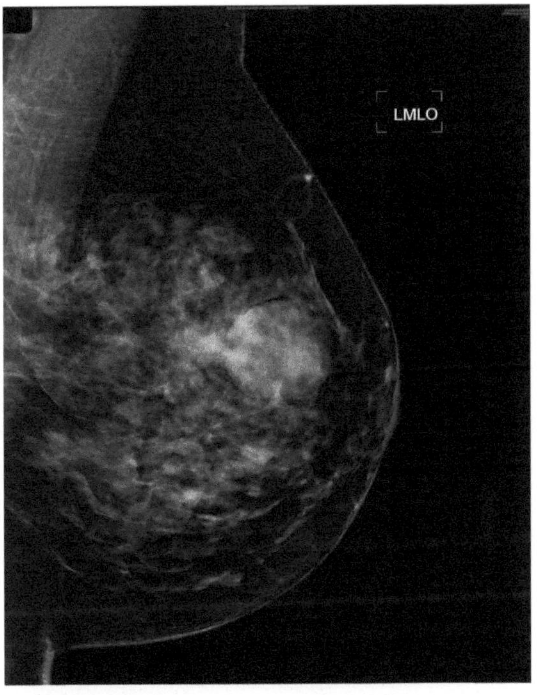

Fig. 2.4 Focal lesion in 'mixed' breast

women because the breast tends to be composed of greater proportions of fatty tissue. There is some evidence to suggest that women with dense breast tissue have a higher than average risk of developing breast cancer. This is because the breast cancer may be obscured in the dense tissue [4, 5].

A high mammographic density is thought to be associated with an increased risk of breast cancer, and is estimated to account for 16 % of all breast cancers [12]. The screening population is also deemed to be at higher risk if breast density is high [13]. However, what is less clearly understood is the breast cancer risk associated with the change in breast density over time; risk increases with age and breast density, but density decreases with age. One study [14] has suggested that the evolution of the density of the breast (as a function of time) may be significant for the risk of developing breast cancer – the faster the changes that occur, the higher the risk. This study does however acknowledge a small sample size and that the cases were not randomly selected. It suggests further research into this. A further study – the PROCAS study – [15] is also presently running, with an aim to recruit 60,000 women to investigate the risk of breast cancer developing over time. This is by using density measurements between routine breast screening, and using these to analyse any risk factors in the screening population.

Nonetheless, regardless of the rate of which breast density changes, sensitivity is reduced in the dense breast [4, 5]. The images, below (Figs. 2.3, 2.4 and 2.5) illustrate a focal lesion which is barely visible in a dense breast, more easily seen in a mixed breast, and clearly seen in a fatty area of the breast.

The images illustrate how the detection of breast cancer through mammography is highly dependent on breast tissue characteristics. A dense breast structure will significantly reduce the detection sensitivity [16].

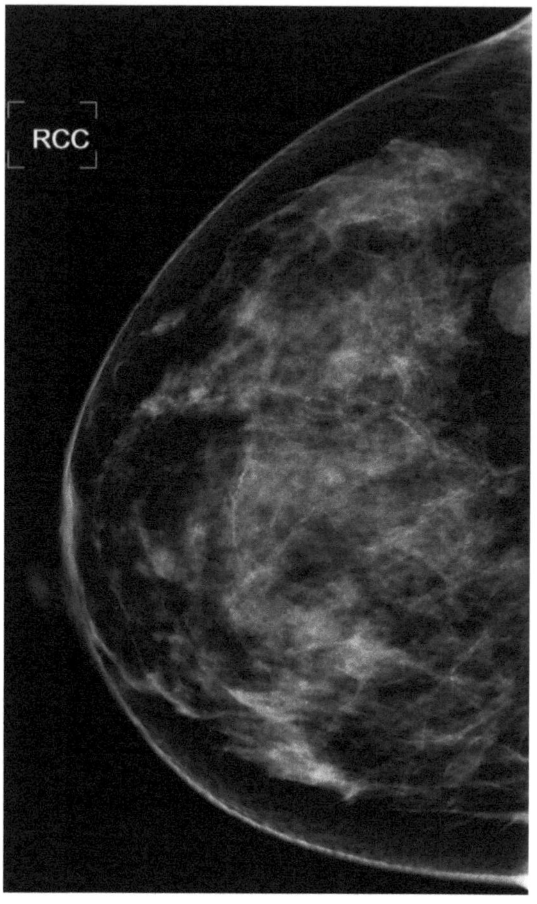

Fig. 2.5 Focal lesion in 'fatty' area of breast

Factors Influencing Breast Density

Age

Age is a factor that influences breast density (Fig. 2.1). A high percentage of women under the age of 30 tend to have dense breasts, – (approximately 90 % dense versus 10 % fatty). The density rate decreases steadily at approximately 1–2 % per year. At 40 years, the ratio is 80/10; 50 years 70/30. It is approximately 50/50 at 65 years [17]. Older women tend to have more of a fatty breast tissue type.

Pregnancy and Lactation

Women with fewer than two pregnancies usually have denser breast types. During pregnancy and breast feeding the number of acini increase with glandular tissue predominating. When lactation ceases, the glandular tissue involutes. The significance of this is that the breast of a woman who has given birth is less glandular than that of a woman of the same age who has not [18].

Hormonal Status

Pre and post hormonal status and reproductive factors have an effect on the density of the breast. Oestrogen levels, which decline with age and menopausal status, can lead to a decline in mammographic density. Oestrogen, post menopause, is positively associated with Body Mass Index (BMI). Tamoxifen ('*****an anti-oestrogen drug that is widely used to treat breast cancer***...' [19]) is also said to reduce density in premenopausal women [7].

Body Mass Index

Women with a large body mass index, (BMI) tend to have large breasts with significant fatty tissue, and with an associated loss in breast density. The breast is a store for fat and as a woman gains or loses weight, this will have an effect in the percentage of dense breast tissue [17]. Consequently weight gain/loss is associated with significant change in breast density.

Lifestyle Factors

Literature, in 2006, suggests that physical activity is associated with the reduction of the incidence of breast cancer quoting a 20–30 % reduction in women who are active in comparison to their non-active colleagues [20]. This is slightly in contradiction to more recent data which suggests that while increasing alcohol consumption is thought to be associated with an increase in density, smoking and physical activity are thought not to be associated [21]. Despite the more recent data, it is widely seen that weight loss is likely to be reflected in a reduced breast density. The health benefits of physical activity are commonly known to be beneficial.

Malignant and Benign Breast Disease

The skin in the breast can sometimes appear to be thickened, manifesting as increased density on the mammogram [1]. This inflammation – or oedema – can be caused by primary breast cancer, axillary lymph node metastases, abscess, congestive heart failure, or radiotherapy [22]. Diffuse increase in the density of breast tissue is caused by oedema, or an increase in glandular and/or fibrous tissue. This is also commonly seen in benign breast changes (BBC).

Benign breast change may be accompanied by evidence of cysts, and women taking hormone replacement therapy (HRT) for menopausal symptoms. Benign breast disease and high breast density are thought to be high risk factor for the future development of breast cancer. A low breast density appears to reduce this risk [23].

Summary

The overall significance of breast density and related factors is that the accuracy of mammography is variable according to the nature of the underlying breast tissue. Dense breast may obscure a focal abnormality, demonstrated in Fig. 2.1, [24]. Fatty breast tissue is less likely to do so. The risk of breast cancer is therefore higher in women who have dense breast tissue, and any way to reduce this risk is beneficial. HRT, pregnancy, lactation and inflammation are amongst the factors that are suggestive of being significant in increasing the density of breast tissue. Ageing, some medications (e.g. Tamoxifen), and a decrease in oestrogen levels, are among the factors thought to be significant in reducing the density of the breast. It is well documented that there appears to be a correlation between fatty breast tissue and the prevalence of cancer. This may be indicated by older women who demonstrate a tendency towards fatty breasts, and experience an increased risk of breast cancer.

References

1. Tabar L. Teaching course in diagnostic breast imaging, multimodality approach to the detection and diagnosis of occult breast cancer. Mammography Education, Inc; Cave Creek, Az, 2008.
2. Hughes LE, Mansel RE. Breast anatomy and physiology. In: Hughes LE, Mansel RE, Webster DJT, editors. Benign disorders and diseases of the breast: concepts and clinical management. London: W.B. Saunders; 2000. p. 7–20.
3. Vorrherr H. The breast: morphology, physiology, and lactation. New York: Academic; 1974.
4. Ghosh K, Hartmann LC, Reynolds C, Visscher DW, Brandt KR, Vierkant RA, Scott CG, Radisky DC, Sellers TA, Pankratz VS, Vachon CM. Association between mammographic density and age-related lobular involution of the breast. J Clin Oncol. 2009; 28(13):2207–12.
5. Grainger RG, Allison DJ, Adam A, Dixon AK. Grainger and Allison's diagnostic radiology, a textbook of medical imaging, vol. 2. 5th ed. Philadelphia: Churchill Livingstone; 2008.
6. Wolfe JN. A study of breast parenchyma by mammography in the normal woman and those with benign and malignant disease of the breast. Radiology. 1967;89(2):201.
7. Ursin G, Qureshi S. Mammographic density- a useful biomark for breast cancer risk in epidemiologic studies. Norsk Epidemiologi. 2009;19(1):59–68.
8. Boyd NF, O'Sullivan B, Campbell JE, Fishell E, Simor I, Cooke G, Germanson T. Mammographic signs as risk factors for breast cancer. Br J Cancer. 1982;45(2):185–93.
9. Gram IT, Funkhouse E, Tabar L. The Tabar classification of mammographic parenchymal patterns. Eur J Radiol. 1997;24(2):131–6.
10. Sickles EA, D'Orsi CJ, Bassett LW, et al. ACR BI-RADS® mammography. In: ACR BI-RADS® atlas, breast imaging reporting and data system. Reston: American College of Radiology; 2013.
11. Sir FP, Dept of Health and Social Security. Breast cancer screening, report to the Health Ministers of England, Wales, Scotland and Northern Ireland. London: Her Majesty's Stationery Office; 1986.
12. Assi V, Warwick J, Cuzick J, Duffy S. Clinical and epidemiological issues in mammographic density. Clin Oncol. 2012;9(1):33–40.
13. Boyd NF, Guo H, Martin LJ, Sun L, Stone J, Fishell E, Jong RA, Hislop G, Chiarelli A, Minkin S, Yaffe MJ. Mammographic density and the risk and detection of breast cancer. N Engl J Med. 2007;356(3): 227–36.
14. Ting C, Astley SM, Morris J, Stavrinos P, Wilson M, Barr N, Boggis C, Sergeant JC. Longitudinal change in mammographic density and association with breast cancer risk: a case-controlled study; Int Workshop on Digital Mammography vol 7361, In: Maidment ADA, Bakic PR, Gavenonis S, editors. IWDM. 2012: LNCS: 7361. Berlin/Heidelberg: Springer; 2012. p. 205–12.

15. Sergeant JC, Warwick J, Evans G, Howell A, Berks M, et al. Volumetric and area based breast density measurement in the predicting risk of cancer at screening (PROCAS) study. IWDM LNCS. 2012;7361:228–35.
16. Oliver A. A novel breast tissue density classification methodology. Inf Technol Biomed. 2008;12(1):55–65.
17. Kopans DB. Breast imaging. 2nd ed. Philadelphia: Lippincott Williams and Wilkins; 1998.
18. Ryan S, McNicholas M, Eustace S. Anatomy for diagnostic imaging. 2nd ed. WB Saunders, London; 2007.
19. Macmillan. Tamoxifen. [Online]. 2013. http://www.macmillan.org.uk/Cancerinformation/Cancertreatment/Treatmenttypes/Hormonaltherapies/Individualhormonaltherapies/Tamoxifen.aspx. Accessed 21 Mar 2014.
20. Warburton ER, Nicol CW, Bredin SSD. Health benefits of physical activity: the evidence. CMAJ. 2006;174(6):801–9.
21. Brand JS, Czene K, Eriksson L, Trinh T, Bhoo-Pathy N, et al. Influence of lifestyle factors on mammographic density in postmenopausal women. Plos One. 2013;8(12):81876.
22. Sutton D. Textbook of radiology and imaging, vol. 2, 7th ed. New York: Churchill Livingstone; 2003. Kopans DB. Basic Physics and Doubts about Relationship between Mammographic Determined Tissue Density and Breast Cancer Risk. Radiology 2008;246(2).
23. Tice JA, O'Meara ES, Weaver DL, Vachon C, Ballard-Barbash R, Kerlikowsk EK. Benign breast disease, mammographic breast density, and the risk of breast cancer. J Cancer Inst. 2013;105(14):1043–9, Oxford University Press.
24. Liste DA. Imaging for students. 3rd ed. London: Hodder Arnold; 2007.

3 Aetiology and Epidemiology of Breast Cancer

Lisa Hackney

Many risk factors are considered attributable to increasing an individual's chance of developing breast cancer, but it is not yet completely understood how these risk factors cause cells to become cancerous.

An oncogene is a gene with the potential to initiate a cancer [1] and in tumour cells they are frequently over-expressed or mutated [2]. Normal cells undergo apoptosis, often referred to as a "programmed form of death". Under certain circumstances, e.g. environmental influences, activated oncogenes cause cells that would have undergone apoptosis to survive and proliferate, developing into a carcinoma [3].

How Common Is Breast Cancer?

Breast cancer is the commonest invasive malignancy in females worldwide [4], with incidence rates being higher in Western Europe and lowest in Middle and Eastern Africa. It is undoubtedly the commonest cancer in UK women (see Fig. 3.1), with 49,961 newly diagnosed cases in 2010, and accounting for 30 % of all new female cancer cases that year [5–8].

L. Hackney
Consultant Radiographer, Breast Care Unit, University Hospital of North Staffordshire, Newcastle Road, Stoke-on-Trent ST4 6QG, UK
e-mail: Lisa.hackney@uhns.nhs.uk

Breast cancer accounted for 15 % (11,684) of UK female deaths in 2011, but interestingly it is no longer the commonest cause of female cancer deaths, which is now attributable to lung cancer [9–11]. A number of factors are responsible for the decline in mortality rates over the past decade. These include: earlier detection via breast screening programmes; increased public awareness; improved treatments (surgical, radiotherapy/chemotherapy regimes and hormonal therapies) and improved delivery of specialist care by multidisciplinary teams [12].

Lifetime Risk (Females)

Lifetime risk refers to the chance a person has of developing or dying from cancer over the course of his or her lifetime (from birth to death). Risk estimates are based upon current incidence and mortality rates but an individual's risk may be higher or lower than the population risk as genetic and lifestyle factors are influential. Cancer research UK reported that in 2010 (UK) the lifetime risk of developing breast cancer is 1 in 8 for women and 1 in 868 for men [13].

Risk Factors for Breast Cancer

Risk factors are merely an indicator and not a certainty that an individual will develop the disease. Some women may have multiple risk factors and

P. Hogg et al. (eds.), *Digital Mammography: A Holistic Approach*,
DOI 10.1007/978-3-319-04831-4_3,

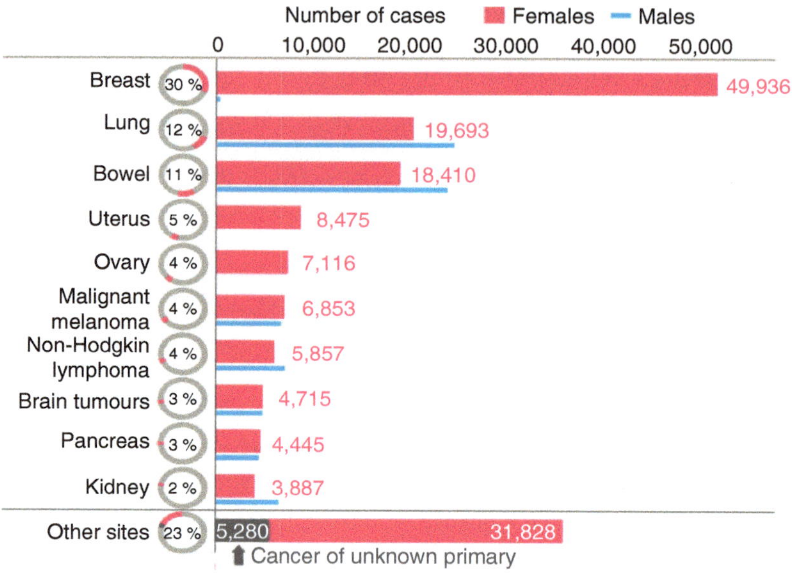

Fig. 3.1 The 10 most common cancers in females, UK, 2011 (Cancer Research UK, www.cancerresearchuk.org/cancer-info/cancerstats/incidence/commoncancers/ October 2014)

never have breast cancer, whilst many of the women diagnosed have no attributable risk factors. Some risk factors are unalterable (e.g. gender or age), but others are controllable and linked to the environment and personal lifestyle. Certain risk factors are more influential than others, and an individual's risk for breast cancer will change over time.

Unchangeable Risk Factors

Gender

Being female is the main risk factor for developing breast cancer. Although men do develop breast cancer the incidence rates are very low in comparison and have remained stable over the last 40 years [4–6]. Cancer research UK reports that in the UK 397 men were diagnosed with breast cancer in 2010. As with females, breast cancer incidence is strongly associated with increasing age [4–6].

Age

In women, the strongest risk factor for breast cancer is age; the older a woman gets, the higher her risk. Data demonstrates that almost half (48 %) of female breast cancer cases are diagnosed in women in the 50–69 age group [4–8]. This contributed to the original rationale underpinning the UK NHS breast screening programme [14], which invites women in the 50–70 age group for screening every 3 years. At the time of writing this chapter, in England there is currently a trial "phasing-in" the age extension from 47 to 50 and 70 to 73. The trial aims to produce data on the incidence and mortality rates from extending the age range for screening.

Although the incidence of breast cancer in young women (i.e. teenager until 30 years old) is uncommon, it remains the main cancer diagnosed in women under the age of 39. Overall, there has been an increase in female breast cancer rates across all age ranges in the past 40 years [4, 6–8].

Genetic Risk Factors

Family History

It is important to remember that the majority of breast cancers are not hereditary, as fewer than 15 % of women with breast cancer have a family member with the disease [15]. Analysis of data [15, 16] shows that having one first –degree relative (sister, mother or daughter) diagnosed with breast cancer almost doubles a woman's risk of developing the disease compared to an individual with no family history. This risk increases further (3-fold) if two first degree relatives are affected and the age at diagnosis is also an important factor as risk is greater if the relative is under 50.

An increased risk does not mean that an individual will develop the disease as more than 85 % of women with a first degree relative with breast cancer will never develop the disease [15]. A very minor proportion of women are at a very high risk of familial breast or ovarian cancer and this is assigned to mutations in the breast cancer susceptibility genes Breast Cancer Gene 1 (BRCA1) and Breast Cancer Gene 2 (BRCA2) [17]. The estimated prevalence of mutations mean this will affect approximately 1 in 450 women who as a result have a high (45–65 %) chance of developing the disease by the age of 70 [18].

Mutations in the BRCA genes are identified as high-penetrance, and confer the greatest increase in risk (10-fold), but there are very rare genes e.g. Tumour Protein 53 (TP53) (Li Fraumeni syndrome) that also lie within this group [19]. There are also a number of intermediate-penetrance gene variants that give a 2–3 fold increase in risk such as Checkpoint kinase 2(CHEK2), Ataxia Telangiectasia Mutated (ATM), BRCA1 interacting protein C-terminal helicase 1 (BRIP1) and Partner And Localizer of BRCA2 (PALB2). A number of low-penetrance gene variants have also been identified [19].

Personal History of Breast Cancer

Women with a prior history of a breast cancer have an increased risk of developing a new cancer in the contralateral breast. Studies [20–22] report a variance from a 3- to almost 5-fold risk increase. This risk is not the same as the risk of recurrence (return) from the primary cancer.

The risk of a contralateral breast cancer is stated to be higher for individuals in whom the primary tumour was hormone-receptor negative compared to a hormone-receptor positive tumour [23] and also if the primary diagnosis was under the age of 40 [24].

Breast Density

There is strong evidence to show that there is an interdependent link between breast density and the risk of developing breast cancer [25, 26]. The greater the density of breast tissue, the greater the chance of developing breast cancer. Research shows that women with a Breast Imaging-Reporting and Data System (BI-RADS) breast density of category 4(d) (Appendix 1) have approximately a four times greater risk of breast cancer comparative to the category 1(a) group [27–29]. There are a number of contributory factors that affect breast density e.g. age, endogenous hormones [26, 30], menopausal status, body weight, pregnancy.) Further information about breast density can be found in Chap. 16.

Socio-economic Status

Data demonstrates that female breast cancer rates are much higher in women from developed countries compared to women from developing nations [31, 32], with rates rising in continents where incidence was historically much lower [33–35]. There are several causative factors for this. Life expectancy is greater in economically developed countries (risk of breast cancer increases with age) together with different lifestyles e.g. use of hormone replacement therapy (HRT), increasing body mass index (BMI), alcohol consumption [36, 37].

Historically South Asian women and those in lower socio-economic groups were considered at lower risk of developing breast cancer, but recent data [38] reports this is no longer the case.

Recent evidence shows that deprivation is one of the most significant factors associated with poor uptake rates at breast screening, which is anticipated to result in poorer outcomes [39].

Reproductive Factors That Influence Breast Cancer Risk

Menstrual Periods

Early age at menarche (before age 12) [40] and and/or late menopause (after age 55) infer a slightly higher risk of breast cancer [41]. The increase in risk may be due to a longer lifetime exposure to the hormones oestrogen and progesterone.

Parity

Childbearing reduces the risk of breast cancer, but this is also relative to maternal age at first live birth and number of full-term pregnancies [42]. Having children lowers individual risk compared to a nulliparous woman [42–44].

Some studies suggest that breastfeeding can slightly lower breast cancer risk, but this is proportional to the amount of time spent breastfeeding [42].

Exogenous Hormones

Oral Contraceptives/HRT

Studies have found that women who currently or recently used oral contraceptives have a slightly greater risk of breast cancer than non-users, but the risk diminishes over time after stopping use. Ten years post use there does not appear to be a residual risk [45]. Similar findings are reported from studies that have looked at Depot-medroxyprogesterone acetate (DMPA; Depo-Provera®) the injectable form of birth control.

Using combined hormone therapy (oestrogen and progesterone) after the menopause is associated with an increased risk (66 %) of developing breast cancer compared to non-users [46]. This increase can be seen with as little as 2 years of use. Again, the increased risk appears to apply only to current and recent users with risk returning to that of the general population within 5 years of ceasing [46].

Previous Benign Breast Disease

Certain benign breast conditions confer an increased risk for breast cancer.

Lesions classified as non-proliferative infer no extra risk. They include:

- Fibrosis and/or simple cysts
- Mild hyperplasia
- Non sclerosing adenosis
- Duct ectasia
- Benign Phyllodes tumour
- Solitary papilloma
- Fat necrosis
- Other benign tumours (lipoma, hamartoma, haemangioma, neurofibroma)

Proliferative lesions without atypia appear to slightly raise (1½–2 fold increase) risk. They include ductal hyperplasia, fibroadenoma, sclerosing adenosis, papillomatosis and radial scar. Proliferative lesions with atypia imply a greater risk (3½–5 fold) and include atypical ductal hyperplasia (ADH) and Atypical lobular hyperplasia (ALH).

Ductal carcinoma in situ (DCIS) and lobular carcinoma in situ (LCIS) have the potential to develop into invasive carcinoma, more probable with high grade rather than low grade disease [47]. Previous in-situ disease is recognised to double an individual's risk of developing an invasive breast tumour [48].

Medical Radiation Exposure

Exposure to ionising radiation is a known risk factor associated with any carcinoma [49]. Young female adults or children who received mantle radiotherapy to the chest area as treatment for Hodgkin's Lymphoma have a significantly increased risk for breast cancer. Studies [49, 50] report a 12–25 fold increased risk dependent on the age at exposure, with the greater risk in adolescents.

Recent data concludes that breast cancer patients have a "small but significantly excess" risk of developing a second cancer close to prior radiotherapy treatment fields [51]. Studies also report an increased risk (3 fold) of breast cancer in females under the age of 30 who received diagnostic doses of radiation whilst undergoing chest x-rays for tuberculosis or pneumonia [49].

Risk associated with radiation exposure from 3 yearly breast screening mammograms is reported to be minimal [52].

Lifestyle Related Risk Factors

Being overweight or obese is one of the few risk factors that is amenable to change. However, the association between body weight and breast cancer risk is multifaceted.

Pre-menopausal women produce most of their oestrogen from the ovaries, with a small amount produced by fatty tissue. Post-menopause a woman's oestrogen mainly comes from the conversion of hormones in fat tissue. Overweight post-menopausal women are reported to have a 10–20 % increased risk of breast cancer, which escalates to 30 % in women categorised as obese [53, 54].

However, the complexity lies in that the risk appears relative as to whether the weight gain is as a child or as an adult. Risk appears greater for women who gained excess weight as an adult but does not appear to have the same implications for those who have been overweight from childhood.

Physical Activity

Evidence supports that exercise can reduce an individual's breast cancer risk. However, this appears to be relative to the intensity and duration of the exercise undertaken. The most significant findings are for vigorous activity in postmenopausal women where studies have reported a 15–20 % risk reduction [55, 56], believed to be due to the associated decreased levels of oestrogen and progesterone [57].

Alcohol Consumption

There is an association between alcohol consumption and an increased risk of developing breast cancer. A Lancet report in 2007 concluded that this association is causal [58], with relative risk increasing with the increasing amount of alcohol consumed.

Uncertain Risk Factors

Diet

Numerous studies have been undertaken to identify if there an association between dietary factors and breast cancer risk, but currently the results are conflicting [59, 60].

Intake of fibre, fruit, vegetables and meat has been studied but the most significant factor appears to relate to fat intake. Higher intakes of saturated fat appear to correlate with an increased risk [61–63].

Smoking and Passive Smoke

Historically there has been no evidence to support a link between cigarette smoking and breast cancer. Larger studies undertaken in 2011 [64, 65] have demonstrated that long-term heavy smoking is associated with a higher risk of breast cancer particularly for certain cohorts i.e. women who started smoking when they were young (under the age of 20) and before their first birth.

There is no consistent evidence to authenticate an association between smoking and breast cancer after the menopause [65].

Passive smoke exposure and breast cancer risk remains controversial [66, 67], with no conclusive evidence.

Night/Shift Work

Several studies show some evidence relating the risk of developing breast cancer to women who work night shifts [68], and those with disrupted or shorter duration sleep patterns [69, 70]. The hypothesis relates this to varying levels of the hormone melatonin which has anti-carcinogenic effects.

Medications and Medical Conditions

Certain medications have been associated with reducing breast cancer risk, mainly aspirin and non-steroidal anti-inflammatory drugs [71–76].

Other medications e.g. diethylstilboestrol (synthetic oestrogen) and long-term use of antihypertensive medications suggest an increased risk [77, 78].

A number of medical conditions are also associated with a higher risk of breast cancer e.g. Graves' Disease (hyperthyroidism) [79] and diabetes although this may be dependent on the type of diabetes, menopausal status and treatment received [80–86].

Appendix 1

The American College of Radiology BI-RADS [87]

1(a). The breasts are almost entirely fatty
2(b). There are scattered areas of fibroglandular density
3(c). The breasts are heterogeneously dense, which may obscure small masses
4(d). The breasts are extremely dense, which lowers the sensitivity of mammography

References

1. Wilbur B, editor. The World of the cell, Becker WM, et al., 7th ed. San Francisco; 2009. Benjamin Cummings
2. Kimball's Biology Pages. "Oncogenes". "Cancer: Disease of Altered Gene Expression." Boundless Biology. Boundless, 03 Jul 2014. Retrieved 26 Nov 2014 from https://www.boundless.com/biology/textbooks/boundless-biology-textbook/gene-expression-16/cancer-and-gene-regulation-118/cancer-disease-of-altered-gene-expression-470-11690/
3. The Nobel Prize in Physiology or Medicine 2002. Illustrated presentation. Nobelprize.org. Nobel Media AB 2014. Web. 27 Nov 2014. http://www.nobelprize.org/nobel_prizes/medicine/laureates/2002/
4. Data were provided by the Office for National Statistics on request, June 2012. Similar data can be found here. http://www.ons.gov.uk/ons/search/index.html?newquery=cancer+registrations.
5. Ferlay J, Shin HR, Bray F, Forman D, Mathers C, Parkin DM. GLOBOCAN 2008 v1.2, Cancer Incidence and Mortality Worldwide: IARC CancerBase No. 10 [Internet]. Lyon: International Agency for Research on Cancer. 2010. http://globocan.iarc.fr. Accessed May 2011.
6. Data were provided by the Northern Ireland Cancer Registry on request, June 2012. Similar data can be found here. http://www.qub.ac.uk/research-centres/nicr/CancerData/OnlineStatistics/.
7. Data were provided by the Welsh Cancer Intelligence and Surveillance Unit on request, April 2012. Similar data can be found here. http://www.wales.nhs.uk/sites3/page.cfm?orgid=242&pid=51358.
8. Data were provided by ISD Scotland on request, April 2012. Similar data can be found here. http://www.isdscotland.org/Health-Topics/Cancer/Publications/index.asp#605.
9. Data were provided by the Office for National Statistics on request, March 2013. Similar data can be found here. http://www.ons.gov.uk/ons/publications/all-releases.html?definition=tcm%3A77-27475.
10. Data were provided by ISD Scotland on request, March 2013. Similar data can be found here. http://gro-scotland.gov.uk/statistics/theme/vital-events/general/ref-tables/index.html.
11. Data were provided by the Northern Ireland Cancer Registry on request, May 2013. Similar data can be found here. http://www.nisra.gov.uk/demography/default.asp22.htm.
12. Kingsmore D, Ssemwogerere A, Hole D, et al. Specialisation and breast cancer survival in the screening era. Br J Cancer. 2003;88(11):1708–12.
13. Lifetime risk was calculated using 2010 data for females and 2008-2010 data for males by the Statistical Information Team at Cancer Research UK, 2012. www.cancerresearchuk.org/cancer.../cancerstats/.../uk-breast-cancer-incidence-statistics.
14. UK National Screening Committee. UK Screening Portal: Breast screening across the UK. Accessed Oct 2012.
15. Collaborative group on hormonal factors in breast cancer. Familial breast cancer: collaborative reanalysis of individual data from 52 epidemiological studies including 58,209 women with breast cancer and 101,986 without the disease. Lancet. 2001;358:1389–99.
16. Pharoah PD, Day NE, Duffy S, et al. Family history and the risk of breast cancer: a systematic review and meta-analysis. Int J Cancer. 1997;71:800–9.
17. Ford D, Easton DF, Stratton M, et al. Genetic heterogeneity and penetrance analysis of the BRCA1 and BRCA2 genes in breast cancer families. The Breast Cancer Linkage Consortium. Am J Hum Genet. 1998;62(3):676–89.
18. Antoniou A, Pharoah PD, Narod S, et al. Average risks of breast and ovarian cancer associated with BRCA1 or BRCA2 mutations detected in case Series unselected for family history: a combined analysis of 22 studies. Am J Hum Genet. 2003;72(5):1117–30.

19. Turnbull C, Rahman N. Genetic predisposition to breast cancer: past, present, and future. Annu Rev Genomics Hum Genet. 2008;9:321–45.
20. Volk N, Pompe-Kim V. Second primary cancers in breast cancer patients in Slovenia. Cancer Causes Control. 1997;8:764–70.
21. Levi F, Randimbison L, Te VC, et al. Cancer risk after radiotherapy for breast cancer. Br J Cancer. 2006;95:390.
22. Soerjomataram I, Louwman WJ, Lemmens VA, et al. Risks of second primary breast cancer and urogenital cancer following female breast cancer in the south of The Netherlands, 1972-2001. Eur J cancer. 2005;41: 2331–7.
23. Kurian AW, McClure LA, John EM, et al. Second primary breast cancer occurrence according to hormone receptor status. J Natl Cancer Inst. 2009;101(15): 1058–65.
24. Rubino C, Arriagada R, Delaloge S, et al. Relation of risk of contralateral breast cancer to the interval since the first primary tumour. Br J Cancer. 2010;102(1): 213–9.
25. Oza AM, Boyd NF. Mammographic parenchymal patterns: a marker of breast cancer risk. Epidemiol Rev. 1993;15:196–208.
26. Tamimi RM, Byrne C, Colditz GA, et al. Endogenous hormone levels, mammographic density, and subsequent risk of breast cancer in postmenopausal women. J Natl Cancer Inst. 2007;99:1178–87.
27. McCormack VA, dos Santos Silva I. Breast density and parenchymal patterns as markers of breast cancer risk: a meta-analysis. Cancer Epidemiol Biomarkers Prev. 2006;15:1159–69.
28. Boyd NF, Guo H, Martin LJ, et al. Mammographic density and the risk and detection of breast cancer. N Engl J Med. 2007;356(3):227–36.
29. Bertrand KA, Tamimi RM, Scott CG, et al. Mammographic density and risk of breast cancer by age and tumor characteristics. Breast Cancer Res. 2013;15(6):R104.
30. Varghese JS, Smith PL, Folkerd E, et al. The heritability of mammographic breast density and circulating sex-hormone levels: two independent breast cancer risk factors. Cancer Epidemiol Biomarkers Prev. 2012;21(12):2167–75.
31. Beral V, Million Women Study Collaborators. Breast cancer and hormone-replacement therapy in the Million Women Study. Lancet. 2003;362(9382): 419–27.
32. Hery C, Ferlay J, Boniol M, Autier P. Changes in breast cancer incidence and mortality in middle-aged and elderly women in 28 countries with Caucasian majority populations. Ann Oncol. 2008;19(5): 1009–18.
33. Hery C, Ferlay J, Boniol M, Autier P. Quantification of changes in breast cancer incidence and mortality since 1990 in 35 countries with Caucasian-majority populations. Ann Oncol. 2008;19:1187–94.
34. Leung GM, Thach TQ, Lam TH, et al. Trends in breast cancer incidence in Hong Kong between 1973 and 1999: an age-period-cohort analysis. Br J Cancer. 2002;87:982–8.
35. Nagata C, Kawakami N, Shimzu H. Trends in the incidence rate and risk factors for breast cancer in Japan. Breast Cancer Res Treat. 1997;44:75–82.
36. Ziegler RG, Hoover RN, Pike MC, et al. Migration patterns and breast cancer risk in Asian-American women. J Natl Cancer Inst. 1993;85(22):1819–27.
37. Deapen D, Liu L, Perkins C, Bernstein L, Ross RK. Rapidly rising breast cancer incidence rates among Asian-American women. Intl J Cancer. 2002;99: 747–50.
38. Levels of socio-economic deprivation affect screening uptake for breast cancer. Press release. Public Health England, 14 June 2013. https://www.gov.uk/government/organisations/public-health-england.
39. Khan H, Meraj S, Wilbraham A, Cox D, Bhatt R, Yates J, Waldron J, Powell A. Review of the determinants of poor screening uptake at City, Sandwell and Walsall Breast Screening Units and the steps taken to improve attendance. Breast Cancer Res. 2013;15 Suppl 1:P43.
40. Garcia-Closas M, Brinton LA, Lissowska J, et al. Established breast cancer risk factors by clinically important tumour characteristics. Br J Cancer. 2006;360:187–95.
41. Collaborative Group on Hormonal Factors in Breast Cancer. Breast cancer and hormone replacement therapy: collaborative reanalysis of data from 51 epidemiological studies of 52,705 women with breast cancer and 108,411 women without breast cancer. Lancet. 1997;350(9084):1047–59.
42. Collaborative Group on Hormonal Factors in Breast Cancer. Breast cancer and breastfeeding: collaborative reanalysis of individual data from 47 epidemiological studies in 30 countries, including 50302 women with breast cancer and 96973 women without the disease. Lancet. 2002;360(9328):187–95.
43. Ma H, Bernstein L, Pike MC, et al. Reproductive factors and breast cancer risk according to joint estrogen and progesterone receptor status: a meta-analysis of epidemiological studies. Breast Cancer Res. 2006;8: R43.
44. Ma H, Bernstein L, Pike MC, et al. Age at first birth, parity and risk of breast cancer: a meta-analysis of 8 studies from the Nordic countries. Int J Cancer. 1990;46(4):597–603.
45. Collaborative Group on Hormonal Factors in Breast Cancer. Breast cancer and hormonal contraceptives: collaborative reanalysis of individual data on 53 297 women with breast cancer and 100 239 women without breast cancer from 54 epidemiological studies. Lancet. 1996;347:1713–27.
46. Beral V. Breast cancer and hormone-replacement therapy in the Million Women Study. The Lancet. 2003;362(9382):419–27.

47. Kerlikowske K, Molinaro A, Cha I, et al. Characteristics associated with recurrence among women with ductal carcinoma in situ treated by lumpectomy. J Natl Cancer Inst. 2003;95:1692–702.
48. Robinson D, Holmberg L, Møller H. The occurrence of invasive cancers following a diagnosis of breast carcinoma in situ. Br J Cancer. 2008;99(4):611–5.
49. John EM, Phipps AI, Knight JA, et al. Medical radiation exposure and breast cancer risk: findings from the Breast Cancer Family Registry. Int J Cancer. 2007;121: 386–94.
50. Alm El-Din MA, Hughes KS, Finkelstein DM, et al. Breast cancer after treatments of Hodgkin's lymphoma: risk factors that really matter. Int J Radiat Oncol Biol Phys. 2008;72(5):1291–7.
51. Grantzau T, Mellemkjær L, Overgaard J. Second primary cancers after adjuvant radiotherapy in early breast cancer patients: A national population based study under the Danish Breast Cancer Cooperative Group (DBCG). Radiother Oncol. 2013;106(1): 42–9.
52. Ryste Hauge IH, Pedersen K, Hole EO, Hofvind S. The risk of radiation-induced breast cancers due to biennial mammographic screening in women aged 50–69 years is minimal. Acta Radiol. 2013.
53. Key TJ, Appleby PN, Reeves GK, et al. Body mass index, serum sex hormones, and breast cancer risk in postmenopausal women. J Natl Cancer Inst. 2003 Aug 20;95(16):1218–26.
54. Parkin DM, Boyd L. Cancers attributable to overweight and obesity in the UK in 2010. Br J Cancer. 2011;105(S2):S34–7.
55. Monninkhof EM, Elias SG, Vlems FA. Physical activity and breast cancer: a systematic review. Epidemiology. 2007;18(1):137–57.
56. Kobayashi LC, Janssen I, Richardson H, et al. A case-control study of lifetime light intensity physical activity and breast cancer risk. Cancer Causes Control. 2013.
57. Chan MF, Dowsett M, Folkerd E, et al. Usual physical activity and endogenous sex hormones in postmenopausal women: the European prospective investigation into cancer-norfolk population study. Cancer Epidemiol Biomarkers Prev. 2007;16:900–5.
58. Baan R, Straif K, Grosse Y, et al. Carcinogenicity of alcoholic beverages. Lancet Oncol. 2007;8: 292–3.
59. Aune D, Chan DS, Greenwood DC, et al. Dietary fiber and breast cancer risk: a systematic review and meta-analysis of prospective studies. Ann Oncol. 2012;23(6): 1394–402.
60. Aune D, Chan DS, Vieira AR, et al. Fruits, vegetables and breast cancer risk: a systematic review and meta-analysis of prospective studies. Breast Cancer Res Treat. 2012;134(2):479–93.
61. Boyd NF, Stone J, Vogt KN, et al. Dietary fat and breast cancer risk revisited: a meta-analysis of the published literature. Br J Cancer. 2003;89(9): 1672–85.
62. Thiebaut AC, Kipnis V, Chang SC. Dietary fat and post menopausal breast cancer in the National Institutes of Health -AARP Diet and Health Study Cohort. J Natl Cancer Inst. 2007;99:451–62.
63. Bingham SA, Luben R, Welch A, et al. Are imprecise methods obscuring a relation between fat and breast cancer? Lancet. 2003;362:212–4.
64. Luo J, Margolis KL, Wactawski-Wende J, et al. Association of active and passive smoking with risk of breast cancer among postmenopausal women: a prospective cohort study. BMJ. 2011;342:d1016.
65. Xue F, Willett WC, Rosner BA, et al. Cigarette smoking and the incidence of breast cancer. Arch Intern Med. 2011;171(2):125–33.
66. Cogliano VJ, Baan R, Straif K, et al. Preventable exposures associated with human cancers. JNCI. 2012;103(24):1827–39.
67. Pirie K, Beral V, Peto R, et al. Passive smoking and breast cancer in never smokers: prospective study and meta-analysis. Int J Epidemiol. 2008;37:1069–79.
68. Megdal SP, Kroenke CH, Laden F, et al. Nightwork and breast cancer risk: a systematic review and meta-analysis. Eur J Cancer. 2005;41:2023–32.
69. Kakizaki M, Kuriyami S, Sone T, et al. Sleep duration and breast cancer: the Ohsaki Cohort study. Br J Cancer. 2008;99:1502–5.
70. Verkasalo PK, Liliberg K, Stevens RG, et al. Sleep duration and breast cancer: a prospective cohort study. Cancer Res. 2005;65:9595–600.
71. Takkouche B, Regueira-Mendez C, Etminan M. Breast cancer and use of nonsteroidal anti-inflammatory drugs: a meta-analysis. J Natl Cancer Inst. 2008;100:1439–47.
72. Mangiapane S, Biettner M, Schlattman P. Aspirin use and breast cancer risk: a meta-analysis and meta-regression of observational studies from 2001 to 2005. Pharmacoepidemiol Drug Saf. 2008;17: 115–24.
73. Gonzalez-Perez A, Gaarcia Rodriguez LA, Lopez-Ridaura R. Effects of non-steroidal anti-inflammatory drugs on cancer sites other than the colon and rectum: a meta-analysis. BMC Cancer. 2003;3:28.
74. Khuder SA, Mutgi AB. Breast cancer and NSAID use: a meta-analysis. Br J Cancer. 2001;84:1188–92.
75. Hudson AG, Gierach GL, Modugno F, et al. Nonsteroidal anti-inflammatory drug use and serum total estradiol in postmenopausal women. Cancer Epidemiol Biomarkers Prev. 2008;17:680–7.
76. Gates MA, Tworoger SS, Eliassen AH, et al. Analgesic use and sex steroid hormone concentrations in postmenopausal women. Cancer Epidemiol Biomarkers Prev. 2010;19(4):1033–41.
77. Largent JA, Bernstein L, Horn-Ross PL, et al. Hypertension, antihypertensive medication use, and breast cancer risk in the California Teachers Study

cohort. Cancer Causes Control. 2010;21(10): 1615–24.
78. Titus-Ernstoff L, Hatch EE, Hoover RN, et al. Long-term cancer risk in women given diethylstilbestrol (DES) during pregnancy. Br J Cancer. 2001;84(1): 126–33.
79. Shu X, Ji J, Li X, et al. Cancer risk in patients hospitalised for Graves' disease: a population-based cohort study in Sweden. Br J Cancer. 2010;102(9):1397–9.
80. De Bruijn KM, Arends LR, Hansen BE, et al. Systematic review and meta-analysis of the association between diabetes mellitus and incidence and mortality in breast and colorectal cancer. Br J Surg. 2013;100(11):1421–9.
81. Boyle P, Boniol M, Koechlin A, et al. Diabetes and breast cancer risk: a meta-analysis. Br J Cancer. 2012;107(9):1608–17.
82. Monami M, Dicembrini I, Mannucci E. Thiazolidinediones and cancer: results of a meta-analysis of randomized clinical trials. Acta Diabetol. 2013.
83. Colmers IN, Bowker SL, Johnson JA. Thiazolidinedione use and cancer incidence in type 2 diabetes: a systematic review and meta-analysis. Diabetes Metab. 2012;38(6):475–84.
84. Col NF, Ochs L, Springmann V, et al. Metformin and breast cancer risk: a meta-analysis and critical literature review. Breast Cancer Res Treat. 2012;135(3):639–46.
85. Zhang P, Li H, Tan X, et al. Association of metformin use with cancer incidence and mortality: a meta-analysis. Cancer Epidemiol. 2013;37(3):207–18.
86. Starup-Linde J, Karlstad O, Eriksen SA, et al. CARING (CAncer Risk and INsulin analoGues): the Association of Diabetes Mellitus and Cancer Risk with Focus on Possible Determinants- a Systematic Review and a Meta-Analysis. Curr Drug Saf. 2013; 8(5):296–332.
87. D'Orsi CJ, Sickles EA, Mendelson EB, Morris EA. Breast Imaging Reporting and Data System (BI-RADS). 5th ed. Reston, VA: American College of Radiology, 2013.

Other Breast Diseases

4

Lisa Hackney and Susan Williams

Breast cancer is not the only finding in mammography. There are numerous other pathologies ranging from the benign to significant risk factors for the subsequent development of a breast cancer. This section describes some of the more common diseases.

Cysts

Breast cysts are formed when there is an accumulation of fluid within the terminal ductal lobular unit. This distension results in ovoid or circular structures that may be evident on mammography dependent on their size. Cysts are most common in pre-menopausal women in their 30s or 40s. They are less common after the menopause, but may persist or reappear in HRT users [1]. Cysts may be unilateral, but are frequently bilateral and multifocal. They can be classified according to size, a microcyst being <3 mm and a macrocyst >3 mm.

L. Hackney (✉)
Consultant Radiographer, Breast Care Unit, University Hospital of North Staffordshire, Newcastle Road, Stoke-on-Trent ST4 6QG, UK
e-mail: Lisa.hackney@uhns.nhs.uk

S. Williams
Consultant Radiographer, Breast Imaging Treatment Centre, Royal Shrewsbury Hospital, Mytton Oak Road, Shrewsbury, SY3 8XQ, UK
e-mail: Susan.williams2@sath.nhs.uk

Simple cysts are benign and do not require any treatment or further diagnostic workup unless painful when aspiration can relieve symptoms. Complex cysts require aspiration or needle core biopsy to exclude intracystic disease [2] (Fig. 4.1).

Fibroadenoma

Fibroadenomas are benign fibroepithelial tumours. They are most common in adolescent girls and young women [3]. Fibroadenomas typically present as smooth, mobile, firm masses but may also be impalpable and detected via mammographic imaging. It is not uncommon for individuals to have multiple fibroadenomata.

On mammography fibroadenomas appear as well-defined round, ovoid, or lobulated masses (Fig. 4.2). The masses may calcify over time and develop a typical popcorn-shaped pattern (Figs. 4.3 and 4.4). A typical benign calcified fibroadenoma requires no further work-up. If non-calcified, ultrasound is required to characterise the lesion and dependent upon the age of the patient histological sampling (needle core biopsy) may be performed.

There are also special types of fibroadenoma to include: lactating adenomas, tubular adenomas and juvenile fibroadenomas. Occasionally in adolescent girls and young women these masses grow to a large size and are termed juvenile giant fibroadenomas.

P. Hogg et al. (eds.), *Digital Mammography: A Holistic Approach*,
DOI 10.1007/978-3-319-04831-4_4,

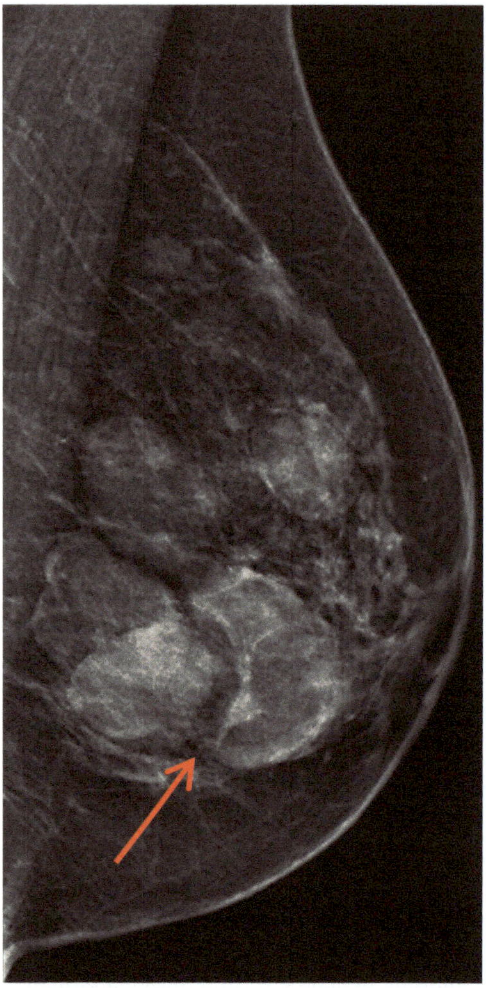

Fig. 4.1 Cysts. Medio-Lateral Oblique (MLO) view showing multiple ovoid/lobulated lesions (*arrow*). Parenchymal structures can be seen through the lesion. The low density, ovoid shape and partial halo suggest a benign lesion, but ultrasound is required to differentiate a cyst from a solid lesion

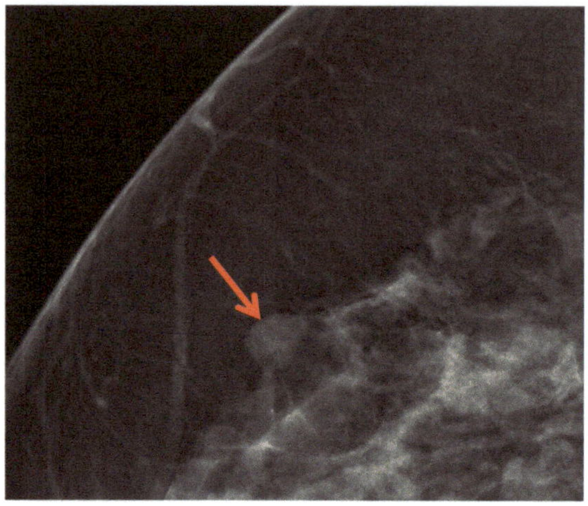

Fig. 4.2 Fibroadenoma. Cranio-caudal (CC) view showing a well-defined lesion (*arrow*) in the outer aspect of the right breast

Phyllodes Tumours

Phyllodes tumours are also fibroepithelial tumours of the breast which have some similarities to a fibroadenoma, but are rare in comparison accounting for less than 1 % of all breast tumours [4]. They most commonly occur between the ages of 40 and 60. Clinically they commonly present as a large rapidly growing lump.

Mammographically, most phyllodes tumours are large, circumscribed masses that are round, oval, or lobulated [5] (Fig. 4.5).

Phyllodes tumours are classified as *benign* (non-cancerous), *malignant* (cancerous), or *borderline.* Benign Phyllodes tumours require excision with a good clear histological margin as they have a likelihood of local recurrence after excision.

Borderline or malignant tumours and those of a large size are considered significant risk factors for local recurrence. For these lesions mastectomy and immediate breast reconstruction may be advocated as the role of adjuvant treatments remain unproven [6].

Haemangioma

Breast haemangiomas are benign vascular tumours, which fall into two categories (capillary and cavernous) dependent upon vessel size [7]. Clinical manifestation is a palpable lump but they are often incidental findings on screening mammography.

Haemangiomas appear as well-defined, ovoid or lobulated masses located within the superficial tissues of the breast (Figs. 4.6 and 4.7), and based

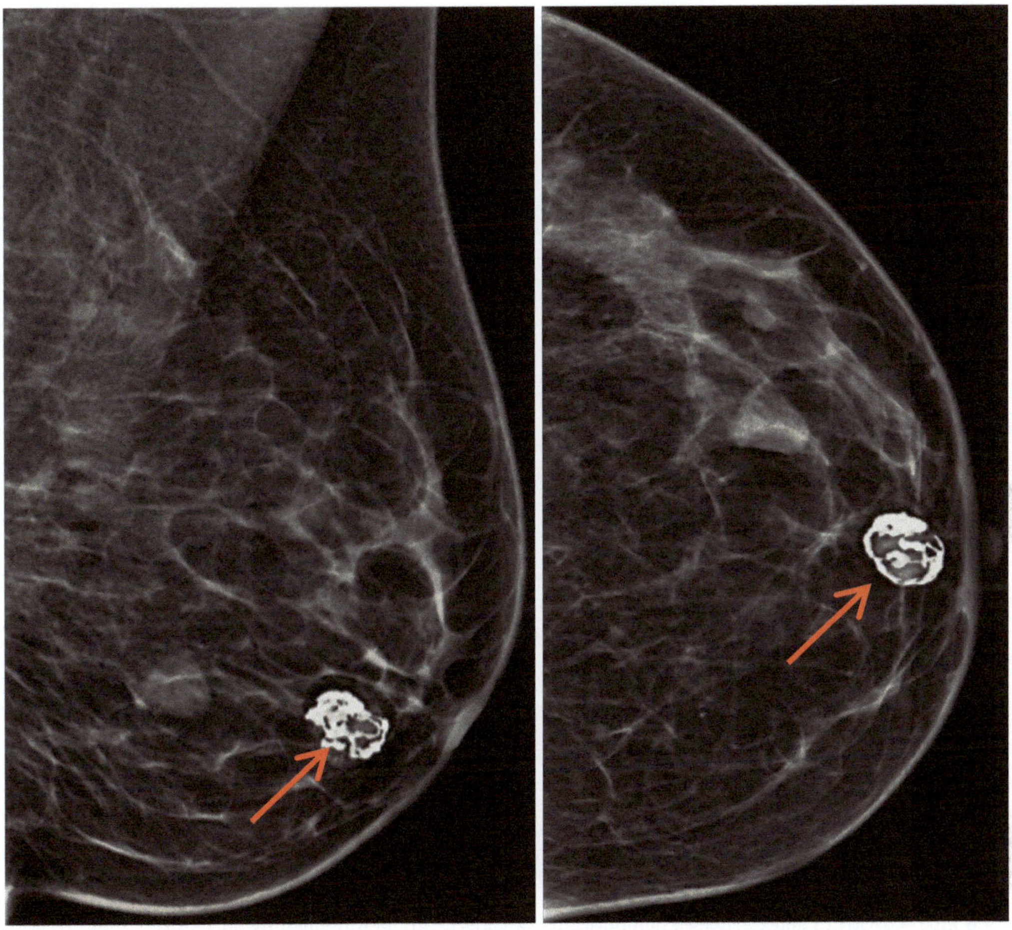

Figs. 4.3 and 4.4 Fibroadenoma: MLO and CC mammogram show several circumscribed masses. The anterior mass (*arrow*) contains course heterogenous "popcorn" calcifications typical for fibroadenoma

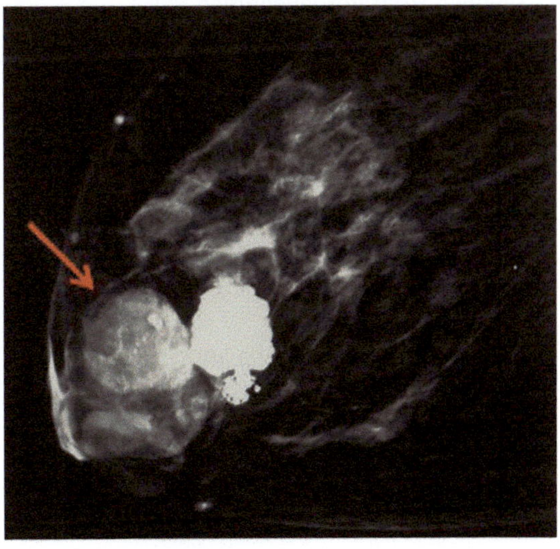

Fig. 4.5 Phyllodes. MLO view shows a heterogeneously dense breast with a rounded, well-circumscribed, 5-cm mass (*arrow*) in the retro-areolar region of the right breast

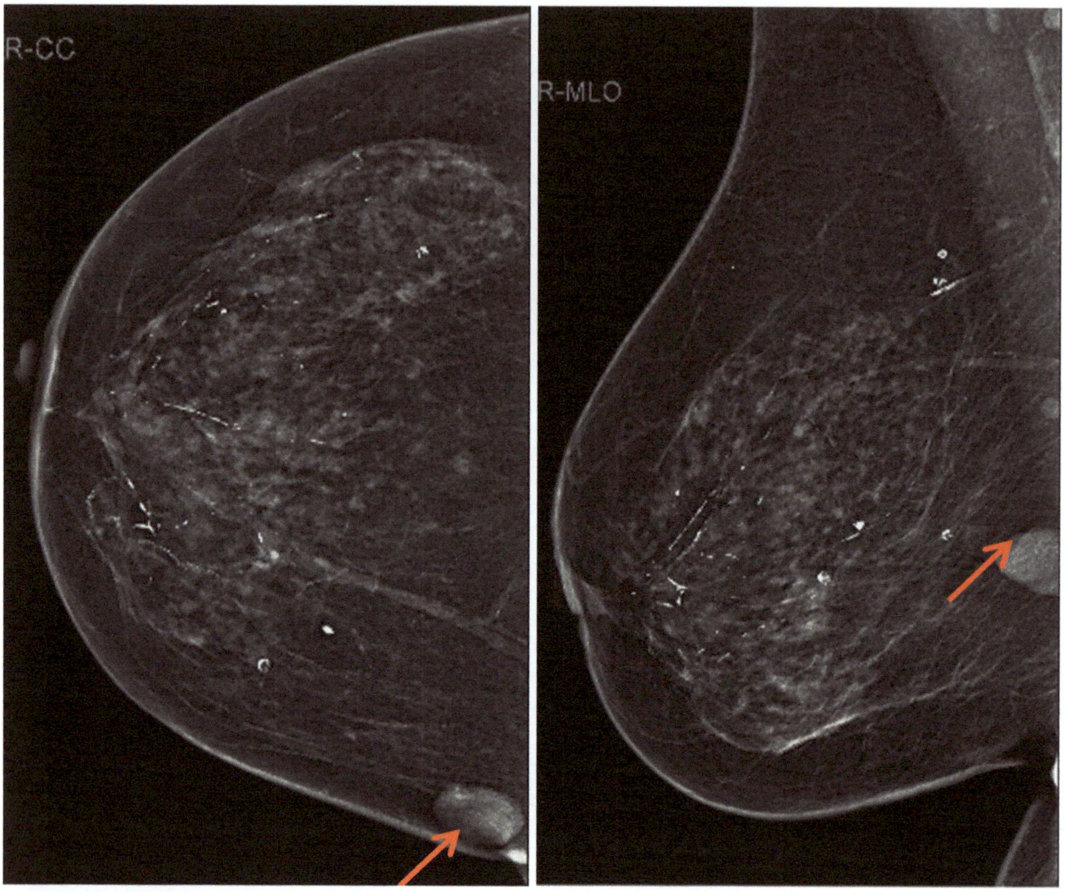

Figs. 4.6 and 4.7 MLO and CC views demonstrating a superficial, well defined ovoid lesion (*arrow*) in the inner aspect of the right breast

on mammography alone can also be difficult to distinguish from fibroadenomas.

Gynaecomastia

Gynaecomastia is the commonest benign male breast condition, peaking in adolescence and over 50 years of age. Breast enlargement occurs due to benign ductal and stromal proliferation. There are a wide range of causes including endogenous hormonal imbalance, systemic disease, hormone producing tumours, obesity and an action of some drugs. Gynaecomastia usually presents as a firm, palpable subareolar mass which may be tender and can be unilateral or bilateral.

On mammography, gynaecomastia has three typical patterns [8]: nodular, dendritic, and diffuse.

The early florid phase of gynaecomastia (nodular) is associated with shorter duration of symptoms and is identified on mammography as a large, poorly defined, subareolar density (Fig. 4.8).

The dendritic growth pattern is observed when symptoms are persistent over a longer time period and mammographically manifests as a smaller, spiculated, subareolar density (Fig. 4.9).

The third pattern, diffuse gynaecomastia, is frequently related to oestrogen exposure. Mammographically this mimics a heterogeneously dense female breast (Fig. 4.10).

Pseudogynaecomastia relates to purely fatty enlargement of the breasts simulating

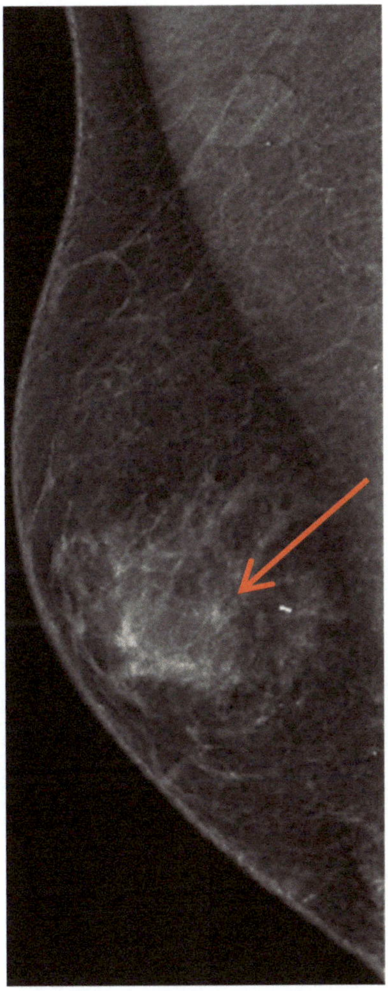

Fig. 4.8 Florid gynaecomastia associated with an acute process

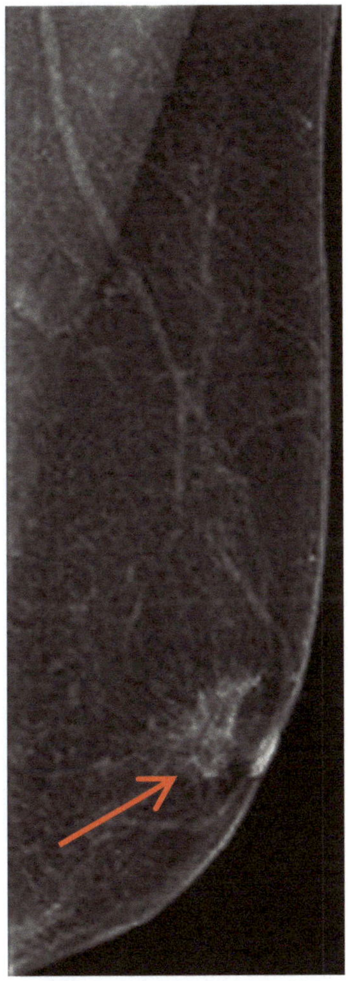

Fig. 4.9 Dendritic gynecomastia representative of a chronic condition

gynaecomastia but there is no glandular tissue (Fig. 4.11).

Schwannoma

The majority of primary tumours of the breast have an epithelial origin. Non-epithelial tumours in the breast are rare [9]. A Schwannoma (Fig. 4.12) develops from 'Schwann' cells of the peripheral nerve sheath, and may also be referred to as a neurilemmoma, or peripheral nerve sheath tumour.

For unknown reasons, Schwann cells can occasionally grow in a neoplastic fashion resulting in a benign tumour. However, there is a remote likelihood of a Schwannoma developing malignant cellular characteristics [10].

Hamartoma

A breast hamartoma is a benign breast lesion resulting from proliferation of fibrous, glandular, and fatty tissue surrounded by a thin capsule of connective tissue [12].

Lesions can be variable in size, and present as painless soft lumps, unilateral breast enlargement without a palpable mass or can be asymptomatic and an incidental finding on mammography.

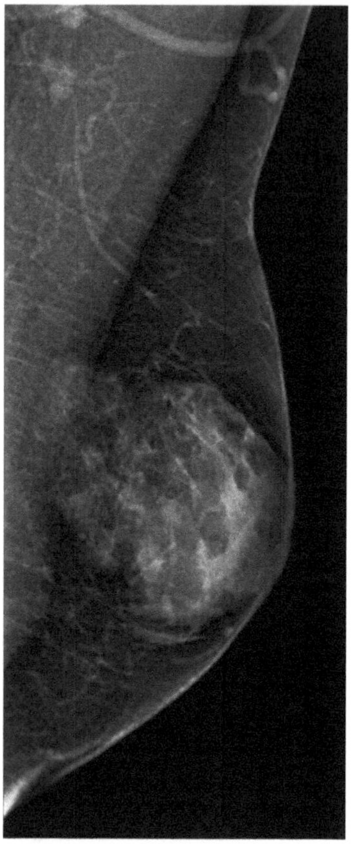

Fig. 4.10 Heterogenously dense breast tissue

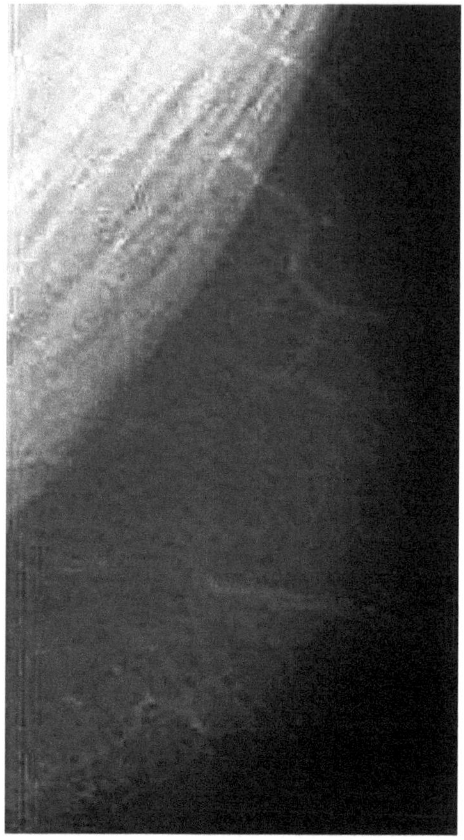

Fig. 4.11 Pseudogynaecomastia, characterised by subcutaneous fat deposition in the breast without a mass or glandular development

Multiple hamartomas are associated with Cowden's syndrome (a rare autosomal dominant inherited disorder), which also carries an associated increased risk of breast carcinoma [13].

Mammographically hamartomas are typically seen as a well circumscribed, round or ovoid masses comprising of both fat and soft-tissue densities (both radiolucent and dense components). Sometimes this is described as a "breast within a breast" appearance [14] (Figs. 4.13 and 4.14).

Lipoma

A lipoma is a benign lesion composed of fat. Generally breast lipomas present as painless, soft, mobile lumps, which are variable in size (ranging from <1 cm to >6 cm) [15].

Mammographically lipomas (Figs. 4.15 and 4.16) are identified as radiolucent masses and are often easier to detect in denser breasts.

Pseudoangiomatous Stromal Hyperplasia (PASH)

Pseudoangiomatous stromal hyperplasia is a benign, uncommon form of stromal (mesenchymal) overgrowth within breast tissue [16].

PASH is typically found in premenopausal women but can be a common incidental finding at breast biopsy. If forming a mass lesion, the presentation is commonly a solitary, circumscribed, firm palpable mass. There is a wide variance of size of PASH mass lesions with diameters

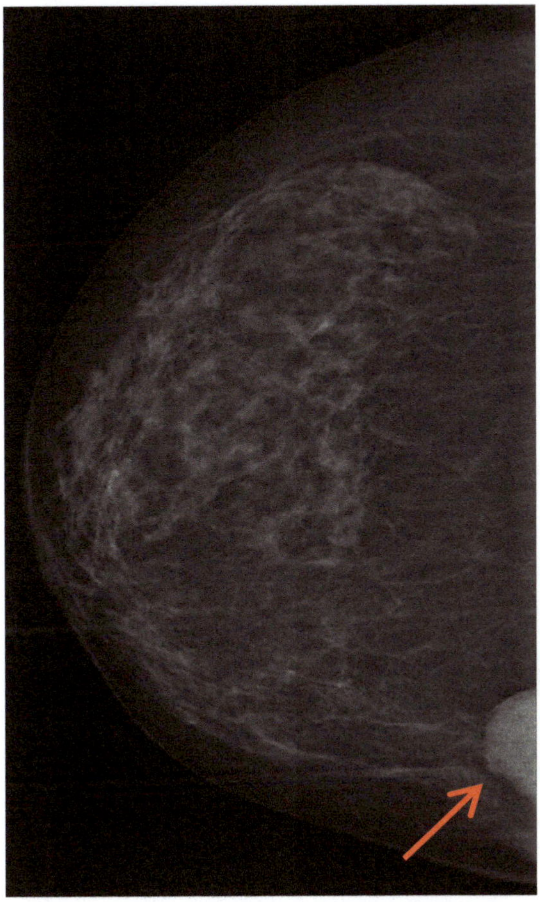

Fig. 4.12 Mammographically schwannomas are most often described as a non-specific well defined round or oval, high-density lesion [11]. The CC view demonstrates the anterior border of a well-defined dense mass in the inner aspect of the right breast (*arrow*). The mass is only partially demonstrated due to its posterior and medial location

ranging from 1 to 12 cm. PASH is not associated with malignancies and is not considered a premalignant lesion [16].

Most frequently they appear on mammography as a circumscribed mass, but variable appearances have also been reported [17].

Galactocele

A galactocele is a benign breast lesion that typically occurs in lactating women or more commonly on cessation of lactation [18]. They occur as a result of ductal obstruction and inspissation of the milk

Galactoceles have differing proportions of water, proteins, fat, and lactose and this is reflected as variable mammographic appearances [19]. Based on this galactoceles could appear radiolucent, have a fat/fluid level or appear of mixed density.

Typical presentation is that of a painless breast lump that may be solitary and unilateral, but multiple and bilateral nodules have also been reported.

Spontaneous resolution occurs in the majority of cases, but if there is diagnostic uncertainty aspiration can be performed which will classically yield milky fluid of variable viscosity dependent on how old the liquid is.

Haematoma

A haematoma is a collection of blood, which usually results from a preceding direct trauma, surgery, or biopsy but can spontaneously occur in those on anticoagulants. Clinical correlation is essential to avoid misinterpretation with breast malignancy.

Dependent on the stage of haematoma formation they have variable mammographic appearances; the most common being an area of diffusely increased glandular density [20]. If more localised a relatively well-defined mass may also be seen (Fig. 4.17).

The majority of haematomas resolve within 2–4 weeks and no further evaluation is required. Some haematomas may liquefy and develop into a breast seroma or over time may evolve into fat necrosis.

Papilloma

An intraductal papilloma is a benign tumour that grows within the breast ducts. They are wart-like growths of glandular tissue with fibrous tissue and blood vessels.

Intra ductal papillomas are classified into two categories. Central – are typically solitary lesions

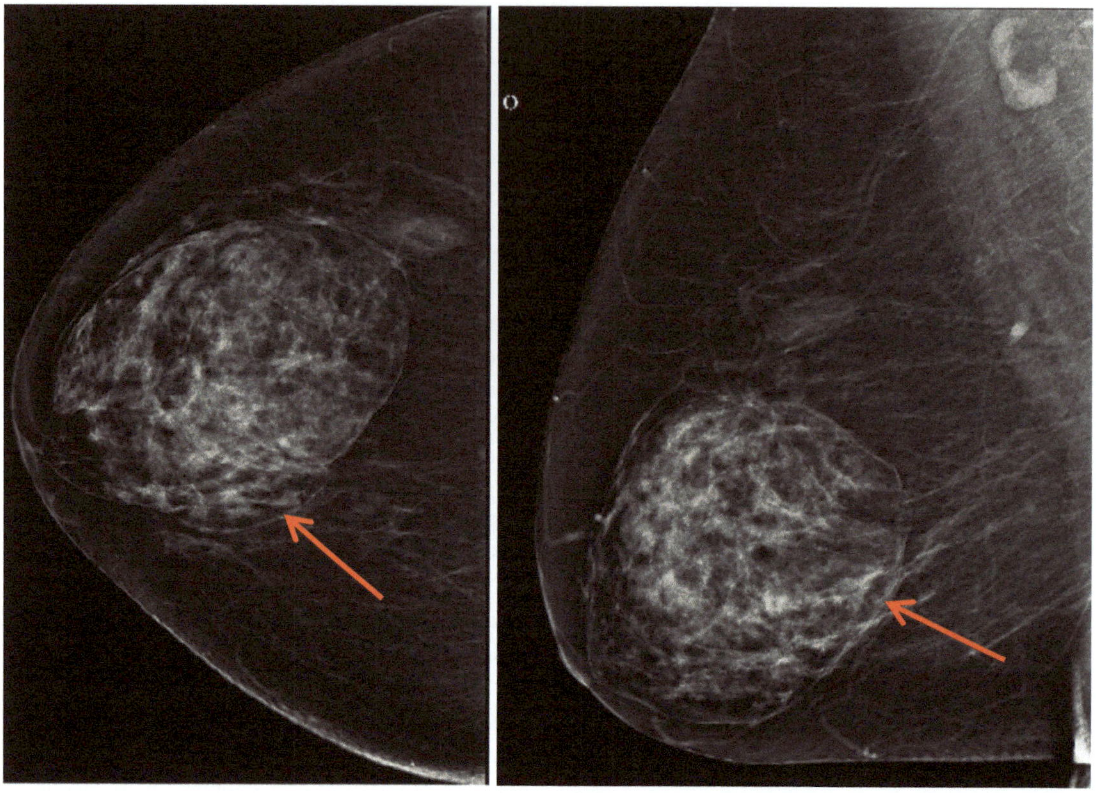

Figs. 4.13 and 4.14 Hamartoma. On mammography hamartomas have a typical appearance. An encapsulated lucent lesion (*arrow*) containing varying amounts of fat, fibrous and adenomatous elements

within a large duct in the subareolar region. These may be felt as a small lump and are typically associated with a clear or bloody nipple discharge. Peripheral papillomas are likely to be multiple and located within smaller ducts.

Mammograms are often normal particularly if the papillomas are small. When imaging findings are present, they are identified as a circumscribed subareolar mass or a solitary dilated retroareolar duct [21] (Fig. 4.18).

Papillomas are considered heterogeneous lesions with variable pathological features and therefore large volume core sampling (Vacuum Assisted Biopsy) or surgical excision is required to exclude atypia.

Multiple papillomatosis is defined as an abnormal overgrowth of cells within the ducts and is more frequently associated with hyperplasia, atypia, DCIS, sclerosing adenosis, and radial scar [22]. Mammographic findings of multiple papillomatosis are variable from well-defined masses with or without calcification, foci of microcalcification, clusters of nodules, and asymmetric densities.

Amyloid Tumour

Amyloidosis results from the abnormal deposition of a protein, called amyloid, in various tissues of the body. Breast amyloidosis is rare and can be part of a systemic disease or it may be localised to the breast [23] (Fig. 4.19). The typical clinical presentation is a unilateral, painless, solitary breast mass, which may have associated microcalcifications.

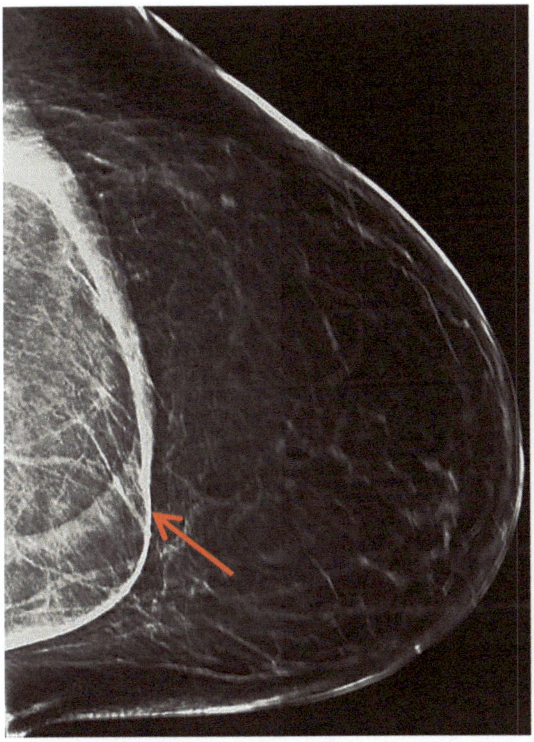

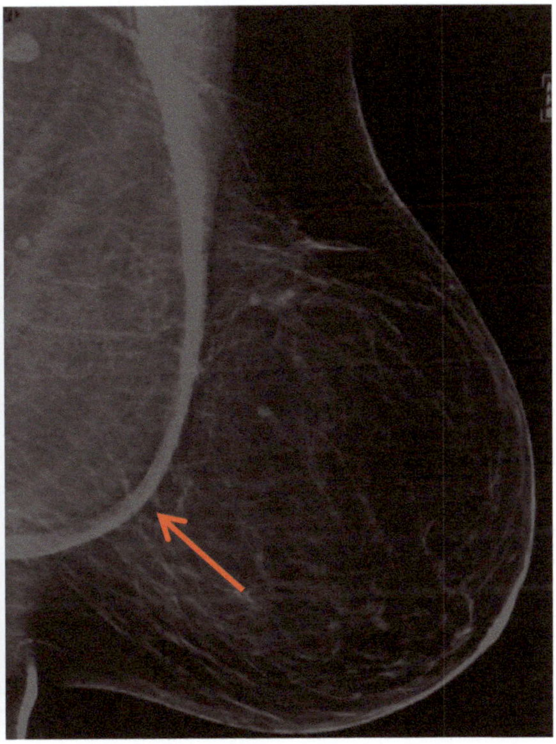

Figs. 4.15 and 4.16 Intra-muscular lipoma visualised as a smooth radiolucent lesion with a surrounding capsule of fibrous tissue (*arrow*)

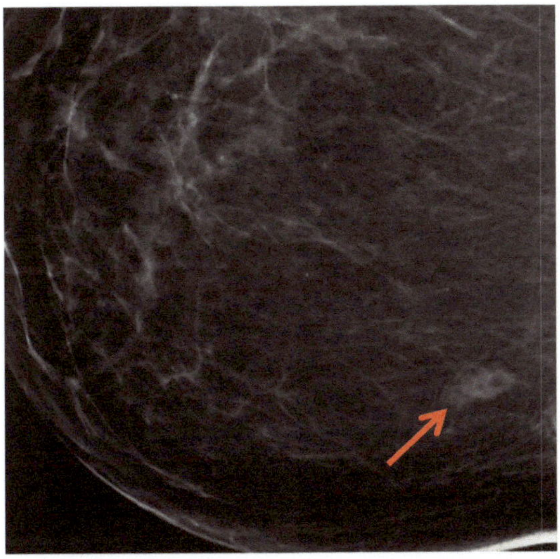

Fig. 4.17 Haematoma. Right CC view shows a relatively well-defined lesion of variable density (*arrow*)

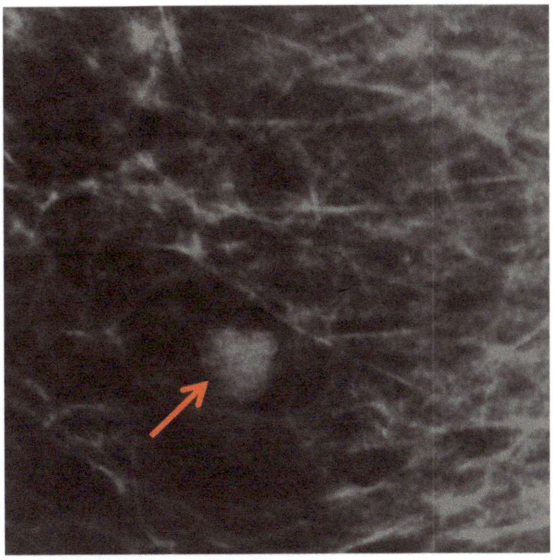

Fig. 4.18 Papilloma. CC view showing a circumscribed solitary subareolar mass (*arrow*)

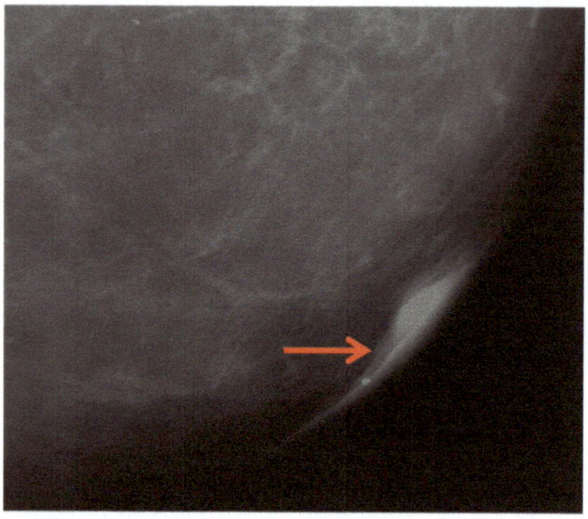

Fig. 4.19 Amyloid tumour. A unilateral, solitary superficial breast mass with associated microcalcification (*arrow*)

Mastitis/Abscess

Mastitis refers to inflammation of breast tissue. Early stages of mastitis typically present as localised pain, redness, swelling, and warmth with a fairly rapid onset.

Puerperal

Puerperal mastitis refers to inflammation of the breast in connection with pregnancy, breastfeeding or weaning and is considered to be a result of blocked milk ducts or excess milk [19].

Non-puerperal

The term non-puerperal mastitis refers to inflammation of the breast unrelated to pregnancy and breastfeeding. Women with diabetes, chronic illness, or an impaired immune system may be more susceptible to developing mastitis [24].

Later stages of mastitis may have associated systemic symptoms and abscess formation (collection of pus).

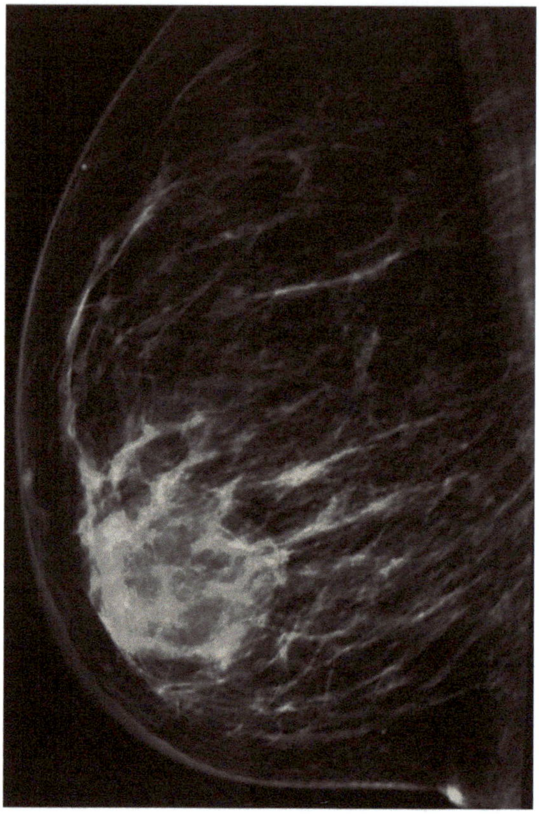

Fig. 4.20 Abscess. Diffuse asymmetric density in the central right breast

Abscesses are managed with antibiotic treatment, aspiration if amenable and irrigation of the abscess cavity. In a certain number of cases incision and surgical drainage is required.

Mammography is rarely indicated but may be undertaken to exclude the possibility of malignancy in non-puerperal abscesses, and in puerperal abscesses that are non-responsive to treatment. Inflammatory breast cancer presents with similar symptoms to mastitis and is an aggressive form of the disease.

Mammographic appearances of an abscess are often non- specific but include

- Skin thickening
- Asymmetric density (Fig. 4.20), or a focal mass

Breast Metastases

Metastases to the breast are rare. The most frequent source of a metastatic breast lesion is the contralateral breast but may also arise from:

Lymphoma/leukaemia, melanoma, sarcomas, prostate cancer, lung cancer, gastric cancer, ovarian cancer and renal cell cancer [25].

Metastases to the breast tend to be rounded, well defined and located in the subcutaneous fat and are much more likely to be multiple and/or bilateral.

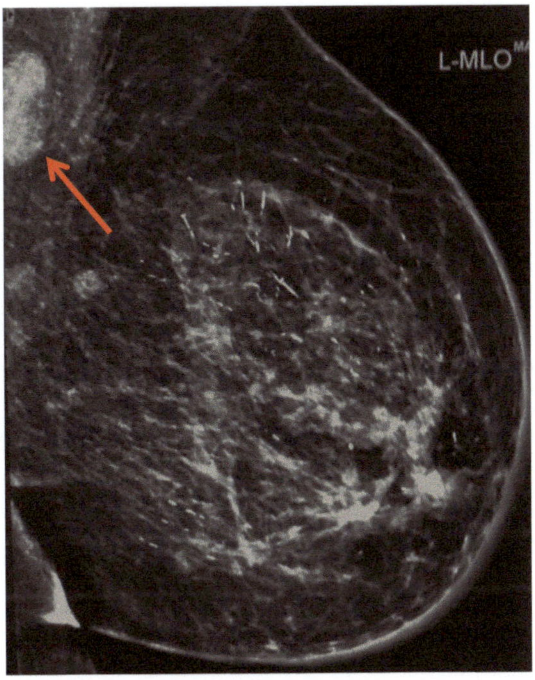

Fig. 4.21 Lymphoma. Diffuse increased reticular pattern with skin thickening and oedema secondary to lymphatic obstruction. Enlarged axillary lymph nodes are evident (*arrow*)

Breast Lymphoma

Breast lymphomas are comprised of lymphoid tissue and breast tissue. They can be primary or secondary lesions, but both are uncommon [26].

Presentation may be as a palpable mass or as diffuse thickening of the breast, with enlarged axillary lymph nodes.

Lymphomas have variable mammographic appearances but typically manifest with a diffuse increase in parenchymal density (Fig. 4.21).

Breast Sarcoma

A breast sarcoma is a rare nonepithelial cancer that develops from connective tissue. They can develop as a primary lesion, occasionally after radiation therapy (therapy related), or after treatment of another malignancy (secondary) when breast or arm lymphoedema is present [27].

Duct Ectasia

Duct ectasia is an involutionary condition characterised by dilated ducts and chronic inflammation resulting in debris within the duct. Inspissation of the debris and secretions can lead to calcification of the ductal contents. It usually coexists with periductal mastitis as the fluid often sets up an irritant reaction in surrounding tissue leading to periductal mastitis or even abscess and fistula formation. It is more common in females aged 50–60 years. Plasma cell mastitis is often used as an interchangeable term with duct ectasia but tends to refer to a more extreme form of the disease process [28]. A common mammographic feature is calcification of variable morphology including calcified ring, oval shapes or elongated, very dense calcification with central lucency. The calcifications are usually of a higher density and wider calibre than malignant type casting calcification and directed towards the nipple as shown in Fig. 4.22 [29]. The symptomatic features include nipple discharge, nipple retraction, non-cyclical mastalgia and subareolar masses, which all mimic breast cancer. It is a feature commonly seen on screening mammograms.

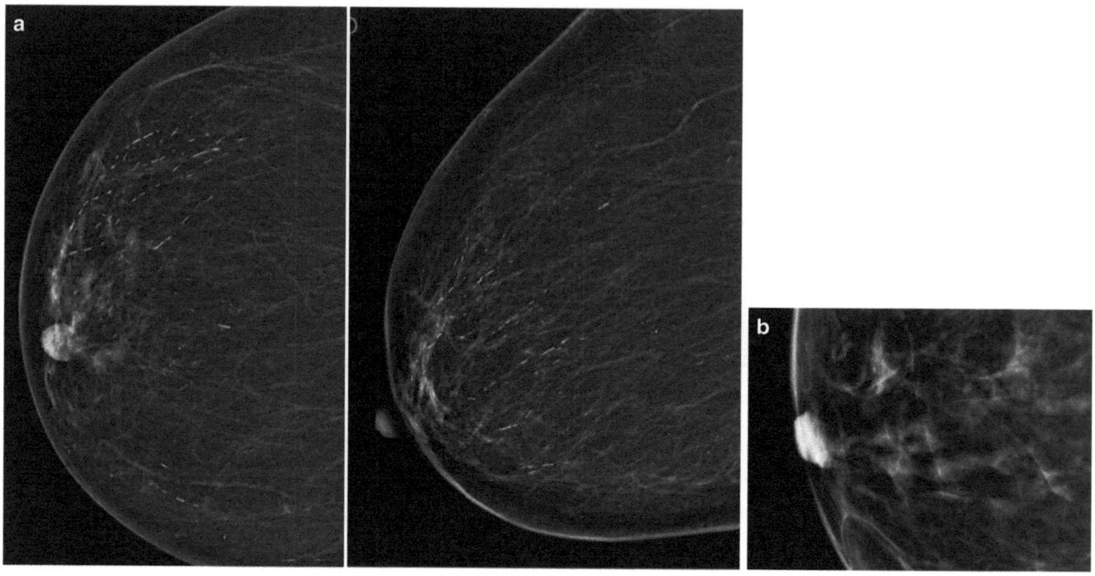

Fig. 4.22 Duct ectasia. Typical mammographic features (**a**) showing thick linear rod-like calcification orientated with the long axes directed towards the nipple, (**b**) dilated ducts in the retroareolar region

Radial Scar/Complex Sclerosing Lesion

Radial scars and complex sclerosing lesions are considered to be the same clinical feature, the differentiation lying in their respective sizes – a radial scar being <10 mm in diameter [30]. Although it is a scarring process, radial scars are not related to trauma. A radial scar is a benign lesion but is important because it can be linked with DCIS and tubular cancers [31]. It is a stellate lesion (Fig. 4.23) which can mimic an invasive carcinoma on a mammogram but their appearance often varies on different projections. Typical mammographic features are a lesion with a radiolucent centre from which multiple long thin spicules radiate [32]. Although they can be palpable [33] they are more frequently a screen-detected or incidental finding. The mammographic appearances are also similar to a post-surgical breast scar. Correlation with the clinical breast examination, an ultrasound scan and a needle core biopsy will assist with the differentiation between a radial scar and an invasive carcinoma.

Fat Necrosis

Fat necrosis is a benign condition resulting from trauma, however, most cases are diagnosed after surgery. Following breast trauma, haemorrhage occurs which may extravasate into the parenchyma causing oedema and disruptions to the fat cells creating intracellular vacuoles filled with necrotic lipid material [34, 35]. Apoptosis and necrosis of the cells also occur in the tissue and a greater necrotic component results in changes to the breast which can mimic more sinister conditions. Mammographically, fat necrosis can range from clearly benign, to malignant appearing masses or calcifications. The most common mammographic finding is dystrophic calcifications followed by a radiolucent oil cyst. An oil cyst is a benign lesion where an area of focal fat necrosis becomes walled by fibrous tissue which can calcify. On mammography it is typically seen as a radiolucent rounded mass of fat density with or without wall calcification (Fig. 4.24a, b). Oil cysts are the only mammographic finding that reliably indicates fat necrosis [36]. Suspicious spiculate masses and focal areas of architectural distortion can also

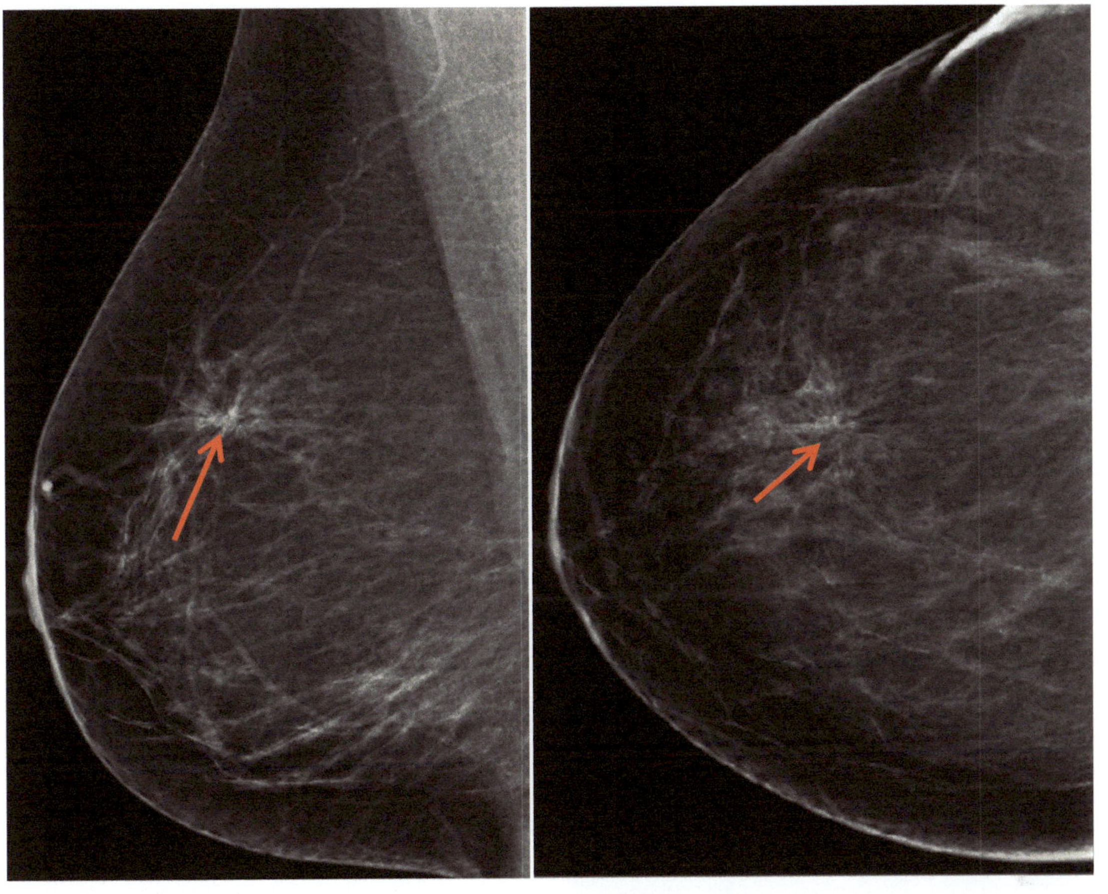

Fig. 4.23 Right MLO view (**a**) and Right CC view (**b**) demonstrating a Radial scar (*arrow*) with long spicules radiating from a radiolucent centre

occur, resembling carcinoma. The calcification of fat necrosis is typically peripheral with a stippled curvilinear appearance creating the appearance of lucent "bubbles" in the breast parenchyma (Fig. 4.24c). Fat necrosis of the breast can change, regressing, or resolving over time [37].

Surgical Scar

A benign complication of postsurgical mammography is scar tissue at the site of surgery. The dense fibrous tissue that develops in a postsurgical scar often appears as an irregular mass with spiculate margins, often with retraction of the surrounding tissue (Fig. 4.25). The mammographic appearances are difficult to differentiate from cancer particularly for the first mammogram after surgery as distortion and increased density may persist for many months post-surgery [34]. Other mammographic appearances include architectural distortion, a poorly marginated soft-tissue mass with interspersed radiolucent areas or a spiculate lesion all of these may have associated calcification. Postsurgical scarring usually has some relationship to the skin scar or site of previous surgery and is either stable or decreases in size over time [34].

Treatment for breast cancer does not necessarily only involve the removal of the tumour. Other interventions such as radiotherapy and axillary surgery will impact on the mammographic appearances (Fig. 4.26) including generalised tissue oedema, skin thickening and a change in shape and texture of the breast parenchyma [38].

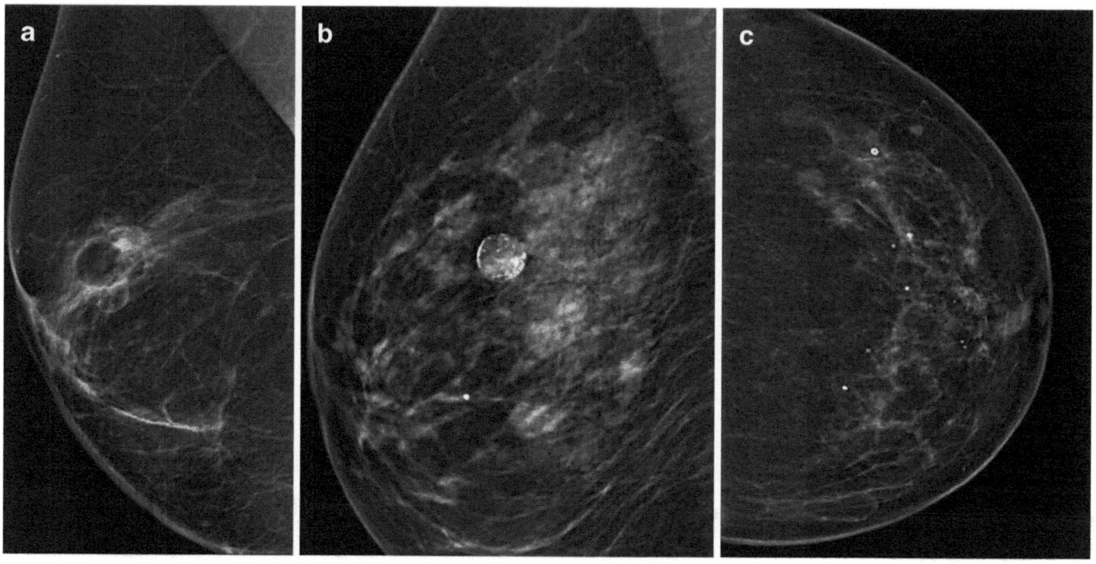

Fig. 4.24 Shows fat necrosis of the breast (**a**) shows the typical mammographic features of an oil cyst (**b**) coarse calcifications in peripheral and central portions of mass with lucent centres (**c**) lucent "bubbles"

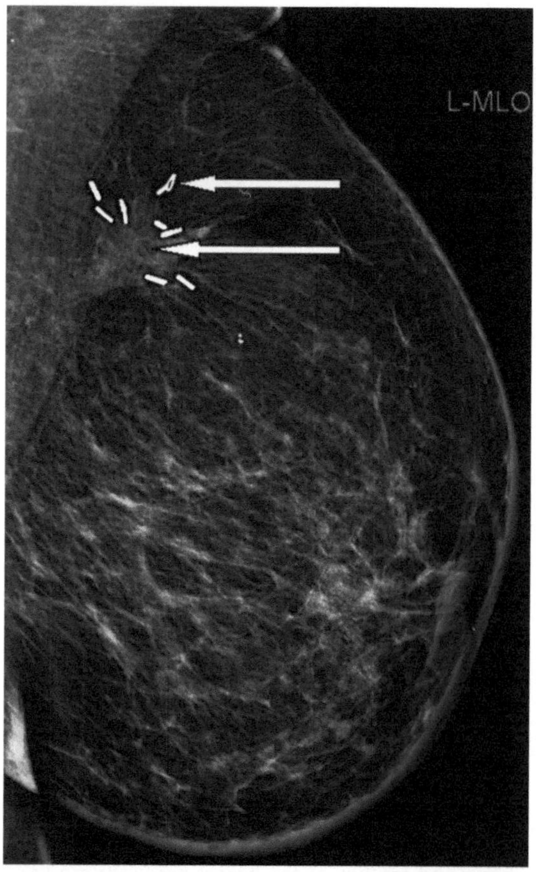

Fig. 4.25 MLO view post-surgery although the scarring appears spiculate there are areas of lucency at the centre. Surgical clips can also be useful to correlate the lesion with the site of surgery (*arrow*)

Postsurgical changes can render mammography technically difficult. Thorough history taking is important including accurate recording of the site of surgery when imaging the client.

Calcifications

Microcalcification on a mammogram is an important finding as it can be associated with tumours but is more often seen as part of benign processes. Calcification can be located in the breast lobules, ducts, blood vessels, skin, stroma, other breast lesions or can be artefactual [39, 40]. The distribution of the calcification is important. It can appear scattered (or diffuse), clustered or linear. The number, size and form the calcification takes is important and can be rounded/punctate, granular, coarse/popcorn, powderish or linear. All of these characteristics inform the underlying biological process and hence the diagnosis [32, 41].

Benign Calcification

Lobular calcifications are usually smooth and round they may be single, loosely grouped (Fig. 4.27) or scattered widely throughout the

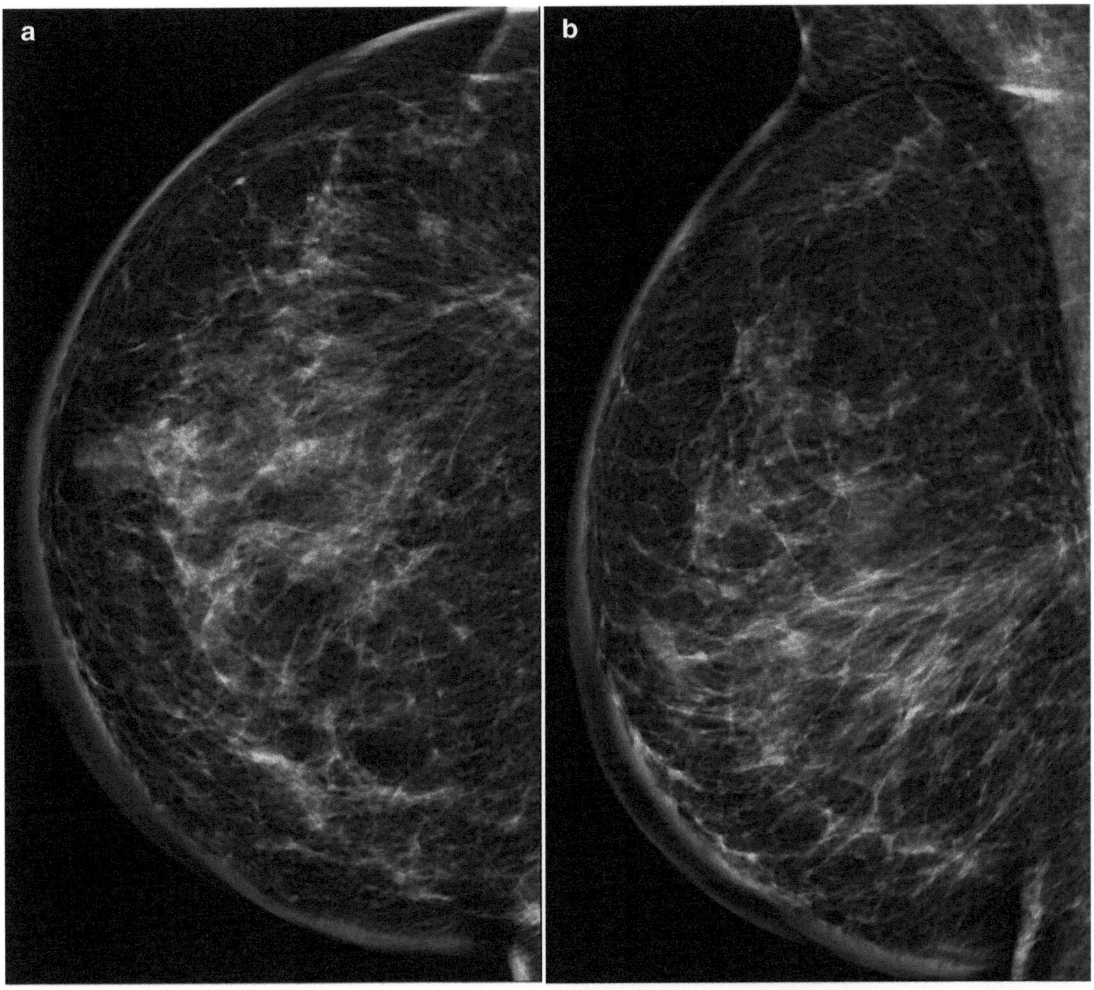

Fig. 4.26 Right cc (**a**) and Right MLO view (**b**) Show generalised treatment changes of the breast post treatment for breast cancer. These include skin thickening, tissue oedema and distortion of the breast contour

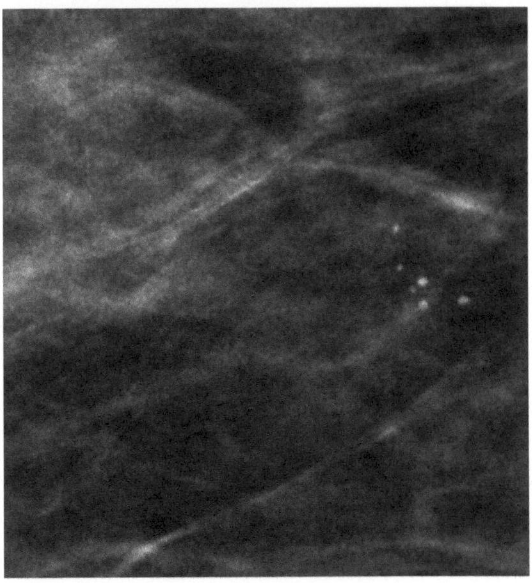

Fig. 4.27 Lobular calcification the individual flecks are rounded, smooth and loosely grouped together

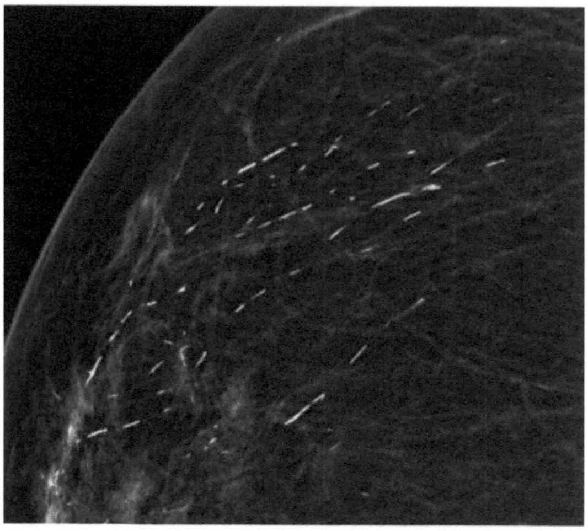

Fig. 4.28 Ductal calcification the calcification is linear and large and forms in the ducts and so has a tendency to direct towards the nipple

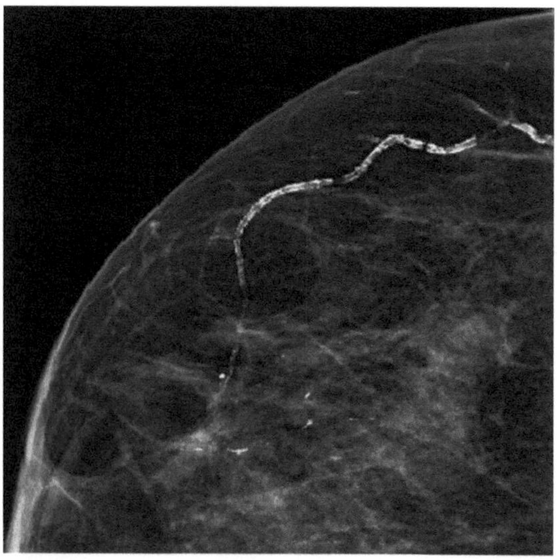

Fig. 4.29 Vascular calcification can be seen to line the blood vessels of the breast and often have a meandering pattern

breast. They usually form in the acini of microcystic dilated lobules [34].

Ductal calcifications form in the duct lumen (Fig. 4.28). In benign processes this is often caused by calcification of the debris in the duct lumen and they are usually much larger than suspicious or malignant calcification [34].

Vascular calcifications (Fig. 4.29) in the breast are associated with blood vessels and are most often seen in post menopausal women with arteriosclerotic heart disease. They are typically seen on mammograms as dense, linear, parallel, circuitous or tram-track like calcifications and are usually not oriented in the direction of the duct towards the nipple-areolar complex [34].

Skin calcifications (Fig. 4.30) in the breast usually form in dermal sweat glands following processes such as low grade folliculitis or inspissation of sebaceous material. Often, these calcifications are seen in groups as they extend into small glands in the skin. Skin calcifications are often round or oval in shape with lucent centres. Calcifications may also form in skin lesions such as moles which can have a lacelike pattern on mammography.

Calcification can be associated with other benign breast lesions and coarse or popcorn calcifications are often seen with involuting fibroadenomas (Fig. 4.31) [14]. The calcifications are usually very dense and much larger than microcalcification.

'Calcification' can also be artefactual from products such as deodorant.

Benign Breast Changes

Aberrations in the Normal Development and Involution of the breast (ANDI) is used to describe a wide spectrum of the benign breast diseases [42]. It is based on the theory that most of the encountered benign breast disorders are essentially minor aberrations in the normal development process, hormonal response and involution of the breast. Processes such as fibrosis, fibrocystic change and sclerosing adenosis are considered disorders of involution. It is less common for post menopausal women to have benign breast disease [43].

Focal fibrosis of the breast is a benign entity composed of dense collagenous stroma with sparse glandular and vascular elements and presents as localised areas of fibrous tissue. Focal fibrosis may appear as a either a well circumscribed mass, an

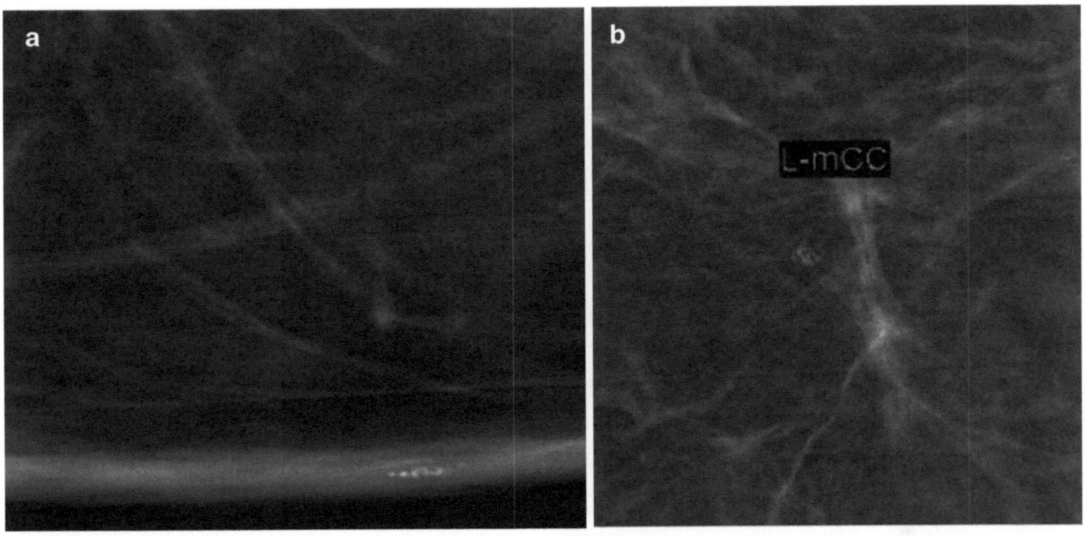

Fig. 4.30 Tangential view (**a**) and magnification view (**b**) demonstrating skin calcification

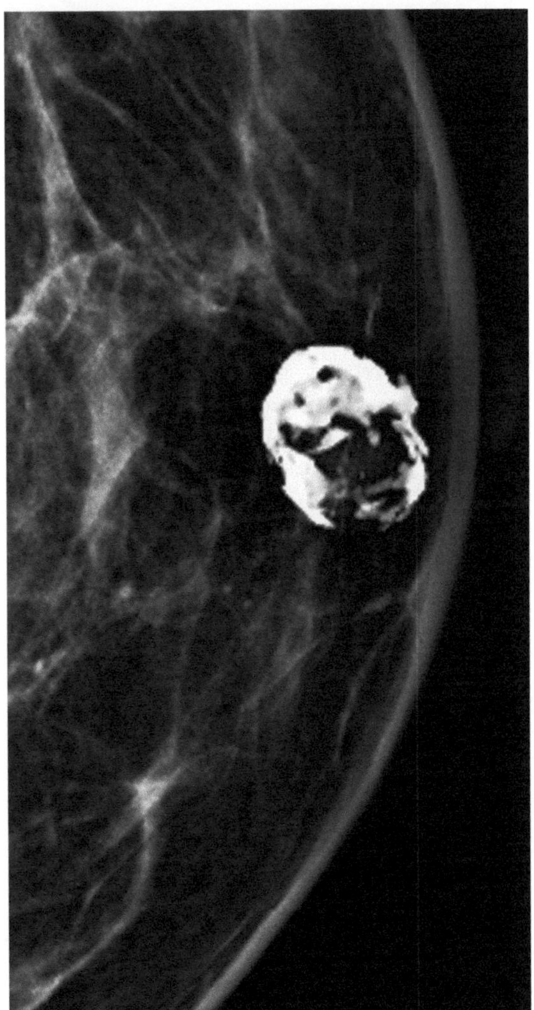

Fig. 4.31 Popcorn calcification. Very coarse and dense calcification associated with a longstanding fibroadenoma

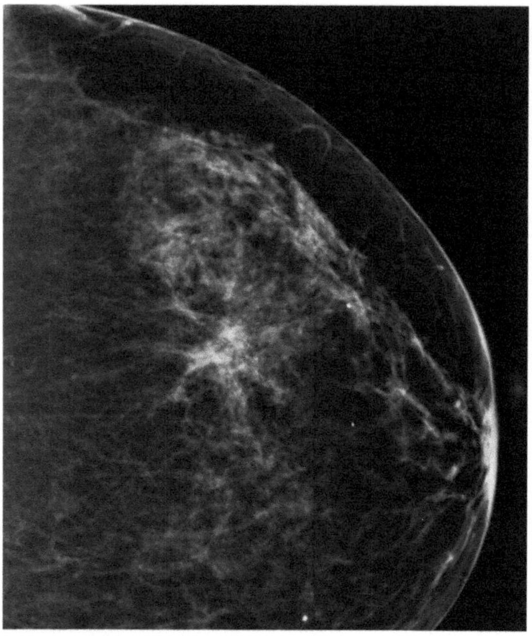

Fig. 4.32 Focal fibrosis showing as an area of possible architectural distortion a needle core biopsy confirmed this was fibrosis

irregular mass or as focal asymmetry mammographically (Fig. 4.32).

Fibrocystic change is a benign process affecting the terminal duct-lobular unit and is thought to be associated with involutionary or hormone changes or related genetic abnormalities. It includes gross and microscopic changes that are often asymptomatic but can present as nodularity and pain. It affects women 20–50 and declines post-menopause. It can be diffuse, patchy or focal and can form a well or poorly defined mass that can be seen on mammography as an increased density (Fig. 4.33). It is seen as a wide spectrum of altered morphology from innocuous to those associated with risk of carcinoma.

Sclerosing adenosis is usually an incidental finding but may show as a mammographic abnormality such as microcalcification or architectural distortion. It is seen more commonly in a slightly older age group. It is a benign condition in which extra tissue develops within the breast lobules forming multiple small, firm, tender lumps, fibrous tissue and sometimes small cysts in the breast. Presentation is frequently recurring pain that tends to be linked to the menstrual cycle.

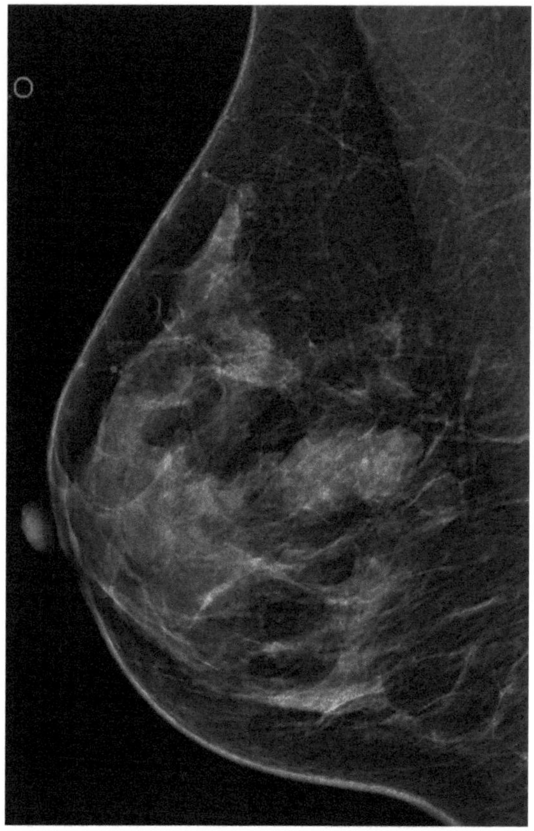

Fig. 4.33 Fibrocystic breast change with multiple well defined masses (cysts) in a background of fibrous breast tissue. Ultrasound is a good adjunct investigation to confirm the mammographic findings

Sclerosing adenosis is usually detected during routine mammograms or following breast surgery. Biopsy usually confirms the diagnosis, because the condition is otherwise difficult to distinguish from breast cancer.

Atypia

Atypical ductal and lobular hyperplasia.

There are two types of atypia namely atypical ductal hyperplasia (ADH) or atypical lobular hyperplasia (ALH). Neither usually shows on a mammogram and they are often diagnosed as an incidental finding to another mammographic concern following core biopsies. ADH and ALH are controversial due to the poorly understood biology but are considered a high risk premalignant lesion holding a bridging position between benign and malignant disease. It is unclear if these lesions are a precursor or histological manifestation of a tissue bed at increased risk. ADH has some, but not all the features of ductal carcinoma in situ (DCIS). The distinction between ALH and lobular carcinoma in situ (LCIS) is that ALH occurs in a non-distended lobule or small lobular duct, whereas LCIS is characterised by distension of the lobules [44].

LCIS

LCIS represents the next step up from ALH along the malignant spectrum of lobular breast carcinoma. LCIS has no macroscopic features, is usually mammographically occult and the diagnosis is often made as an incidental finding making the true incidence of LCIS in the general population unknown. Characteristically LCIS is both multifocal and bilateral. It originates in the terminal ductal lobular unit but leaves the basement membrane intact [44].

DCIS

Ductal carcinoma in situ (DCIS) is a breast carcinoma limited to the ducts which does not extend beyond the basement membrane and so cannot metastasize. Although it is often a mammographic finding some patients do present with a palpable abnormality of the breast or nipple changes. DCIS is associated with a spectrum of disease and has varied mammographic appearances although calcification is the most common (Fig. 4.34) it may present as a simple mass or asymmetry without calcification [34]. The calcifications may have varied appearances but are often linear or granular. DCIS is likely the precursor of invasive ductal carcinoma.

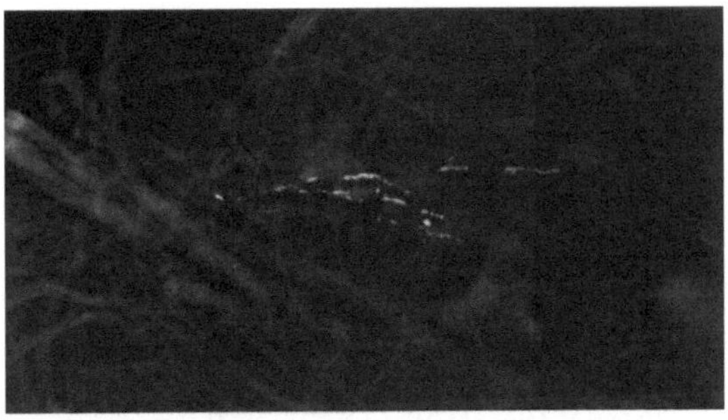

Fig. 4.34 DCIS presenting as focal calcification on a screening mammogram. The calcification has formed in the ducts in a focal linear pattern

Pagets

Pagets disease of the nipple is usually DCIS that initially grows from the terminal ducts and progresses by intraepidermal spread to the nipple skin. It is not demonstrated mammographically. Presentation is often with nipple changes including redness, itching or a burning sensation.

References

1. Devang J, Doshi MD, March DE, Crisi GM, Coughlin BF. Complex cystic breast masses: diagnostic approach and imaging-pathologic correlation. Radiographics. 2007;27 Suppl 1:S53–64.
2. Rinaldi P, Lerardi C, Costantini M, Magno S, Giuliani M, Belli P, Bonomo L. Cystic breast lesions. Sonographic findings and clinical management. J Ultrasound Med. 2010;29(11):1617–26.
3. Chung EM, Cube R, Hall GJ, Gonzalez C, Stocker JT, Glassman LM. From the archives of the AFIP: breast masses in children and adolescents: radiologic-pathologic correlation. Radiographics. 2009;29(3): 907–31.
4. Walter HS, Esmail F, Krupa J, Ahmed SI. Phyllodes tumour of the breast: a retrospective analysis of 87 cases. Cancer Res. 2012;72(24 Suppl 3):P4-14-14.
5. Tan H, Zhang S, Liu H, et al. Imaging findings in phyllodes tumors of the breast. Eur J Radiol. 2012; 81(1):e62–9.

6. Guillot E, Couturaud B, Reyal F, Curnier A, Ravinet J, Laé M, Bollet M, Pierga JY, Salmon R, Fitoussi A, Breast Cancer Study Group of the Institut Curie. Management of phyllodes breast tumors. Breast J. 2011;17:129–37.
7. Mesurolle B, Sygal V, Lalonde L, Lisbona A, Dufresne MP, Gagnon JH, Kao E. Sonographic and mammographic appearances of breast hemangioma. Am J Roentgenol. 2008;191(1):W17–22.
8. Frazier AA. Three patterns of male gynaecomastia. Radiographics. 2013;33(2):460.
9. Dialani V, Hines N, Wang Y, Slanetz P. Breast schwannoma. Case Rep Med. 2011;2011, 930841.
10. Yi JM, Moon EJ, Oh SJ, Lee A, Suh YJ, Baek JM, Choi SH, Jung SS. Malignant peripheral nerve sheath tumor of the breast in a patient without neurofibromatosis: a case report. J Breast Cancer. 2009;12(3):223–6.
11. Balci P, Pekcevik YT, Caferova S, Canda T, Sevinc A, Saydam S. A case of benign schwannoma of the breast: mammographic, ultrasonographic and color doppler ultrasonographic findings. Breast J. 2009;15(4):417–8.
12. Tse GMK, Law BKB, Ma TKF, Chan ABW, Pang LM, Chu WCW, Cheung HS. Hamartoma of the breast: a clinicopathological review. J Clin Pathol. 2002;55:951–4.
13. Ni Y, He X, Chen J, Moline J, Mester J, Orloff MS, Ringel MD, Eng C. Germline SDHx variants modify breast and thyroid cancer risks in Cowden and Cowden-like syndrome via FAD/NAD-dependant destabilization of p53. Hum Mol Genet. 2012;21(2):300–10.
14. Farrokh D, Hashemi J, Ansaripour E. Breast hamartoma: mammographic findings. Iran J Radiol. 2011;8(4):258–60.
15. Lanng C, Erikson BØ, Hoffmann J. Lipoma of the breast: a diagnostic dilemma. Breast. 2004;13(5):408–11.
16. Jones KN, Glazebrook KN, Reynolds C. Pseudoangiomatous stromal hyperplasia: imaging findings with pathologic and clinical correlation. Am J Roentgenol. 2010;195(4):1036–42.
17. Jesinger RA, Johnson T, Demartini S, et al. Radiology case (# 53) and image: pseudoangiomatous stromal hyperplasia. Mil Med. 2010;175(11):935–6.
18. Sabate JM, Clotet M, Torrubia S, et al. Radiologic evaluation of breast disorders related to pregnancy and lactation. Radiographics. 2007;27 Suppl 1:S101–24.
19. Son EJ, Oh KK, Kim EK. Pregnancy-associated breast disease: radiologic features and diagnostic dilemmas. Yonsei Med J. 2006;47(1):34–42.
20. Okcu ÖS, Bilgen IG, Oktay A, İzmir TR. Radiologic appearance of changes in breast after trauma, surgery and radiation therapy: a pictorial review, ECR 2012/C-2145.
21. Muttarak M, Lerttumnongtum P, Chaiwun B, Peh WCG. Spectrum of papillary lesions of the breast: clinical, imaging, and pathologic correlation. Am J Roentgenol. 2008;191(3):700–7.
22. Debnath D, Al-Okati D, Ismail W. Multiple papillomatosis of breast and patient's choice of treatment. Pathol Res Int. 2010;2010, 540590.
23. Charlot M, Seldin DC, O'hara C, et al. Localized amyloidosis of the breast: a case series. Amyloid. 2011;18:72–5.
24. Trop I, Dugas A, David J, et al. Breast abscesses: evidence-based algorithms for diagnosis, management, and follow-up. Radiographics. 2011;31(6):1683–99.
25. Klein RL, Brown AR, Gomez-Castro CM, Chambers SK, Cragun JM, Grasso-LeBeau L, Lang JE. Ovarian cancer metastatic to the breast presenting as inflammatory breast cancer: a case report and literature review. J Cancer. 2010;1:27–31.
26. Joks M, Mysliwiec K, Lewandowski K. Primary breast lymphoma – a review of the literature and report of three cases. Arch Med Sci. 2011;7(1):27–33.
27. Chugh R, Sabel MS, Feng M. Breast sarcoma: epidemiology, risk factors, clinical presentation, diagnosis, and staging. 2013. www.uptodate.com/.../breast-sarcoma-epidemiology-risk-factors-clinical-.... Accessed 26 Aug 2013.
28. Rosen PP. Rosen's breast pathology. 3rd ed. Philadelphia: Lippincott Williams & Wilkins; 2009.
29. Chinyama CN. Benign breast disease radiology-pathology-risk assessment. Berlin: Springer; 2004.
30. Patterson JA, Scott M, Anderson N, Kirk SJ. Radial scar, complex sclerosing lesion and risk of breast cancer. Analysis of 175 cases in Northern Ireland. Eur J Surg Oncol. 2004;30(10):1065–8.
31. Douglas-Jones AG, Denson JL, Cox AC, Harries IB, Stevens G. Radial scar lesions of the breast diagnosed by needle core biopsy: analysis of cases containing occult malignancy. J Clin Pathol. 2007;60(3):295–8.
32. Tabar L, Dean DB. Teaching atlas of mammography. 4th ed. New York: Thieme; 2011.
33. Wallis MG, Devakumar R, Hosie KB, James KA, Bishop HM. Complex sclerosing lesions (radial scars) of the breast can be palpable. Clin Radiol. 1993;48(5):319–20.
34. Kopans DB. Breast imaging. 3rd ed. Philadelphia: Lippincott Williams & Wilkins; 2007.
35. Jorge L, Taboada JL, Stephens TW, Krishnamurthy S, Brandt KR, Whitman GJ. The many faces of fat necrosis in the breast. Am J Roetgenol. 2009;192:815–25.
36. Harris JR, Lippman ME, Morrow M, Osborne CK. Diseases of the breast. 3rd ed. Philadelphia: Lippincott Williams & Wilkins; 2004.
37. Aqel NM, Howard A, Collier DS. Fat necrosis of the breast: a cytological and clinical study. Breast. 2001;10:342–5.
38. Dershaw DD, Shank B, Reisinger S. Mammographic findings after treatment with local excision and definitive irradiation. Radiology. 1987;164(2):455–61.
39. Muttarak M, Kongmebhol P, Sukamwang N. Breast calcification: which are malignant? Singapore Med J. 2009;50(9):907–14.
40. Nalawade YV. Evaluation of breast calcifications. Indian J Radiol Imaging. 2009;19(4):282–6.

41. Pilnik S. Common breast lesions – a photographic guide to diagnosis and treatment. Cambridge: Cambridge University Press; 2003.
42. Hughes LE, Mansel RE, Webster DJT. Benign disorders and disease of breast. 3rd ed. Philadelphia: Saunders Elsevier; 2009.
43. Osuch JR. Breast health and disease over a lifetime. Clin Obstet Gynecol. 2002;45(4):1140–61.
44. Hartmann LC, Radisky DC, Frost MH, Santen RJ, Vierkant RA, Benetti LL, Tarabishy Y, Ghosh K, Visscher DW, Degnim AC. Understanding the premalignant potential of atypical hyperplasia through its natural history: a longitudinal cohort study. Am Assoc Cancer Res. 2014;7(2):211–7.

Bibliography

Chinyama CN. Benign breast disease radiology-pathology-risk assessment. Berlin: Springer; 2004.

Kopans DB. Breast imaging. 3rd ed. Philadelphia: Lippincott Williams & Wilkins; 2007.

Rosen PP. Rosen's breast pathology. 3rd ed. Philadelphia: Lippincott Williams & Wilkins; 2009.

Tabar L, Dean DB. Teaching atlas of mammography. 4th ed. New York: Thieme; 2011.

5 Signs and Symptoms of Breast Cancer with Management Pathways

Zebby Rees and Susan E. Garnett

Introduction

The majority of breast cancers are found by clients noticing unusual changes in their breast or axilla and visiting their general practitioner [1].

Clinical Signs and Symptoms

Clients may present with the following symptoms which require investigation to rule out or confirm breast cancer [2].

- Discrete hard lump with fixation – there may be skin tethering, dimpling, altered colour or contour of the breast.
- A lump that has enlarged.
- A new, discrete breast lump.
- A new lump in pre-existing nodularity.
- A persistent focal area of lumpiness or a focal change in breast texture.
- Progressive change in breast size with signs of oedema.
- Asymmetrical nodularity persisting after menstruation.
- Skin distortion.
- Previous history of breast cancer with a new lump or suspicious symptoms.
- Nipple discharge or inversion of the nipple.
- Nipple eczema or change that does not respond to topical treatments.
- Axillary lump or lymphadenopathy
- Ulceration of the breast skin may indicate locally advanced breast cancer

All the above are symptoms requiring specialist referral and most of them are clinical indications for mammography and/or ultrasound. Further criteria for mammograms are clients with a strong family history of breast or ovarian cancer, any new signs or symptoms in patients with a previous history of breast cancer and unilateral breast pain.

However, mammography is not recommended in women under 35 years with the exception of clinically suspicious or malignant findings. Younger women have denser, more glandular breast tissue and consequently mammography is less sensitive in detecting breast cancer [3]. Ultrasound is the imaging method of choice for the majority of women aged <35 years and during pregnancy and lactation.

Z. Rees (✉)
The Breast Centre, University Hospital Llandough, Penlan Road, Cardiff CF64 2XX, UK
e-mail: Zebby.rees@wales.nhs.uk

S.E. Garnett
Breast Unit, Ground Floor West Wing University Hospital, Clifford Bridge Road, Coventry CV2 2DX, UK
e-mail: sue.garnett@uhcw.nhs.uk

P. Hogg et al. (eds.), *Digital Mammography: A Holistic Approach*,
DOI 10.1007/978-3-319-04831-4_5, © Springer International Publishing Switzerland 2015

Location of Cancers in the Breast

Research [4, 5] has shown that the majority of cancers are found in the upper outer quadrants of the breast, this is an area of the breast that has the most glandular breast tissue. The lower outer quadrant of the breast is another glandular area that is predisposed to breast cancer. Studies have found this to be the case in women of all ages and ethnic groups.

Breast tumours are less commonly found in the medial (inner) quadrants of the breast.

However, infiltrating ductal and lobular carcinomas (often seen on mammograms as a dense spiculated mass), calcification, distortions and well defined lesions may all be found anywhere within the breast parenchyma [6]. Patients should not be falsely reassured by the location of abnormalities in the breast and seek a referral to a specialist breast centre for assessment for any of the aforementioned signs and symptoms [16].

Referrals

Referrals to a breast unit often come from general practitioners. Some breast abnormalities may be identified when patients are in hospital under investigation for other medical conditions. Clients may also be referred from A & E departments with breast infections, often these are post natal breast infections or abscess [7]. Occasionally presentations are made following an incidental breast finding during another imaging investigation for example CT and MRI scans.

Surgical patients are sometimes referred from the ward with post-surgical seromas' or infections that may require aspiration [8].

Triple Assessment

Triple assessment by a multidisciplinary team comprising clinical and radiological examination, supplemented with tissue diagnosis, is the standard of care for evaluating patients with potential breast cancer in symptomatic and screening breast clinics in the UK. (Breast services may be configured differently in other countries.) Studies [7, 9, 10] have shown an overall sensitivity for triple assessment of 99.6 %; multi-disciplinary 'triple' assessment is currently considered the 'Gold Standard' for evaluating clients with potential breast cancer.

Many UK breast units are organised so that all appropriate tests can be carried out on the same visit (triple assessment), the so called 'fast track' or 'one stop' model. Triple assessment consists of:

- Clinical breast examination and patient medical history.
- Imaging/radiological assessment – mammography and/or ultrasound.
- Pathology assessment – Needle biopsy or fine needle aspiration (FNA).

The imaging component of the triple assessment should include:

- Mammography
- High frequency ultrasound with probes suitable for breast imaging

Breast MRI does not form part of the initial imaging assessment but it is useful in the further investigation of some breast lesions and in the evaluation of patients with confirmed breast cancer [11].

Within most triple assessment clinics there are clear links between breast imaging and the breast clinic, this will ensure:

- Efficient service delivery
- Best use of resources
- Clear and rapid communication for clinic scheduling
- Rapid exchange of information and test results
- Effective liaison between all members of the multidisciplinary team

The clinical assessment and appropriate imaging and needle biopsy should be carried out during the same clinic appointment. This helps to alleviate client anxiety and stress due to periods of waiting [14, 15, 17].

The Treatment Team

The specialist healthcare professionals in a multi-disciplinary team will usually include the following staff groups [12]:

- Consultant surgeons
- Consultant clinical oncologists
- Consultant radiologists/radiographers
- Advanced practitioner radiographers
- Breast clinicians
- Breast care nurses
- Chemotherapy nurses
- Consultant histopathologists/cytologists
- Diagnostic radiographers and assistant practitioners
- Therapy radiographers
- Research nurses

The NHS Cancer Plan [10, 13] states *'the care of all patients with cancer should be formally reviewed by a specialist team'*. It also notes that this would help ensure that *'all patients have the benefit of the range of expert advice needed for high quality care.'*

Multi-disciplinary teams (MDTs) need to bring together staff with the necessary knowledge, skills and experience to ensure high quality diagnosis, treatment and care. The MDT meeting considers the holistic needs of the patient, not just the cancer treatment. To support this, an MDT should take account of the patient's views, preferences and circumstances wherever possible when considering the advice on the care that is most appropriate for the patient's condition.

An MDT makes recommendations and decisions which are reliant on the information available to the MDT at the meeting. The final decision on the way forward needs to be made by the patient in conjunction with their clinicians. MDTs should be alerted if there are significant changes to their recommendations and the reason for this, so they have the opportunity to review and learn from these cases.

The initial focus of the MDT is a patient's primary treatment. However, it is for organisations to decide locally if/and how patient cases should be reconsidered put; in light of any additional findings taking into account any relevant guidance recommendations by appropriate bodies.

References

1. Mansel RE, Webster DJT, Sweetland HM. Benign disorders and diseases of the breast. Philadelphia: Elsevier; 2009.
2. Willet AM, Michel MJ, Lee MJR. Best practice diagnostic guidelines for patients presenting with breast symptoms. 2010. www.associationofbreastsurgery.org.uk
3. Britton PD, Forouhi P, O'Neil A, Wallis M, Sinnetamby R, Gaskarth M, Sue B, Kohn BC, Wishart GC. The sensitivity of multidisciplinary triple assessment for diagnosing breast cancer in a symptomatic clinic. J Cancer Res. 2009;69(2 Suppl 1):6009.
4. Jackson VP. Diagnostic mammography. Radiol Clin North Am. 2004;42:853–70.
5. Kwong S. Laterality, detailed site, and histology of female breast cancer, California. Breast cancer in California. 2003. Chapter 9.
6. Berg W, Birdwell R, Gombos E, Wang S, Parkinson B, Raza S, Green G, Kennedy A, Kettler M. Diagnostic imaging breast. Chapter IV.2. 122. Pub: AMIRSYS. Inc. Utah & Canada; 2006.
7. The Characteristics of an effective multidisciplinary team (MDT). National Cancer Action Team. 2010.
8. Faculty of Clinical Radiology. Guidance on screening and symptomatic breast imaging. 3rd ed. London: Faculty of Clinical Radiology; 2013. www.rcr.ac.uk
9. Wilson R, Liston J. Quality assurance guidelines for breast cancer screening radiology. 2nd ed. NHSBSP publication No: 59. Sheffield: National Health Service Cancer Screening Programme; 2011.
10. The NHS Cancer Plan. The characteristics of an effective multidisciplinary team (MDT). 2000. www.nationalarchives.gov.uk
11. CG 27. Referral for suspected cancer. Nice guidelines. National Institute for Health & Care Excellence. Pub: NICE.CG27; 2005.
12. Veronisi U, Boyle P, Goldhrrsh A, Orachia R, Viale G. Breast cancer. Lancet. 2005;365(9472):1727–41.
13. The NHS Cancer Plan. Progress report. 2006. www.publications.parliament.uk/pa/cm200506/cmselect.
14. CG80. Early and locally advanced breast cancer guidelines. National Institute for Health and Care Excellence. Pub: NICE. CG80; 2009.
15. Barlow WE, Lehman CD, Zheng Y, Ballard R, Barbash B, Yankaskas B, Cotter G, Carney P, Geller B, Rosenburg R, Kerlikowske K, Weaver D, Taplin

S. Performance of diagnostic mammography for women with signs and symptoms of breast cancer. J Natl Cancer Inst. 2002;94(15):1151–9.
16. Magnus MC, Ping M, Shen MM, Bourguois J, Magnus JH. Effectiveness of mammography screening in reducing breast cancer mortality in women aged 39–49 years: a meta-analysis. J Women's Health (Larchmt). 2011;20(6):845–52.
17. Taggart FM, Donelly PK, Dunn JA. Options for early breast cancer follow up in primary and secondary care – a systematic review. BMC Cancer. 2012;12(1):238.

Disease Progression: Local and Distal Spread (Mechanisms)

6

Susan Williams

Introduction

A normal cell has a clearly defined well regulated life cycle. Chemical and biological mechanisms manage the normal regeneration, life and death (apoptosis) of the cell. This process is required to replace worn out cells. Normal cells communicate with each other and regulate proliferation (division) of cells through chemical signals transmitted by specific proteins [1]. A cancer cell does not respond to this communication or regulation and proliferates without limits. The change from a normal cell to a cancerous cell is complex and involves damage to the genes that regulate the normal cell function. Multiple permanent mutations are needed for cancer to develop and this often occurs over a long period of time.

The Influence of Genes

At the cellular level cancer is fundamentally a genetic disease. Cancer results from a disruption of the normal genetic programme. Regulatory genes involved are growth promoting proto-oncogenes, growth inhibiting tumour suppressor genes, genes that regulate apoptosis and genes involved in gene repair. These genes encode many kinds of proteins that help control cell growth and proliferation; mutations in these genes can contribute to the development of cancer.

- Oncogenes are a mutation of a proto-oncogene which promote the specialisation and division of normal cells. The resultant oncogenes expressed at abnormally high levels contribute to converting a normal cell to a cancer cell [2].
- Tumour suppressor genes inhibit mitosis of the cell. They regulate uncontrolled cell division by applying the brakes to cell proliferation. Tumour suppressor genes cause cancer when they are inactive [2].
- Neoplastic cells form from mutation in genes controlling apoptosis, initiated through either extrinsic or intrinsic factors.

The Mutated Cell

Cancer formation is a difficult process and a mutated cell is usually unable to reproduce restricting damage to the individual cell, others will divide but the daughter cells are too damaged to divide. However, if the daughter cells are able to divide the mutation will be replicated and probably undergo further mutation. Oncc the cell is a cancer cell its behaviour is altered in five main areas:

S. Williams
Consultant Radiographer, Breast Imaging, Treatment Centre Royal Shrewsbury Hospital, Mytton Oak Road, Shrewsbury SY3 8XQ, UK
e-mail: susan.williams2@sath.nhs.uk

P. Hogg et al. (eds.), *Digital Mammography: A Holistic Approach*,
DOI 10.1007/978-3-319-04831-4_6, © Springer International Publishing Switzerland 2015

- Cell Reproduction: The normal reproductive process is disrupted resulting in unchecked growth and reproduction.
- Cell Communication: Cancer cells lose the ability to communicate with other cells and do not respond to chemical signals telling them when to reproduce or stop reproducing.
- Cell Adhesion: Cells have adhesion molecules on their surface allowing them to stick to neighbouring cells and keep them in their proper place. Cell to cell contact is required to suppress proliferation. Loss of the adhesion molecules allows the cells to spread to distant areas of the body through the lymphatic and blood circulatory systems.
- Cell Specialisation: Normal cells have the ability to differentiate or develop into specialised cells. Cancer cells are unspecialised and do not develop into cells of a specific type.
- Cell Death: Cell damage goes undetected and the cell will not undergo programmed cell death.

Hallmarks of Cancer

All of the cells produced by division of the first mutated, ancestral cell will display inappropriate proliferation. The uncontrolled altered cell behaviour results in a primary tumour. The fundamental changes in cell physiology dictate the malignant phenotype but the resultant cancer cells display hallmark features. Mutation of genes that regulate some or all of these cellular traits are seen in every cancer.

- The growth pattern is unregulated by physiological cues – cancer cells ignore signals telling them how to behave.
- Lack response to growth inhibitory signals – cancer cells do not respond to signals instructing them to stop their inappropriate behaviour.
- The avoidance of cell death – the gateway in the normal cell cycle inducing apoptosis is missed.
- Immortality – cancer cells will continue to divide indefinitely.
- Development of angiogenesis to sustain the growth of cancer cells – tumour cells develop their own blood supply
- The ability to invade local and distant sites – they have the capacity to infiltrate, invade or metastasise to distant sites.
- Programming pathways – Tumour cells undergo reprogramming of energy metabolisms marking them as superior in the survival game as they become more resilient in their local environment.
- Ability to avoid the immune system – Tumours may avoid the immune system by mechanisms that allow them to go undetected.

Establishing the Tumour

Tumours are made up of two basic components

- The parenchyma – made up of neoplastic cells, this determines the tumours biology
- The supporting host –derived non-neoplastic stroma comprising of connective tissue, blood supply and host derived inflammatory cells.

The differentiation of parenchymal tumour cells is the extent to which they resemble their equivalent normal cells morphologically and functionally. Poorly differentiated cells lose the functional capabilities of their normal counterparts and tend to grow more rapidly. The site of the primary tumour will dictate the biology of the tumour. The tumour may remain within the originating tissue, invade nearby tissues or distant tissue sites. Most cancers begin as localised growths confined to the epithelium in which they arise. As long as the tumour does not penetrate the basement membrane on which the epithelium rests they are termed carcinoma in situ.

The proliferating cancer cells, are supported by a stroma of connective tissue and a blood supply influencing the growth pattern, differentiation and biological behaviour of the developing tumour, promoting or preventing tumorigenesis [3]. Two theories of tumour progression include predisposition of the tumour to progress or the interaction of the tumour cells and the surrounding stroma, it seems likely both occur. The microenvironment is composed of the extracellular matrix, numerous types of stromal cells including endothelial and immune cells, fibroblasts and adipocytes, and is an important participant of tumour progression [4].

Tumour cells need oxygen, nutrients and removal of waste products. Tumours cannot grow beyond 1–2 mm without vascularisation. Cancer cells can stimulate angiogenesis, during which new vessels sprout from previously existing capillaries these abnormal vessels are leaky and dilated, with a haphazard pattern of connection. Angiogenesis is required for the cancer to grow and metastasise.

Lymphangiogenesis, the growth of new lymphatic vessels, can be induced in pathological process such as cancer. These lymphatic vessels will transport cancer cells to the lymphatic system [5]. Although the system is currently poorly understood lymph members of the vascular endothelial growth factor family play major roles in both lymphangiogenesis and angiogenesis. The vascular and lymphatic anatomy influences the pattern of metastatic spread. The seed and soil needs a suitable microenvironment in which to grow [3, 5, 7].

Local Invasion

Tumours exert local effects including compression and displacement of adjacent tissues to effect invasion. Malignant tumour growth pattern is often disorganised and random. Malignant tumours enlarge and infiltrate the normal tissues of their origin but may extend directly beyond the confines of that organ to involve adjacent tissues.

At the molecular level continued mutations cause heterogeneity in the tumour, generating subclones with different characteristics. Thus although cancer origins are monoclonal by the time they are clinical detectable they can be extremely heterogeneous. During progression the tumour cells are subject to selection processes with the more resilient subclones selected for survival. The genetic evolution and selection processes make tumours become more aggressive and acquire greater malignant potential – tumour progression.

Metastasising

Metastasis is the migration of malignant cells from one site to another remote site. Metastases tend to resemble the primary tumour histologically. Tumour spread is a complex process involving a series of sequential steps which can be interrupted at any stage by host or tumour related factors. Figure 6.1 shows a summary of the metastasis cascade.

A lack of adhesion between cells facilitates loosening of the tumour cells allowing them to move away from the tumour body. Enzymes secreted by the tumour cells cause local degradation of the basement membrane and interstitial connective tissue. Breach of the basement membrane is the first event in cell invasion. The tumour cells attach to the extracellular matrix proteins causing modification to the matrix that promotes invasion and metastasis and allowing the tumour cells to enter the circulatory system. Tumour cells are quite inefficient at colonising distant organs and most tumour cells circulate as micrometastases undetected in the system for prolonged periods of time.

Extravasation of the tumour cells involves adhesion to the vascular endothelium followed by egression through the basement membrane into the organ parenchyma by mechanisms similar to those involved in invasion.

The site of extravasation and the organ distribution of metastases can be predicted by the site of the primary tumour and its vascular or lymphatic drainage. This may be the first capillary bed they encounter. Other influences may include expression of adhesion molecules by tumour cells whose ligands are expressed preferentially on the endothelium of the target organ. They are also influenced by the expression of proteins that direct movement. Once the cancer cells reach a target the tumour cells must be able to colonise to continue growth. Tumour cells appear to secrete cytokines, growth factors and proteases that act

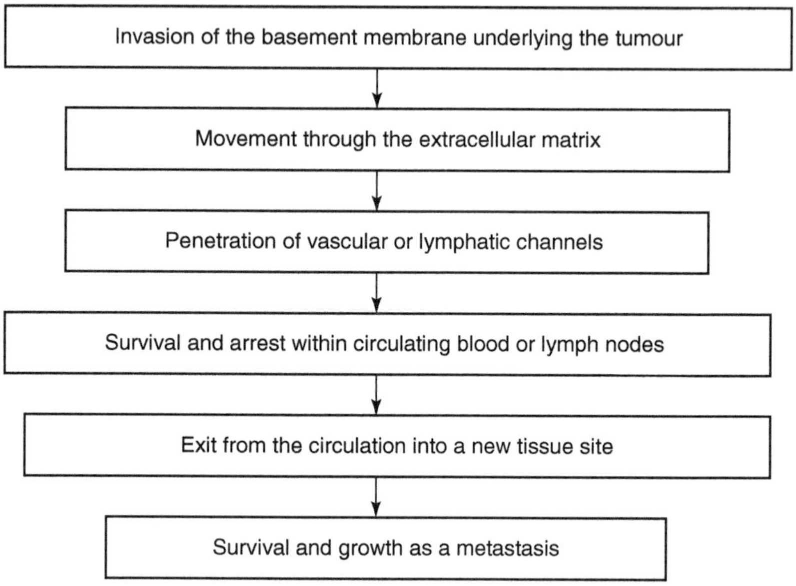

Fig. 6.1 The mechanism of tumour invasion and metastasis

on the resident stromal cells to make the site habitable.

Tumour cells arising in tissue with a rich lymphatic network such as the breast often metastasise by this route. Invasive tumours may penetrate lymphatic channels more readily than blood vessels. Lymph formation occurs at the microscopic level. During the exchange of fluid and molecules between the blood circulation and body tissues, blood capillaries may not reabsorb all of the fluid; surrounding lymphatic capillaries absorb the excess fluid and cancer cells. This is then filtered and carried to the sentinel lymph node and from there to distal nodes and other organs [5].

Breast Cancer

The biology of breast cancer is complicated and little understood making it difficult to predict and manage [4, 6–10]. Breast cancer is a heterogeneous process with very variable appearances, biology and clinical behaviour. However, the cancer cells develop from the epithelium of lobules and ducts.

There are many ways that breast cancer can develop [8] and a theoretical typical progression may be:

- Atypical and In situ disease
- Invasive tumour
- Regional metastases to sentinel lymph nodes
- Involvement of other regional lymph nodes
- Metastatic spread to distant sites

Atypia and In Situ Disease

During this phase tumour growth is restricted to the lobules and ducts which are delineated by a continuous basal membrane and are therefore non-invasive [11]. Although controversial atypical ductal and lobular hyperplasia are often considered to be a precursor or risk indicator for subsequent breast cancers [6, 7]. Lobular carcinoma in situ (LCIS) has cells with the morphology of invasive lobular carcinoma but is contained within the basement membrane. Ductal carcinoma in situ (DCIS) grows within the duct system of the breast and can vary in size and extent. High grade DCIS is a more inherently high-risk disease in terms of progression into invasive breast cancer. All of these conditions are confined within the boundaries of the normal structures of the breast and therefore cannot metastasise [1–3].

Invasive Tumour

The transition from in-situ to invasive disease of the breast is poorly understood but is defined by the loss of the myoepithelial cell layer and basement membrane of the terminal ductal lobular units [4]. The infiltration of the surrounding stromal tissue means there is the potential to spread to lympho-vascular spaces and to metastasise. Some invasive breast cancers are more aggressive and may spread earlier to distant sites. There are a variety of methods for classifying invasive breast cancer; most are based on the architectural microscopic pattern and nature of the cancerous cells and indicate differing clinical behaviours and prognoses. The combination of the physical and physiological properties of the tumour such as size, grade, location and histological features will give an indication of predicted disease progression and prognosis.

Although the growth pattern of the breast tumour is influenced by the biology of the tumour as the cancer starts to grow it takes up more space and forces itself through the normal tissue often taking the path of least resistance. The space occupying lesion will block small blood vessels causing death of the normal cells making it easier for the tumour to continue growing. The cancer cells invade the nearby surrounding breast tissue or nearby structures such as the pectoral muscle and ribs.

Regional Nodes

Breast cancer spread occurs through lymphatic and haematogenous channels. The lymphatic system collects excess fluid in the body's tissues and returns it to the bloodstream. The breast has a rich lymphatic network and the initial metastases are almost always lymphatic. Tumours located laterally and centrally typically spread first to the axillary nodes. Those in the medial inner quadrants often travel first to the lymph nodes along the internal mammary arteries. The assessment of lymph nodes in the axilla is crucial to staging and prognosis of patients with operable breast cancer. The sentinel lymph node(s) are the primary nodes that drain the breast parenchyma. A sentinel lymph node free of cancer is highly predictive of absence of cancer in the remaining nodes.

Metastatic Spread

More distant dissemination eventually ensues and can involve virtually any organ or tissue. Common sites for metastases of the breast are lungs, skeleton, liver, adrenals and (less commonly) brain but can involve virtually any organ or body tissue. Metastases have histological properties similar to the primary tumour. Metastases may come to clinical attention many years after the apparent control of the primary tumour.

References

1. Lodish H, Berk A, Zipursky SL, Matsudaira P, Baltimore D, Darnell J. Molecular cell biology. Chapter 1. In: The dynamic cell 1.4 – the life cycle of cells. 4th ed. New York: WH Freeman; 2000.
2. Lodish H, Berk A, Zipursky SL, Matsudaira P, Baltimore D, Darnell J. Molecular cell biology. Chapter 24 Cancer 24.2. In: Proto-oncogenes and tumor-suppressor genes. 4th ed. New York: WH Freeman; 2000.
3. Tot T, Tabar L, Dean PB. Practical breast pathology. New York: Thieme; 2002.
4. Place AE, Huh SJ, Polyak K. The microenvironment in breast cancer progression: biology and implications for treatment. Breast Cancer Res. 2011;13:227. http://breast-cancer-research.com/content/13/6/227.
5. Alitalo A, Detmar M. Interaction of tumour cells and lymphatic vessels in cancer progression. Oncogene. 2012;31(42):4499–508.
6. Hartmann LC, Radisky DC, Frost MH, Santen RJ, Vierkant RA, Benetti LL, Tarabishy Y, Ghosh K, Visscher DW, Degnim AC. Understanding the premalignant potential of atypical hyperplasia through its natural history: a longitudinal Cohort study. Am Assoc Cancer Res. 2014;7(2):211–17.
7. Lakhani SR, Audretsch W, Cleton-Jenson A-M, Cutuli B, Ellis I, Eusebi V, Greco M, Houslton RS, Kuhl CK, Kurtz J, Palacios J, Peterse H, Rochard F, Rutgers E. The management of lobular carcinoma in

situ (LCIS). Is LCIS the same as ductal carcinoma in situ (DCIS)? Eur J Cancer. 2006;42(2006): 2205–11.
8. Bombonati A, Sgroi DC. The molecular pathology of breast cancer progression. J Pathol. 2011;223:307–17.
9. Heimann R, Hellman S. Clinical progression of breast cancer malignant behaviour: what to expect and when to expect it. J Clin Oncol. 2000;18(3):591–99.
10. Geyer FC, Weigelt B, Natrajan R, de Lambros MBK, Biase D, Vatcheva R, Savage K, Mackay A, Ashworth A, Reis-Filho JS. Molecular analysis reveals a genetic basis for the phenotypic diversity of metaplastic breast carcinomas. J Pathol. 2010;220:562–73.
11. Tavassoli FA, Hoeffler H, Rosai J, Holland R, Ellis I, Schnitt S, Lakhani SR, Boeker W, Heywang-Kobrunner SH, Moinfar F, Peterse J. Intraductal proliferative lesions. In: World Health Organization classification of tumours, editor. Pathology and genetics of tumours of the breast and female genital organs. Lyon: IARC Press; 2003. p. 63–73.

Bibliography

Cross SS. Underwood's pathology a clinical approach. 6th ed. Edinburgh: Churchill Livingstone; 2013.

Kumar V, Abbas AK, Aster JC. Robbins basic pathology. 9th ed. Elsevier: Philadelphia; 2013.

Rosen PP. Rosen's breast pathology. 3rd ed. Philadelphia: Lippincott Williams & Wilkins; 2009.

Rubin E, Reisner HM. Essentials of Rubin's pathology. 6th ed. Philadelphia: Lippincott, Williams & Wilkins; 2014.

Mammography Screening: Philosophy – Evidence for and against

7

John A. Dewar

Introduction

The concept of screening for cancer is simple – one uses a diagnostic test that detects the cancer "early" so that it can be successfully treated and the patient "cured". Unfortunately, the reality is not as straight forward as that. Amongst the questions one needs to know are: how reliable is the test? Does it have any side-effects? Are the "cancers detected" really cancers? Can all the cancers be successfully treated? It is therefore necessary to examine the principles underlying screening for any disease [1]; such principles might include

1. the disease should pose an important health problem
2. the natural history of the disease should be well understood
3. there should be a recognisable early stage
4. treatment of the disease at an early stage should be of more benefit than treatment started at a later stage
5. there should be a suitable diagnostic test
6. the test should be acceptable to the population
7. there should be adequate facilities for the diagnosis and treatment of abnormalities detected
8. for diseases of insidious onset, screening should be repeated at intervals determined by the natural history of the disease
9. the chance of physical or psychological harm to those screened should be less than chance of benefit
10. the cost of screening should be balanced against the benefit it provides

This chapter will examine some of these principles in relation to mammographic screening for breast cancer, focussing on the potential benefits and risks of such screening.

Benefits of Screening

As mentioned above, screening presupposes that mammography detects breast cancer at a stage when treatment will reduce the risk of dying from breast cancer compared to not screening (i.e. symptomatic presentation only). How can we measure whether this occurs? Progress in cancer treatment is often measured by calculating survival figures – for example 5 year survival is the proportion of women alive at 5 years from the date of diagnosis. For screening to be effective, it must detect the cancer at an earlier stage of its development, so the time of diagnosis (from which survival is calculated) is brought forward. Thus, even if screening had no overall effect on the risk of dying from breast cancer, because the time of diagnosis is brought forward, the women would have lived longer from diagnosis to death.

J.A. Dewar
Department of Surgery and Molecular Oncology,
University of Dundee,
Hays House, Church St Kingham,
Chipping Norton OX7 6YA, UK
e-mail: johndewar60@gmail.com

P. Hogg et al. (eds.), *Digital Mammography: A Holistic Approach*,
DOI 10.1007/978-3-319-04831-4_7,

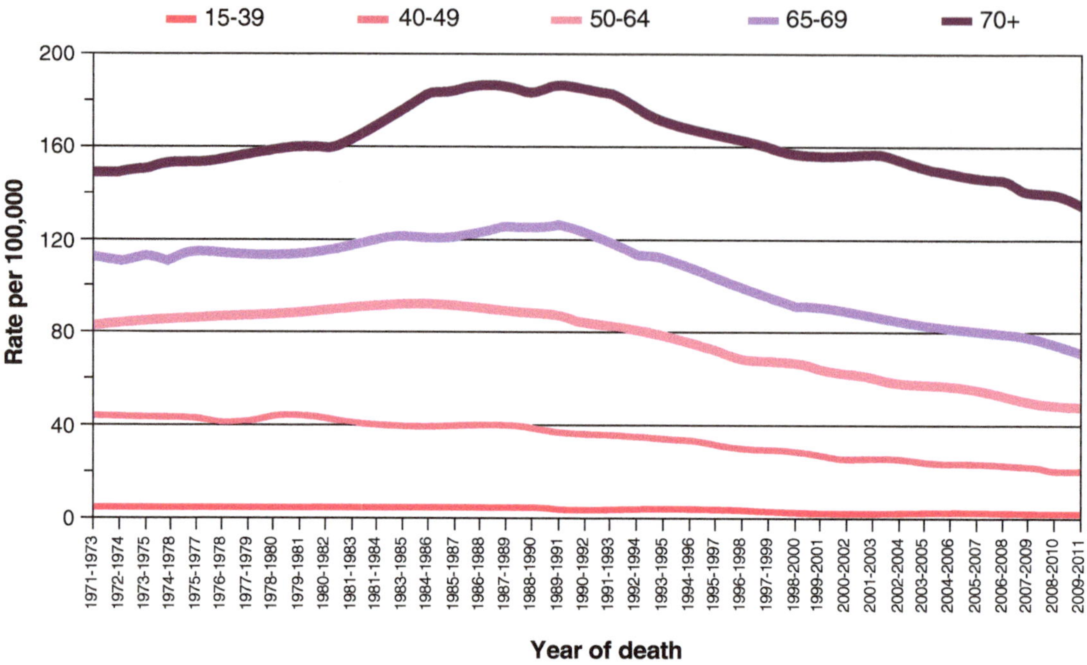

Fig. 7.1 Changes in breast cancer mortality by age group, expressed as European age standardised mortality rates per 100,000 population, by age, females, UK. 1971–2011 (Cancer Research UK, http://www.cancerresearchuk.org/cancer-info/cancerstats/types/skin/incidence, March 2014)

This is called "lead time bias". An example may make this clearer:

If a woman was diagnosed symptomatically with breast cancer in 2005 and died from breast cancer 4 years later in 2009, she would appear as a death in the 5 year survival figures. If she had been screened and the cancer detected (say) 2 years earlier in 2003, but supposing screening didn't affect her prognosis, then she would still die in 2009 – but this would be 6 years from diagnosis, so she would appear as a 5 year survivor. In other words, because screening brings forward the date of diagnosis, 5 year survival will appear to improve even if there is no effect on the risk of dying of breast cancer.

Thus survival cannot be used to assess whether screening works because of lead time bias.

Any benefit from screening must therefore be determined by measuring breast cancer mortality, which is the number of women dying of breast cancer in a given year. This is usually expressed as the number dying per 100,000 women in a population and may be further subdivided by age groups (e.g. 50–59, 60–69 etc.), as shown in Fig. 7.1. Mammographic screening for breast cancer was introduced in the UK in 1988 for women aged 50–64. Figure 7.1 shows a clear reduction in breast cancer mortality for this age group since then. Does this mean screening works? Unfortunately, assessment of benefit is not as straightforward as that. Firstly, if screening is effective, any benefit would take some time to be reflected in mortality figures (at least 5 and probably nearer 10 years, see later). Thus any effect would be seen from 1993 onwards and would be seen in women aged 65–75 as well as 50–64. Secondly, there are clearly factors other than breast screening affecting mortality since the beginning of the fall antedates any effect of screening. Further, the under 50s (an age group not exposed to screening) also show a clear reduction in mortality. Thus, simple examination of population figures cannot give a reliable estimate of the impact of screening because of the

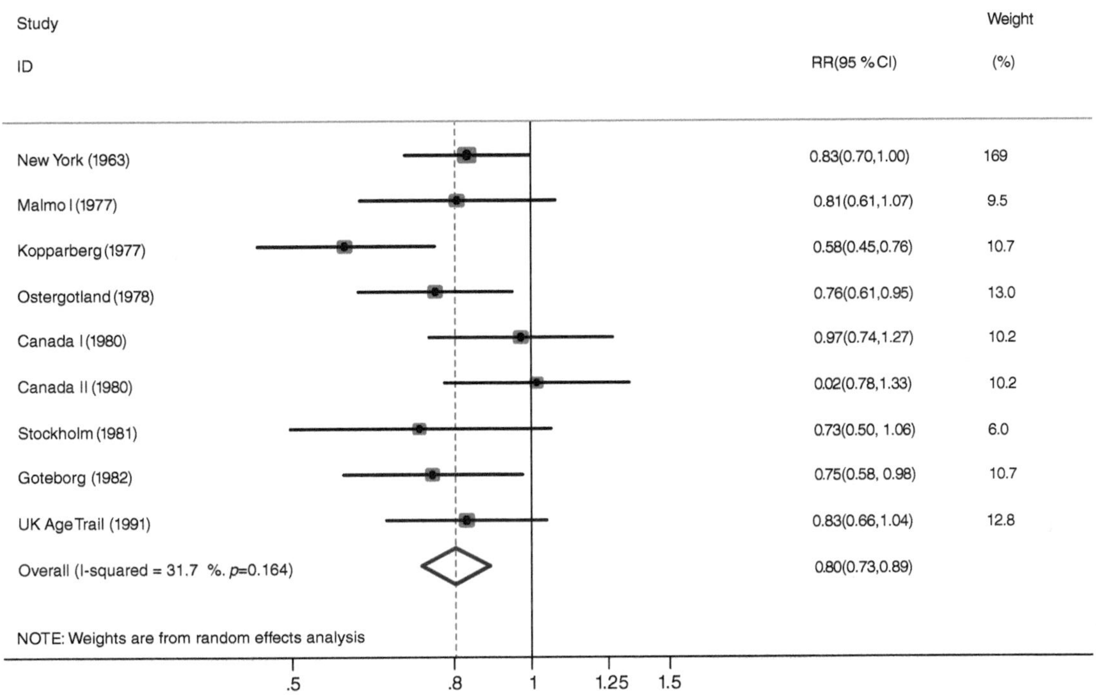

Fig. 7.2 Meta-analysis of the breast cancer screening trials: relative risk (RR) of breast cancer mortality after 13 years of follow-up. Note: Malmö II is excluded because follow-up approximating 13 years was not available; the Swedish Two County (Kopparberg and Östergötland) and Canada I and II trials are split into their component parts; the Edinburgh trial is excluded because of severe imbalances between randomised groups (Reproduced with permission from *British Journal of Cancer* [2])

impact of other factors such as changes in treatment – for example, the introduction of effective systemic adjuvant therapies, such as tamoxifen and chemotherapy. In summary, the population mortality figures do not exclude an effect of screening but do not prove it either.

A more useful estimate of the effect of mammographic screening comes from randomised controlled trials (RCTs). Here, populations of women were randomised to either undergo several rounds of screening (mostly about every 2 years) or no screening. The effect on the risk of dying from breast cancer was then measured. Figure 7.2 shows a meta-analysis of the main trials from the Marmot review [2]. This shows a reduction in the risk of dying from breast cancer in the screened women compared to the unscreened of 20 %. This is a relative risk reduction; the absolute benefit depends on the risk of dying of breast cancer. If it is assumed that

- the female UK population aged 50–70 are screened from age 50 for 20 years,
- they gain no benefit for the first 5 years (because of the relatively long natural history of breast cancer)
- the effect on mortality continues up to 10 years after screening (again because of the long natural history of breast cancer)

Then there would be an effect on the mortality of women aged 55–79. The risk of dying of breast cancer (without any effect of screening) for this age group is 2.13 %. A reduction of 20 % in this mortality is 0.43 % which equates to 43 deaths prevented for every 100,000 women invited for screening, corresponding to one breast cancer death prevented for every 235 women invited for screening [2].

There have been numerous publications examining the impact of screening on populations. As mentioned above, they need to allow for the effect of other factors on incidence, changes in treatment, lead time bias etc. and differences in the assumptions to account for these other factors make it difficult to produce a reliable measure of the impact of screening. Thus, the results of RCTs (albeit they were started several decades ago) remain the most reliable measure.

Risks of Screening

The potential risks of screening can be considered under two main headings. Firstly, there is the anticipated (and readily measurable) risk of women being recalled for further investigation if their mammogram is deemed abnormal and secondly the risk of overdiagnosis.

Recall

Figure 7.3 summarises the recall rate, biopsy rate etc. for the UK Breast Screening programme. It shows that, for 100,000 women invited for screening, 2,522 women (3,105 recalled minus the 583 diagnosed with cancer =2,522) were recalled and found not to have cancer. This is called a false positive result (i.e. 3.36 % of all the women screened). Of the women recalled and found not to have cancer, the majority (1,744/2,522 = 69 %) had only further imaging (mammography, ultrasound etc.) but a minority (778/2,522 = 31 %) had a biopsy. This was core biopsy under local anaesthetic in all except 2.3 % (57/2,522) who had an open biopsy under general anaesthetic. The latter group represents only 0.076 % (57/75,057) of all women screened.

There are psychological effects of a false-positive result on women but the studies show conflicting results. A recent systematic review of the literature [3] concluded that, in the population at general risk of breast cancer, a false-positive result can cause breast cancer specific psychological distress which may endure for up to 3 years. The degree of distress is associated with the level of invasiveness of subsequent assessment. Some studies found that the distress caused by a false-positive result deterred some women from re-attending for breast screening which would reduce any benefit they would otherwise

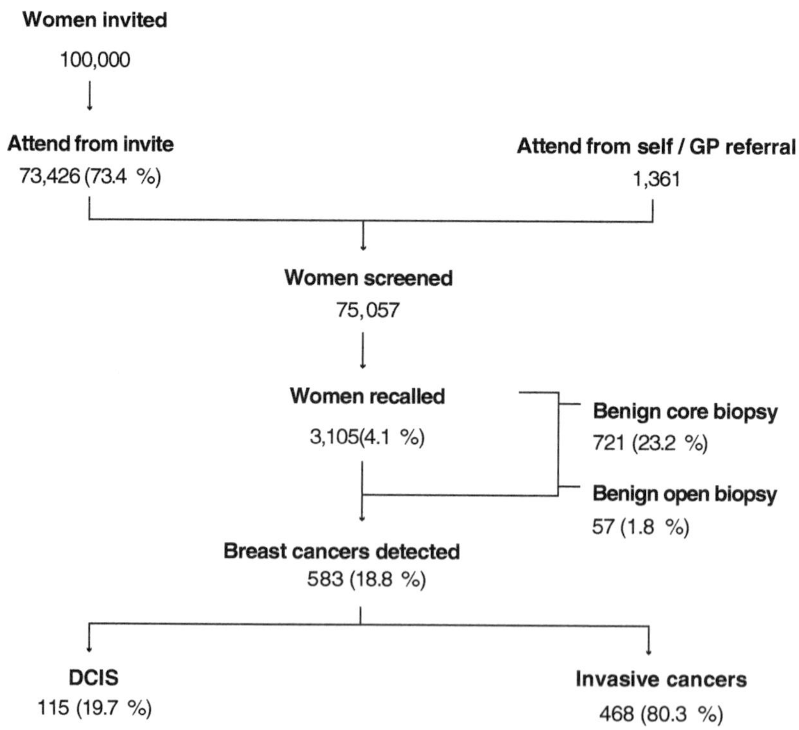

Fig. 7.3 Overall cancer detection rate is 583/75,057 = 7.8 cancers/1,000 women screened. Of the 3105 women recalled, 583 (18.7 %) will be diagnosed with invasive or in-situ cancer. Data extracted for women aged 50–70 for year 2009/10 (*refs. NHS Breast Screening Programme Annual Review 2011 (UK) and the NHS Breast Screening Programme Report, England 2009/10* www.ic.nhs.uk) (Reproduced with permission from *British Journal of Cancer* [2])

have got from being offered screening in the first place. The level of distress can be mitigated by providing women with clearly worded information about the recall and appropriate support from clinical staff before and during assessment [3]. Further information about caring for patients and clients can be found in Part II of this book.

No screening test is completely accurate and sometimes mammography will not detect a cancer. This may be because the cancer is not mammographically visible or develops between screening rounds (referred to as an "interval" cancer) – women are warned of this possibility in screening literature. When women present with an interval cancer, the previous mammograms are reviewed blind to assess whether a suspicious abnormality was visible on the previous screening mammogram. If so, such cases are classified as a true false negative mammogram, i.e. the suspicious abnormality was not detected at the previous screening round. For women attending at three yearly intervals, the false negative rate is estimated as 0.2/1,000 women screened (c.f. the cancer detection rate by screening of 7.8 cancers/1,000 women screened) [2].

Overdiagnosis

Overdiagnosis can be defined as "detection of cancers on screening that would not have become apparent were it not for the screening test" [4]. Screening detects cancers earlier, so that incidence of breast cancer will be higher among screened women during the screening period (because of "lead time"), compared to unscreened women. Once screening stops, one would expect the incidence to reduce (because cancers that would have been detected "earlier" by screening are not being detected) so by the end of the screening period plus lead time, the cumulative incidence in the screened and control populations should be the same (see Fig. 7.4a). If, however, the cancer is so slowly growing that it would never have presented clinically in her lifetime; or the woman were to die (of another cause, e.g. cardiovascular disease) before the cancer would have presented clinically, then she has undergone diagnosis and treatment, with its associated hazards, for no personal benefit. This phenomenon is called overdiagnosis and includes both invasive and in-situ cancers. If overdiagnosis occurs, then the cancer incidence will not reduce after the cessation of screening but will remain elevated (Fig. 7.4b). Overdiagnosis thus depends on a complex interaction between screening, the relative growth rate of cancers detected and other causes of death. It is estimated from studies (see below) but individual cancers cannot be recognised as "overdiagnosed" – they will be invasive or in-situ cancers, histologically indistinguishable from other screen detected cancers.

Quantifying overdiagnosis is not easy. The ideal way would be to measure the incidence of breast cancer in screened and unscreened populations within randomised controlled trials over the lifetime of the women. Unfortunately, the importance of overdiagnosis was not appreciated when the screening trials were set up, so they were not designed to measure the extent of overdiagnosis. In particular, in many trials, following cessation of screening within the trial, the control (unscreened) population was offered screening. This control population is thus exposed to the risk of overdiagnosis and cannot be used as a comparator. A further difficulty is how the rate of overdiagnosis is expressed. There is agreement that the numerator is the number of excess breast cancers in the screened population. Should, however, this be expressed as a percentage of all

(a) the cancers detected over the lifetime of the women screened (or unscreened)?
(b) the cancers detected only during the screening period?
(c) the cancers detected by screening?
(d) or other methods?

[In any fraction, the numerator is the upper number and the denominator the lower (and percentage is this fraction multiplied by 100). Thus if in a screening trial, 100 cancers are detected in the screened group and 80 in the unscreened, the "excess breast cancers" would be 20 (100–80) – this is the numerator. If the denominator is the number of cancers found in the screened population, then the percentage is 20 % ($\{20 \div 100\} \times 100$). If the denominator is

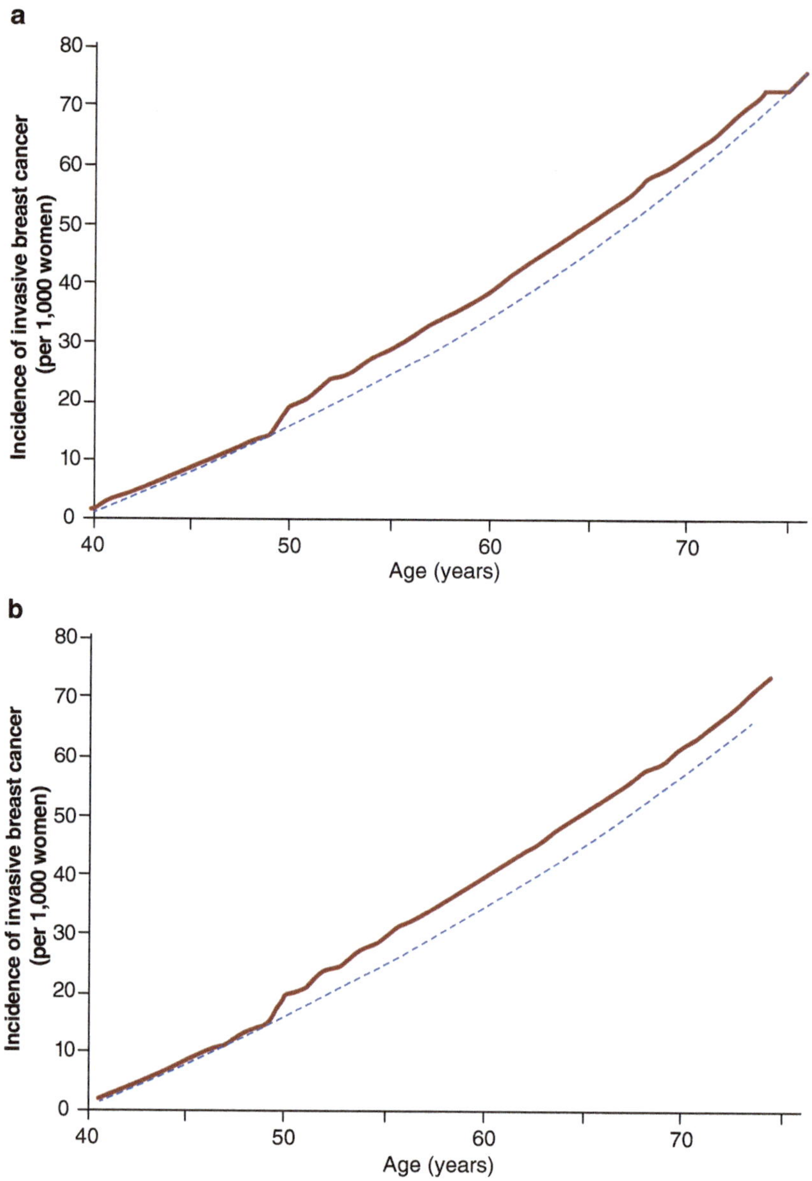

Fig. 7.4 (**a**, **b**) Hypothetical cumulative incidence of breast cancer without (*left*) or with (*right*) overdiagnosis, based on screening women between 50 and 68 years (*red line* shows screened women and *blue line* unscreened women) (Reproduced with permission from *British Journal of Cancer* [2])

the number of cancers found in the unscreened population, then the percentage is 25 % ({20 ÷80} × 100). Thus, even with a constant numerator, changing the denominator changes the percentage figure.]

All of the above are valid methods, but give different results and in measuring overdiagnosis, it needs to be clear which denominator is used. The best estimates of overdiagnosis come from the randomised controlled trials (one Swedish and two Canadian) in which the control population was not offered screening on completion of the trials. Meta-analysis of these trials [2] give an estimate of 11 % of cancers being overdiagnosed if one considers all the cancers diagnosed during screening and subsequently. If one considers overdiagnosed cancers as a proportion of the cancers detected during the screening period only, then the figure is about 19 %. Attempts to estimate the incidence of overdiagnosis from population studies vary widely, in part because of differences in the clinical assumptions made and the statistical methods employed. Thus, population studies have not yielded consistent figures.

In summary, the limited trial data confirms that overdiagnosis occurs but there is some uncertainty as to its magnitude. It is, however, a consequence of screening and women invited for screening need to be aware of it as a potential hazard.

Summary

Mammographic breast screening remains an important part of breast cancer care. In the absence of treatments that can cure all cases of breast cancer, screening remains an important means of decreasing deaths from breast cancer. Overall, it is estimated [2], that for 10,000 women invited to screening from age 50 for 20 years, 681 cancers (invasive and in situ) will be diagnosed and 43 deaths prevented. This is equivalent to 1,300 deaths from breast cancer prevented every year in the UK.

There is, however, a cost to this programme. Some women (3.4 % of those screened) will be recalled and undergo investigations that show they do not have cancer. Of those found to have cancer, some would never have been troubled with it in their lifetime – so called overdiagnosis. Of the 681 cancers diagnosed above (in 10,000 women invited for screening from age 50–70), approximately 19 % (129) will be overdiagnosed. They will be told they have a cancer, will undergo surgery and possibly radiotherapy and systemic therapy, for a cancer that would never have presented clinically in their lifetime.

Currently, we lack any means of differentiating between those cancers that have truly malignant potential (i.e. to metastasise and cause death) and those that would pursue a more indolent course. It may be that advances in pathology, particularly in genetic analysis of the tumours will help in this regard. Similarly, advances in the treatment of breast cancer will tend to reduce the absolute benefit of screening (i.e. factor 4 in the principles of screening becomes relatively less important). Until that time, screening will continue and it is important that the programme is run to the highest standards. In particular, the women invited for screening need to understand the potential advantages and risks of attending for screening before deciding whether to accept their screening invitation.

References

1. Forrest APM. Breast cancer screening, report to the Health Ministers of England, Wales, Scotland and Northern Ireland by a working group. London: HMSO; 1986.
2. Marmot MG, Altmann DG, Cameron DA, Dewar JA, Thompson SG, Wilcox M, Independent UK Panel on Breast Cancer Screening. The benefits and harms of breast cancer screening: an independent review. Br J Cancer. 2013;108:2205–40.
3. Bond M, Pavey T, Welch K, Cooper C, Garside R, Dean S, Hyde CJ. Psychological consequences of false-positive screening mammograms in the UK. Evid Based Med. 2012;18(2):54–61.
4. IARC. IARC handbooks of cancer prevention, breast cancer screening. International Agency for Research on Cancer; World Health Organisation. Lyon: IARC Press; 2002. p. 144.

Screening Programmes for Breast Cancer in Europe

8

Solveig S.H. Hofvind and Chris J.M. de Wolf

Background

Organised screening for breast cancer is offered women aged 50–69 years in most European countries. Two-view mammography at biennial intervals is usually performed at stationary or mobile units by specially trained radiographers. The screening mammograms are usually read by two independent readers according to the European guidelines for quality assurance in breast cancer screening and diagnosis. Continuous quality assurance is necessary to guarantee high quality screening. Results from early performance measures are regularly monitored and compared to desirable and acceptable levels described in the European guidelines, or to guidelines created by the specific country/region. Quality assurance is a team effort of all screening professionals to ensure that all aspects of the screening service achieve optimal quality performance. The key professional personnel must hold the requisite professional qualifications in their own country and have undergone specific training before start working with mammographic screening. The knowledge and the skills have to be maintained. There are pro and cons of mammographic screening and the women invited to the programme need to be informed in a way to make them able to do an informed choice of whether to participate or not.

S.S.H. Hofvind (✉)
Cancer Registry of Norway and Oslo and Akershus University College of Applied Sciences,
Fr Nansens vei 19, Oslo 0304, Norway
e-mail: solveig.hofvind@kreftregisteret.no

C.J.M. de Wolf MD
Swiss Cancer Screening, Effingerstrasse 52,
PB 8219, Bern CH-3001, Switzerland
e-mail: chris@iquat.org

Introduction

Breast cancer mortality is the most frequent cause of death in women 50–70 years of age [1]. Organised mammographic screening is shown to decrease mortality from breast cancer, particularly among screened women aged 50–69 [2, 3]. In 2003, the European Parliament and the Council of Europe, represented by the Health Ministers of the European Union, recommended implementation of organised breast cancer screening programmes [4] based upon European guidelines [5]. These guidelines are based on the development and experience of the Europe Against Cancer programme.

This European Commission programme supported actively screening programmes for breast cancer in the period 1990 and to 2002 [5]. The commission established a European network for breast cancer screening programmes, which was in charge of the establishment and development of the European Guidelines. These guidelines present acceptable and desirable quality levels a screening programme should meet. It does not describe how a screening programme should be run, but rather

P. Hogg et al. (eds.), *Digital Mammography: A Holistic Approach*,
DOI 10.1007/978-3-319-04831-4_8, © Springer International Publishing Switzerland 2015

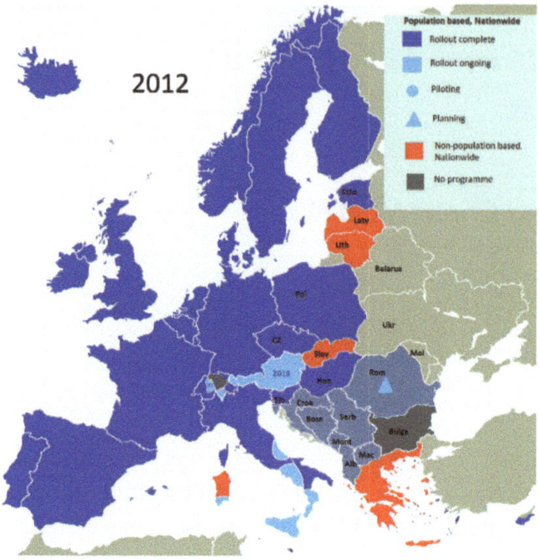

Fig. 8.1 Implementation of screening programmes for breast cancer in Europe (Adapted for year 2012 [6])

support to understand what is the best practice according to implementation, management, monitoring, adaption and modifications. However, the final organisation should be adapted to the health care structure in the actual countries. The guidelines were supported by the European Union in the Council Recommendations in 2003 [4].

According to the 'Report on the implementation of the Council Recommendation on Cancer Screening' [6], over 59 million women residing in the EU states were in the 50–69 target age for breast cancer screening in 2007, and approximately 41 % were offered screening. Eleven member states rolled out population-based programmes in 2007 and an additional seven states had commenced the process. Non-population-based programmes were running in five additional member states, and one country was piloting a population-based programme. The implementation situation of 2012 is illustrated in Fig. 8.1. A survey performed by the European Commission (Joint Research Centre, Institute for Health and Consumer Protection) shows operational mammographic screening in 22 countries, whereas 20 are organised and 18 are population-based [7].

Women aged 50–69 years represent the main target group of mammographic screening programmes in Europe, but some countries/regions offer screening in the age range from 40 to 75 years [6]. The screening interval is in general 2 years, only the UK and Malta perform it every 3 years.

Organisation Models

Healthcare is provided exclusively or mainly by public authorities, reflecting the European tradition of universal public coverage in health care in 88 % of the 25 countries included in the survey performed by the Joint Research Centre [7]. However, each health care system in Europe has a unique composition, which reflects the history, the political context and the financial means of each country. The systems have great influence on how the screening programmes are organised and managed [8]. The Netherlands, Germany, Iceland, Norway, and UK have national population-based screening programmes with national recommendations and organisation, while Belgium, France, Italy, Sweden, Switzerland have regional programmes (administered and run by the region, county or cantons). An organised screening programme requires a high degree of management, in contrast to non-organised services. In organised programmes the target population, screening test and intervals are given and the programme policy specifies the procedures for performance, surveillance, and quality assurance according to guidelines, rules and recommendations.

Most screening programmes for breast cancer in Europe are population-based, in contrast to the U.S. [9]. Population-based means that all women in the target population living in the area, are served by the programme. The target group are identified and personally invited to attend each round of screening.

Some organised programmes send an appointment with a fixed date and time for the examination. The procedure ensures higher participation rates compared to programmes where the women have to schedule her appointment herself. The disadvantage of this system is that there are timeslots that are not used. Overbooking is thus usual to avoid down time and fill up all the timeslots. Other programmes send invitations where the client must make herself an appointment at a specific institute. In this case, clients usually show up for appointments. General practitioners and gynaecologists in some countries (e.g. Germany) play an important role in motivating clients to participate. Participation rates are substantially higher (≈25 % higher) in programmes with appointments with fixed time and places for screening examination. Attending organised mammographic screening is free of charge in most countries. In Norway and Switzerland, a small fee is required. In most countries, the additional work up and eventual further follow-up and treatment is free of charge or paid by the insurance companies. However, sometimes subjects do co-payments.

The screening examination can take place at mobile or stationary units (e.g. dedicated screening units, private radiological institutes, and radiological departments in public hospitals). The mobile units are placed at easy accessible places that facilitate participation. In addition, mobile units do not interfere with patients in hospitals and therefore strengthen the message that screening is offered to healthy clients without symptoms of disease. In the Netherlands, there are 52 mobile units and one fixed unit offering 1.1 million screening examinations every year [11]. The UK, Norway, Sweden, and Germany combine mobile and stationary units, while Belgium, France, and Switzerland use mainly stationary units. France, for instance has one of the highest number of mammography devices per inhabitant, in Europe as illustrated in Fig. 8.2 [10].

Screening programmes for breast cancer have a centralised or decentralised organisation [6]. The annotation is related to the organisation of the screening and reading facilities. If both image readers read the screening mammograms in a reading centre (usually a screening centre), the reporting delay is managed because the image readers discuss and agree on a result on whether to recall the client or not at the center for assessment. In countries were the screening mammograms are read by one image reader at geographically spread units and/or one reader at a breast centre, it is more difficult to organise daily consensus, certainly if the mammograms have to be sent from one place to another. The distinction between centralised and decentralised screening is now fading out due to implementation of digital mammography. Image reading can be done on any high resolution workstation and phone, or video conferences consensus can be held to discuss discrepancy cases.

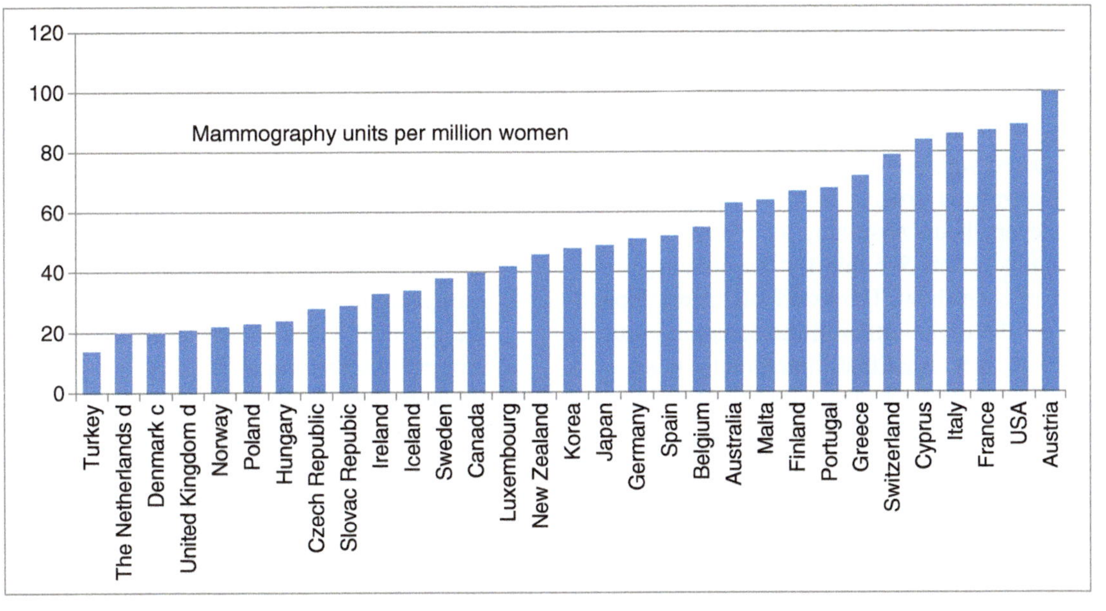

Fig. 8.2 Number of mammographic units in 31 countries [9] by permission of Oxford University Press

Many screening examinations are performed in a diagnostic or clinical context, so-called "grey", "wild," or "opportunistic" screening. Grey screening may or may not be performed according to the public screening policy. Apparently healthy clients, older or younger than the recommended age for mammographic screening use the grey screening. Grey screening might be available as the only possibility or as an additional option in some countries (Norway, Switzerland, Belgium, and France). Some countries and health care systems allow mammographic screening outside an organised programme and consider grey screening a valid earning model. For example, the U.S. does not offer organised screening programmes while this does not fit in their health care system. Grey screening may or may not be public financed, depending on the rules for reimbursement and/or payment of diagnostic mammography in the country. This means that governments, insurance companies, cantons, and private institutions fund the programmes.

The Screening Examination

The screening examination usually includes two-view mammography of each breast. In the early days of screening, only the oblique view was utilised. Most screening programmes changed during the last decade to two-view mammography because it has a higher sensitivity and specificity compared with one-view [5].

Centralised programmes invite up to 15 clients every hour. Assuming a 75 % participation rate, this means 5–6 min for the imaging procedure of each client. The workload differs depending on the organisation in the screening unit. In Norway, it is usual that three practitioners work in a team – one does the registration and checks the questionnaire of the client, the two others performing the image, one the left breast the other the right breast. In other programmes, only one practitioner performs the imaging, while other screening centres prefer one practitioner following the client from her entrance at the screening unit until her examination is completed.

Quality Assurance

A comprehensive quality assurance scheme of the screening programme is necessary to guarantee high quality screening [5]. Quality assurance is a team effort of all screening professionals to ensure that all aspects of the screening service achieve optimal quality performance. Desirable and acceptable quality parameters are defined; standardisation of epidemiological calculations and harmonisation of data collection allows comparison between regions and countries [5]. The implementation of the quality assurance parameters are thus important tools for monitoring, evaluation, identifying weaknesses for improvements and development of screening programmes for breast cancer.

The "European guidelines for quality assurance in breast cancer screening and diagnosis" is probably the most important tool in the implementation of European breast cancer screening services [5]. Most European countries follow the recommendation formulated in these guidelines. The guidelines are not a blueprint of how screening must be organised but rather description of important parameters that should be measured according to acceptable and desirable levels of quality. These quality assurance parameters are required to ensure an optimal service for the clients and to maximise the public health effects. Some countries have created their own version of the guidelines, usually based on the European version, but with national adaptation.

The 4th edition of the European Guideline includes 12 chapters [5]:

1. Epidemiological guidelines for quality assurance in breast cancer screening
2. European protocol for the quality control of the physical and technical aspects of mammography screening
3. Radiographic guidelines
4. Radiological guidelines
5. Multi-disciplinary aspects of quality assurance in the diagnosis of breast disease
6. Quality guidelines for pathology
7. Quality guidelines for surgery
8. Data collection and monitoring in breast cancer screening and care

9. The requirements of a specialist Breast Unit
10. Guidelines for training (epidemiologists, physicist, radiographers, radiologists, pathologists, surgeons, care nurses, oncologists/radiotherapists)
11. Certification protocol for breast screening and breast diagnostic services
12. Guidance for screening communication

A particular important quality parameter is the recall rate. Clients are recalled if the screening mammograms show suspicious findings and further assessment is required to clarify the findings. If it is a breast cancer it is called a true-positive screening result. If the lesion appeared to have a benign origin (cyst, fibroadenoma or a constructed image due to overlapping tissue), it is called a false-positive screening result. True-positive and false-positive screening results are results of the image reader performance and therefore considered important quality parameters for a screening programme.

Another important quality parameter is the interval cancer rate. Interval cancers are cancers detected in between screening rounds, whereas the last screening exam was defined as negative. In retrospect, true interval cancers have no signs on the prior screening mammograms of a suspect lesion, while missed interval cancers are showing significant signs. An interval cancer might also be radiologically occult, which means that the cancer was present in the prior mammogram but due to dense tissue or overlapping tissues, not visible.

Further information about quality assurance can be found in Chap. 17.

Communicating About Screening

Mammographic screening usually involves healthy and asymptomatic women who require adequate information presented in an appropriate and unbiased manner in order to allow a fully informed choice as to whether to attend or not. This information should be adequate, honest, evidence based, accessible, respectful, and tailored.

Communication was included for the first time in the fourth version of the EU guidelines [5]. At that time several countries and regions were updating their information material and strategy due to criticism for not providing complete, objective or sufficient information about the harms of mammographic screening. Results from early performance measures from several screening programmes have created new knowledge and thereby new perspectives and knowledge from organised service screening programmes. The increased attention on communication, information and use of informed consent in mammographic screening is a result of the debate of the efficacy of mammographic screening, but also the availability to information about the topic, as for heath related issues in general.

The intention of the communication and information in mammographic screening is to provide clear, precise and unbiased information. However, the topic is challenging due to the complexity of screening and the different perspectives of the benefits and harms.

The European guidelines recommends that the invitation and accompanying leaflet should include information about [5]:

- the purpose of screening
- the population to be targeted
- the screening interval
- the benefits and disadvantages of screening
- the cost of the test and eventual follow up examinations and treatment
- how to make or change the appointment
- how to obtain the results and interpret them
- the possibility and nature of any necessary further investigation
- how to get further information

The level of literacy skills in the population, poverty, ethnicity and race are factors to consider in the process of developing information. Further, multicultural and multi-linguistic populations require an understanding of the cultural values, beliefs, health practices and communication styles.

Training

The 4th edition of the European guidelines for quality assurance in breast cancer screening and diagnosis made recommendations for training and continuing medical education for all professionals working in a screening programme [5]. The guidelines state that all professionals involved should have knowledge of the principles of breast cancer diagnosis, management and screening. A curriculum of training, including academic and clinical components at approved training centres with a multidisciplinary approach, is recommended. The skills of communication, both between the professionals involved and between the staff and the invited clients should be learned. Records of the academics and training activities represent an important part for the certification review process.

Most countries and regions require and perform training of the personnel at all levels to ensure that the programme is able to deliver high quality screening. The radiographic work, producing high quality mammograms is crucial for the early diagnosis of breast cancer.

The European guidelines recommend, among others, that the radiographers take part in assessment clinics and to be familiar with all investigative procedures carried out at a breast clinic [5]. The guidelines also state that the radiographers should participate in team meetings because of their vital part of the multidisciplinary team. Further, in order to maintain breast screening skills, the minimum requirement with regard to participation for radiographers in the screening programme is 2 days per week. In a similar manner, radiographers participating only in symptomatic breast services should carry out a minimum of 20 mammographic examinations per week. Some programmes have a minimum of 1,000 mammograms per year. The requirements do not make a distinction between diagnostic and screening mammograms. A volume requirement is not the optimal quality parameter. Some countries are using image quality assessment tools such as PGMI, to measure the image quality of practitioners; however that tool is not ideal nor evidence based. A combination of these two parameters might be a reasonable solution.

There is limited documentation in relation to the practical part of the radiographers training, and how the different countries and regions handle the guidelines. There are some studies regarding performance of PGMI and distribution of screening mammograms according to quality classification, but how the radiographers are educated to fulfil the criteria set by the European guidelines is lacking. The requirements and certification used for radiographers, in a randomly selected number of countries and regions is shown in Table 8.1.

Accreditation and Certification

There are several basic determinants of successful implementation to start up and run a screening programme in a country or a region [5]. The 2014 supplement to the 4th edition of the European Guidelines specifies these determinants [15]. Applying minimum requirements and quality indicators is essential to improve organisation, performance and outcome in screening and breast care. Efficacy and compliance need to be constantly monitored to evaluate the quality of client care and to allow appropriate corrective actions leading to improvements. A robust and reliable system of accreditation is thus required for screening and diagnostic units to identify which are operating to a satisfactory standard. Any accreditation system should only recognise centres that employ sufficiently skilled and trained personnel.

With the free movement regulations in the European Union and the standardisation of the qualifications of paramedical trained personnel, it is possible to apply for similar positions in most member states [4]. There will be language requirements that need to be fulfilled, but in principle this exchange is possible. European Free Trade Association (EFTA) countries like Iceland, Norway, and Switzerland have also signed bilateral agreements with the EU and follow the same rules. However the standardisation of qualifications relates to basic training and the specialisation

Table 8.1 Duration and content, proofs of participation/certificates of training programmes for radiographers working in some of the European screening programmes [5, 12–14]

Country	Duration and content	Proof of participation/certificate
Switzerland	French speaking part of Switzerland: 2 days course + half-day internship. If the level of competence is not achieved, the internship is extended	Multiple choice questions internship certificate
	German speaking part: 2 days course + at least 1 week internship at a reference centre	Certificate of course participation and proof of the achievement of the objectives of the internship
France	2 days: organisation of programmes for early detection of breast cancer and quality testing of digital or analogue mammograms. The course is carried out together with the radiologist	Certificate
Germany	2 days: understand the basic principles of the screening programme. Anatomy, pathology, breast imaging	Feedback after each module is finished
	Epidemiology, diagnosis, treatment	
	3 days specific programme for radiographers: practical course: imaging and quality assessment. Communication with the women	
	At least 2 weeks internship at a reference centre	
Great Britain	1 week theory and 1 week practical work +115 h practice	Thesis (master level) + Portfolio, including 500 self performed mammograms and a confirmed evaluation on quality of at least 75 mammograms
	The training is accepted by the University College of Radiography, and is part of the Post Graduate Education	
The Netherlands	3 weeks of practical skills (clinical skill training) for the acquisition of knowledge in anatomy, pathology and physics	Portfolio, including 50 self performed mammograms
	3 weeks of work in a screening centre (perfection)	
	3 days theoretical training: positioning, ergonomics, interpretation of mammography, social competence, physics, breast cancer pathology and diagnosis	
Norway	No specific requirements	
	A 1-week course with a test is recommended	
	Continuous evaluation of the performance with PGMI is recommended	
	A 30 CME in mammography (epidemiology, basic principles of the screening programme, anatomy, pathology, breast imaging, diagnosis, treatment, communication) is offered every 2 years	The 30 CME could be included as a part of a master thesis

(continued)

Table 8.1 (continued)

Country	Duration and content	Proof of participation/certificate
European Guidelines	A minimum of 40 h course and practical exercise At least 75 screening examinations performed with guidance/evaluation Practical work 2–6 weeks where at least 150 examinations should be performed Participation in continuous courses and extern evaluations anatomy, pathology, breast imaging, diagnosis, treatment, communication) is offered every 2 years	About 97 % of the performed mammograms must be able to be interpreted by radiologists and radiographers

as screening practitioner is not available in all countries. National radiography societies are able to provide information on specific requirements related to screening.

References

1. Breast Cancer. Estimated incidence, mortality and prevalence worldwide in 2012. Globocan: IARC; 2014 [cited 14.07.2014]. Available from http://globocan.iarc.fr/Pages/fact_sheets_cancer.aspx.
2. Gøtzsche PC, Jørgensen KJ. Screening for breast cancer with mammography. Cochrane Database Syst Rev. 2013;6:CD001877. pub5. Review.
3. Independent UK Panel on Breast Cancer Screening. The benefits and harms of breast cancer screening: an independent review. Lancet. 2012;380(9855):1778–86. Review.
4. European Commission – health and consumers directorate. European Commission initiative on breast cancer [cited 14.07.2014]. Available from http://ec.europa.eu/health/major_chronic_diseases/docs/eibc_structure_2014_en.pdf.
5. Perry N, Broeders M, de Wolf C, Törnberg S, Holland R, von Karsa L. European guidelines for quality assurance in breast cancer screening and diagnosis, 4th ed. Luxembourg: European Communities; (2006). http://europa.eu.int.
6. Cancer screening in the European Union. Report on the implementation of the Council Recommendation on cancer screening. [cited 14.07.2014]. Available from http://ec.europa.eu/health/ph_determinants/genetics/documents/cancer_screening.pdf.
7. European Commission. Joint Research Centre Report of a European survey on the organisation of breast cancer care services supporting information for the European Commission initiative on breast cancer. [cited 29.08.2014]. Available from http://bookshop.europa.eu/en/report-of-a-european-survey-on-the-organisation-of-breast-cancer-care-services-pbLBNA26593/.
8. Giordano L, von Karsa L, Tomatis M, et al. Mammographic screening programmes in Europe: organization, coverage and participation. J Med Screen. 2012;19 Suppl 1:72–82.
9. Hofvind S, Vacek PM, Skelly J, Weaver DL, Geller BM. Comparing screening mammography for early breast cancer detection in Vermont and Norway. J Natl Cancer Inst. 2008;100(15):1082–91.
10. Broeders MJ, Scharpantgen A, Ascunce N, Gairard B, Olsen AH, Mantellini P, Mota TC, Van Limbergen E, Séradour B, Ponti A, Trejo LS, Nyström L; European Breast Cancer Network. Comparison of early performance indicators for screening projects within the European Breast Cancer Network: 1989–2000. Eur J Cancer Prev. 2005 Apr;14(2):107–16.
11. Heeten D, Broeders M. Nationwide breast cancer screening in the Netherlands [cited 14.07.2014]. Available from National Expert and Training Centre for Breast Cancer Screening.
12. Barreau B, Brault I, Deghaye M, Ceugnart L, Marelle P, Haber S. Effet indirect du dépistage à la française: la formation Indirect results of the French breast cancer screening program: training. The experience of FORCOMED. 7 journée de la SFSPM, Deauville, 2005 FORCOMED, 62, boulevard Latour-Maubourg 75007 Paris.
13. Versorgung im Rahmen des Programms zur Früherkennung von Brustkrebs durch Mammographie-Screening. Anlage 9.2 BMV-Ä/EKV [cited 14.07.2014]. Available from http://www.kbv.de/media/sp/09.2_Mammographie.pdf.
14. NHS Breast Screening Programme (NHSBSP) [cited 14.07.2014]. Available from https://www.google.no/webhp?sourceid=chrome-instant&ion=1&espv=2&ie=UTF-8#q=NHSBSP.
15. Perry N, Broeders M, de Wolf C, Törnberg S, Holland R, von Karsa L. European guidelines for quality assurance in breast cancer screening and diagnosis, 4th ed, supplements. Luxembourg: European Communities; (2013). http://europa.eu.int.

Part II

Caring for Patients and Clients

9 Sue's Story: The Big Journey

Susan Cliffe* and Colin Cliffe*

Acknowledging that breast cancer has a significant impact on the patient, their relatives and their friends, we, the editors, decided to ask Sue to share her story. We spent an evening with Sue and her husband, Colin, to explain about this book and what we wanted from them. They readily agreed to help and during that evening, with the help of Colin, Sue told us her story. It was riveting and moving. Sue and Colin then spent the next few weeks reflecting and making notes, ready for Sue to write her story – the big journey.

Sue's story is a good starting point for this section of the book, as it provides a real example of a patient's experience, prior to diagnosis through treatment and her return to work. With Sue's story in mind, subsequent chapters highlight psychological theories and concepts that might prove valuable in caring for patients. Here is Sue's story…

I would say that life was going particularly well. I had just completed a gruelling interview and been appointed as the Head of one of the largest schools in the borough, my husband was doing well following open-heart surgery 3 years previously, we were established in our new home and my daughters were settled in school and University respectively. I was fit and healthy and we were enjoying life.

I suppose that at the back of my mind I always had a nagging thought about getting breast cancer- my Mum and Aunt both died of the disease and I had first hand experience of its impact. I did think that, like them, I had until my '60s until I was really at risk, however!

It was on New Year's Day 2010 that I discovered a lump. It felt quite hard and unlike the surrounding tissue. As a trained, registered general nurse I suppose I was always a little neurotic about lumps and bumps. With a high level of anxiety, I decided to go to my general practitioner (GP) doctor. I initially saw a male doctor who told me he wouldn't examine me and that I should see a lady doctor the following week. When I saw her she examined me and said that it "Definitely isn't cancer" and that I should return in the future if I was still worried as it might be hormonal and may alter with my periods. This was music to the ears and, I admit, I did try to forget about the lump, convincing myself that that part of my breast had always been rather lumpy.

Three months later I was having a break in a touring caravan busying myself with a spot of vacuuming when the machine bellowed out copious quantities of dust- this made me extremely wheezy and I ended up in the local accident and emergency centre on a Salbutamol nebuliser. This restored me to the joys of normal breathing and I was advised to go to my GP to discuss my diagnosis of Asthma. This event, indirectly, started the treatment for my breast cancer. When I saw my GP I mentioned, almost in passing, that

*S. Cliffe and C. Cliffe: Patients.

P. Hogg et al. (eds.), *Digital Mammography: A Holistic Approach*,
DOI 10.1007/978-3-319-04831-4_9,

the lump in my right breast was still there. She examined me and reiterated her opinion that it wasn't cancer. However, she did suggest that I visit the Breast Clinic at our local hospital.

The appointment was made and I attended on my own as I was sure that there wouldn't be a problem. My visit took the form of a series of experiences. As I was just 50, I had never had a mammogram before and this was the first stage of the visit. I approached the machine with trepidation. The lady performed the procedure in a fairly perfunctory way and I was amazed at the level of pain that the procedure caused. I was so relieved to leave the room and I went out to wait for the next stage – the meeting with the Registrar. She was delightful! She examined me and said she could feel a lump but she was unsure about whether it should cause concern. She said the only way to be sure was to have a biopsy. What was to follow was, I think, one of the worst parts of the visit beaten only by the diagnosis.

I went into a darkened room and was asked to lie on the couch. The radiologist used ultrasound to establish the location of the lump and he let me know that he could see it on the monitor. He told me that he was going to take some core biopsies and that he would give me a local anaesthetic. When this took effect, he cut me (no pain- phew!) and at this point I realised that I was becoming frightened. I asked the nurse who was in attendance if I could hold her hand which she did. I feel that I might have coped better if I had been distracted by small talk rather than waiting and having time to reflect on how awful this experience might be. The nurse merely watched the procedure. The radiologist then pushed a needle (much larger than I imagined – I thought it would be the size of an injection needle!) into my breast and then he told me that there would be a loud click. I think this was a vast understatement. I thought that I'd been shot – the force was quite startling and by the third shot, I had become a little more relaxed, if that was possible. When I was dressing, the nurse told me that I had been very brave. I thanked her for her support.

I went back out into the waiting room. As I sat there, I realised that this trip was far more of an ordeal than I had hoped for and I wished that I had someone with me – even as a distraction to talk to and to put on a brave face for. I read all the booklets I could find (I found a magazine of mastectomy wear particularly disturbing). After what felt like an age, I was called back into one of the Consulting Rooms. I sat on my own in a small room waiting, trying to read as many notices in the room to keep my mind busy. Eventually, the knock on the door came and the very pleasant Registrar came in accompanied by a nurse. They both looked rather sombre. I felt the bottom fall out of my stomach. She said that they were very concerned about what the investigations thus far had shown. She said that I was to return in 1 week for the results and that I should bring someone with me. She said that they could do wonderful things nowadays and that "Our ladies do particularly well at our hospital." I remember thinking, "But I don't want to be one of your ladies!" The rest of what was said was something of a muddle. I heard mention of using chemotherapy before an operation, mastectomies, lumpectomies and reconstructions. I felt totally overwhelmed. I asked how fast things would progress in terms of treatment and she replied, "Very fast."

Bizarrely, my main thought was, "What am I going to do about the new job I've just accepted?" I actually shared my concern with the two staff sitting with me in that room. The registrar simply said, "Let's just wait until we get the definitive diagnosis next week." What followed was the longest week of my life.

On leaving the clinic in something of a daze, I phoned my husband on the way to the car and told him that the doctor was concerned about the results of tests. I don't know how I travelled home along a busy A-road with tears blurring my vision. When I arrived home, I fell into a heap of uncontrollable sobbing feeling that I was the main character in a nightmare. I was still totally fixated on what I was going to do about my new job- it seems amazing that I had such concern for something so relatively trivial but I suppose deep down I wanted my life to be as settled around me whilst I concentrated on the battle ahead. I phoned my good friend from work and told her the news and then I contacted my school Chair of Governors. I explained that I needed to see him urgently. Being the lovely man he is, he immediately told me to come straight over to his house with Colin, my husband.

I was very nervous as I explained my fears to my Chair – he listened attentively. The upshot of me externalising my thoughts was for me to reach the point of saying that, even though I had recently indicated my intention to resign, I really didn't want to embark on this journey away from the school community I felt so at home with. Without hesitation, my Chair said that I should not hand in my formal resignation and give back word to the other school. I felt so relieved and moved at how supportive people could be. This was something that would be impressed on me more and more in the future journey.

I now had the onerous task of telling friends and family of the potential diagnosis. It was at this point that I decided to be as open as possible about facing cancer. I was so fortunate that Colin took on the task of phoning a range of people to warn them of what might be looming. However, I told my daughters. They both responded in a fairly similar way sounding almost detached. With time it became apparent that this was how they managed to handle the situation. Colin faced the future with great positivity – his attitude was that we had coped with the surgery he underwent and that we could face whatever the future flung at us together.

I don't know how I dealt with the wait – it was almost unbearable. The nurse at the clinic said that not knowing was worse than knowing and I am now inclined to agree. I tried to carry on as normal busying myself with work and seeing friends. I found sharing my experience of the clinic visit helped enormously. However, this period was when I became acquainted with the most dangerous of pastimes – looking up articles about breast cancer on the Internet! I began to do this and entered the world of biopsies, cancer types and survival rates. I was to become something of an amateur authority within the year that followed.

After what seemed an age, the day came to go for the results. I was invited into a consulting room with Colin and eventually a knock came on the door and another consultant came in accompanied by a lady who was introduced to me as a breast care nurse. At this point I knew for sure what would be said – why else would a specialist nurse accompany the doctor? After exchanging pleasantries, I was told that they had indeed found a grade 2 tumour about 1.5 cm in size and that there was no reason to believe that there was any spread. A lumpectomy would be performed along with the removal of a sentinel lymph node and nearby lymph nodes which would be checked for cancer spread. Following this, there would be a course of radiotherapy (which I was acquainted with as it had been part of my Mum's treatment) and perhaps a requirement to take Tamoxifen. I was really delighted – which was surreal given that I had just been told I had cancer! I felt positive and able to face what looked like the scenario for treatment. The Lumpectomy would take place in about 3 weeks.

I returned to work later that afternoon and painted a very optimistic picture about my treatment plan and all my friends were caught up in my relief and positive spin. Before I knew it, I was presenting myself at the same hospital for surgery. The staff were very welcoming and I immediately began chatting to a lady who was also going to theatre for a lumpectomy. Sadly, I had starved from midnight and was not due in theatre until the afternoon – I was so hungry and thirsty by the time I went that I think it distracted me from what was going to happen. I went down to have the radioactive injection in preparation for the procedure and the staff were so chatty with me – which is exactly what I needed. I wanted life to continue as before. I didn't want to be labelled. I found it strange walking to theatre and I must confess that I felt rather tempted to escape from the hospital whilst en route. When I arrived in the anaesthetic room, the Registrar who had first seen me in clinic came in to see me and gave me a hug. She said they would look after me and that she was so sorry to meet me again in these circumstances. This made me feel confident and in caring hands. The anaesthetic experience was rather awful – it took a while to find a vein (which was to become a recurring nightmare) and the anaesthetist was talking a medical student through my preparation. One of the drugs injected began to burn up my arm and I said calmly that it really hurt. Then the pain became excruciating burning up into my neck. At this point I tried to exit off the trolley and I was held back by alarmed staff and before I lost consciousness I heard someone shout, "Get some help!" I woke up in a somewhat agitated state and, after being sick a few times, settled into a quick recovery supported by attentive staff. Yet again, I had to endure the colossal stress of waiting for results – the surgeon said that she thought she had removed the entire tumour but the histology would reveal what we were dealing with. Going back to work and living a normal life seemed to be my coping mechanism. I was very concerned about the results as my optimism had waned somewhat. When we were waiting in the consulting room for the feedback following the surgery I was very aware of the discomfort around the wound site but I told myself that it would be worth it to get rid of the troublesome lump. As soon as the Consultant entered the room with the Breast Care Nurse I knew that all was most certainly not well. My worst fears were to be realised. I was told that the tumour was much worse than had been first hoped and that the three lymph nodes removed all showed cancer cells. This meant chemotherapy. Also there was extensive lymphovascular invasion which meant a mastectomy and removal of all of the lymph nodes under my right arm. As radiotherapy would also be needed following surgery, he recommended that an immediate reconstruction should not be done as the appearance of the new breast would be adversely affected. I was stunned. He saw this and said that he realised that I was shocked but that the situation wasn't hopeless. He booked me in for the operation in 3 weeks giving me a chance to come to terms with what faced me. When he left, the Breast Care Nurse spent some time with us and comforted me by saying that, although the bar had been raised in terms of treatment, it would be a more thorough attack. At this point I was happy to throw every form of weapon at the cancer – I'd always thought that my Mum and Aunt might have fared better with more extreme treatment. The Nurse agreed that it would be unwise for me to return to work considering the shock I was in. She also assured me that a mastectomy was an operation which was fairly simple and that they now had good drugs to deal with the side effects of chemotherapy. Her words gave me hope which I now know is the strongest piece of armour. When I returned home I informed my Deputy, Assistant Head and Chair that I could be off work for up to a year! The nurse suggested that working with children whilst having chemotherapy would be too risky in terms of the threat of infection. We were also expecting a school inspection ('Ofsted') which added to our sense of panic at work but I was assured that all would be taken care of at school and that I shouldn't worry about it. From this point on my priorities changed – I focused on the fight. I was so blessed to have such a supportive workplace. I think at this point if I could have retired, I would have done. I was envious of all of the older women who were facing the battle in their retirement without the worry of work.

Before I knew it I was setting off to hospital for the next round of surgery. I went back to the same ward I had had the Lumpectomy on and the staff were as supportive as ever. I walked down to the theatre with Colin who left me at the door of the suite and I waited to be called from a small room where I sat with a nurse who kept me distracted with small talk – another great way of quelling the nerves. On the trolley the Theatre Technician held my hand and stroked my head as they battled to find a vein – the last words I heard were, "Don't worry- we'll look after you." I woke up to drains and bandages. I was just so glad to have survived the operation even during the usual bout of sickness on returning to the ward. I felt strangely euphoric and almost enjoyed the interaction with staff and patients as I began my recovery. The Staff Nurse made me feel so hopeful when she shared that she thought I'd do very well because I was so positive. Small, almost throw away comments make such a difference to your outlook as a patient faced with an illness we all dread.

I was discharged after having one of the two drains removed. I was waited on hand and foot by Colin who continued to be so positive. On return to the surgeon, he said that we had taken the right course of action as the rest of the breast showed many traces of cancer. I was pleased to hear that only one of the remaining removed nodes had cancer cells present – I was by now ready to hear the worst possible feedback! My next stage of treatment loomed with a visit to the Oncologist who suggested that chemotherapy was the correct plan of action. I was to start treatment about three weeks after the mastectomy – time to be sufficiently recovered. Like the Ghost of Christmas Past, this was the treatment that filled me with the most fear. You are always worried about how you will respond to the drugs – especially when you are told that one comes from the yew tree and is highly toxic. I went to the unit at my local hospital which was an outpost of the Christie Hospital to prepare to be given what I saw as poison. They had arranged for me to have an ice cap to prevent hair loss and I went along for my first treatment. I was frankly terrified but I was put at my ease by the fantastically friendly staff who talked me through each step of the treatment. The ice cap was put on – it was excruciatingly cold. The nurse managed to find a vein after two attempts and the infusion started. It stopped flowing after about 20 min and it took seven attempts by different staff to find a vein. As a final shot, they used a vein on my mastectomy side which they didn't really want to do due to the increased risk of lymphoedema in the arm. As time went by, I began to feel rather strange. I began to shiver, not in a conventional way, but with uncontrollable shaking. I thought I was going to pass out. The staff realised that something was going on and they checked my pulse and blood pressure which were hard to find. I was hypothermic. At this point I told them to get the ice cap off me - I didn't care if I lost my hair! This was not possible immediately as the cap was firmly united with my head! They brought lots of blankets and warmed me up. They were very concerned and did their utmost to make me comfortable as the last of the drugs were infused. I felt totally traumatised – the episode with the ice cap had certainly taken my mind off the chemotherapy. A few days later, my hairdresser advised that I should have my head shaved before the hair began to fall out in clumps. We had some fun as I was given a punk style before all my locks were consigned to the bin. My wig was lovely and I had more compliments about my hairstyle than when I had my own head of hair!

I was so lucky with this treatment in that I was never sick. I felt extremely lethargic for a couple of days following treatment. I had to lie down to get my breath back after a shower. I certainly caught up on films and reading I had missed. Many people were so kind during this time – especially the lady who made us lots of pies and cakes to save us from the chore of cooking. I was bolstered by the text messages and little notes sent by friends. Many had put me in touch with others who had endured the same treatment and I felt this was a superb source of support. Just talking to someone who had survived was so uplifting. The eight sessions of chemo were over in just under 6 months – the staff helped me through, especially when I was scared at receiving Taxotere which I had been told can cause anaphylaxis within the first ten minutes. The nurse told me before we began the infusion that the hydrocortisone injection was ready if there were to be a problem and she talked non-stop to me telling me tales of her exploits over Christmas and before I knew it, the infusion was in with no ill effects.

I did, however, develop two infections of unknown origin whilst I was having chemo. The first time my temperature crept above 37° the nurse who I phoned at The Christie advised sympathetically, " You'd better pack your bags and drive down here sweetheart." I couldn't believe how poorly the others on the admissions ward were. In comparison, I felt reasonably alright – just a little 'spaced-out'. The second infection led me to attend our local Accident and Emergency Department. They seemed to be somewhat at a loss about my treatment and didn't realise that I had had a drug (Neulasta) to boost my white cell count making my blood picture appear better than it was. I was discharged and my temperature began to rise further. On phoning The Christie, they wanted to admit me immediately. During both admissions I was pumped full of antibiotics and was discharged swiftly.

I was so relieved to have the chemotherapy behind me and to have coped with all of the maximum doses. I next attended The Christie hospital for preparation for 15 sessions of radiotherapy. My tattoos were done (the most painful part of the procedure) and I attended each week day for three weeks. I usually had the same radiographers which gave the opportunity for 'bonding'. They kept apologising to me about the uncomfortable positions I had to lie in – I assured them that this part of my treatment was bliss compared with what had gone before. On the penultimate day of treatment, one of the radiographers saw me to discuss after care. She went through my pathology report and told me to continue to apply E45 cream to the site of the therapy on the chest wall and above my right clavicle. That evening I was drawn to the Internet and I looked up the type of cancer I knew I had. It was very rare and had a poor prognosis. I read that 40 % of people are dead within 3 years. I was so depressed. I had coped well up to this point. The next day a good friend took me for the final day of radiotherapy. I mentioned to the two radiographers what I had read. They sensed my distress and said they would get an oncologist to come and speak to me. Within half an hour of finishing the treatment an oncologist and radiographer were talking to me about the perils of the Internet. The oncologist told me that I was not a hopeless case and that they would tell me in all honesty if this were the situation. She also said that statistics mean nothing. You could be in either sets of the percentages. If survival was only 5 % you could be one of those. She boosted me by stating, "Susan, you had cancer. We have treated it. As far as we are concerned, it has gone. Just carry on with your life."

And that is what I have attempted to do. I have been back at work as a head teacher in my challenging school for over 2 years. I have enjoyed good health – every day is a blessing and I give thanks every day if I feel well. Colin continues to support me, and my daughters seem to have come through the ordeal relatively unscathed. They handled the situation in their own way and, on reflection, I would rather they were more detached than falling apart around me. They gave us a sense of normality. I do feel that I have less tolerance for those who complain about trivial things. I have been a happier, more grateful person since embarking on this journey and I have learnt how very important human beings are in supporting each other through the challenges of life. This is especially so in the caring professions – a small comment can have a massive impact for good or ill.

Psychological Considerations in Attending for Mammography Screening

10

Anne Pearson and Ashley Weinberg

Introduction

The UK NHS Breast Screening Programme has set a national minimum rate for uptake of routine invitations at 70 % [1]. In 2012–2013, 2.32 million women aged 50–70 were invited to attend for a routine mammogram, 72.2 % of whom complied. This represented a further decrease from previous years in which uptake of routine invitations had fallen (73.4 % in 2010–11 and 73.1 % in 2011–12 [1]). Breast cancer is the most common cancer in women in the UK [2], with more than 80 % survival 5 years after diagnosis [3]. Screening can help reduce breast cancer mortality [4], so why would 27.8 % of women in 2012–2013 fail to accept an invitation for a routine mammogram which may ultimately help to save their lives?

What Can Psychology Offer?

Psychological models have attempted to explain the perceptions and beliefs underlying the decision to attend screening. However research efforts to turn these models into predictors of attendance behaviour have met with varying levels of success [5], suggesting that the theory is relevant, but may not capture the full picture. Additional considerations linked to demographic background, individual differences in psychological attributes, as well as events which cue thoughts about mammography screening are also likely to inform the decision to attend.

With knowledge of working in a location and its particular mix of client groups, the practitioner is well placed to assess which factor(s) is (are) influential in this process. Whilst no single approach will suit all potential attendees, it is hoped that awareness of a range of factors, such as those discussed in this section, will encourage or confirm the practitioner's efforts in understanding what lies behind an individual's decision to attend for a mammogram.

The psychological contributors to a decision to attend for screening or not, may be broken down into specific components. The Health Beliefs Model [6] suggests that we assess the threat posed by a specific cause of illness taking into account our own susceptibility and perceptions of the severity of a potential health problem, calculations about which may be prompted by a cue, such as the arrival of an invitation for an appointment or seeing an awareness raising advertisement. From this starting point, the Model suggests we balance the benefits and barriers provided by the prospect of preventative action. For mammography this means that clients are unlikely to come forward when perceiving there is little chance of developing breast cancer, but are more likely to attend for screening if there is knowledge about highly increased mortality if

A. Pearson (✉) • A. Weinberg
Department of Psychology, University of Salford, Frederick Road, Salford M6 6PU, UK
e-mail: a.pearson1@salford.ac.uk; a.weinberg@salford.ac.uk

P. Hogg et al. (eds.), *Digital Mammography: A Holistic Approach*,
DOI 10.1007/978-3-319-04831-4_10, © Springer International Publishing Switzerland 2015

the cancer remains undetected [7]. Considerable efforts have been made to raise public awareness of breast cancer in recent years, particularly in the UK, resulting in increased availability of information about both of these aspects of threat [3]. However the psychological impact of information concerning breast cancer and screening has also been more carefully considered.

Perceptions of Risk and Pain

Previous research has documented that women tend to overestimate their own breast cancer risk, causing them to suffer high levels of anxiety about developing the disease [8, 9]. Interestingly, Yavan et al. [10] found that in a sample of Turkish women at average risk they actually perceived themselves at 50 % or more risk of developing breast cancer, and this rate increased as they got older; other research such as Jones et al.'s [11] large-scale Australian studies suggest instead that younger women perceive the most elevated risk. Either way the consequence of this inaccurate perception of risk and associated levels of anxiety may adversely affect attendance for regular screening in these women. It is unclear what causes such inaccuracies, and it would seem reasonable to examine the effectiveness of the process of communication of risk itself. Historically, research has documented that international variations in risk communication have made no difference to inaccurate risk perception [12–15].

Recently, the UK's Independent Breast Screening Review Panel [16] indicated a number of policy recommendations to the NHS Breast Screening Programme, one of which concerned the communication of risk and benefit of routine mammograms. It is important that 'clear communication of the harms and benefits of screening to women is essential. It is at the core of how a modern health system should function' [17]. However, it may be that as the risks or harms are more effectively communicated, women who already overestimate their risk may tend to utilise this information and conclude that screening is unsafe, and decline the invitation to attend for routine mammograms. A study in Germany looked at risk information for colorectal screening; they found that risk information was most effective when presented in a traditional format, offering simple advice and general guidelines. Conversely if risk information was presented as evidence-based information that considered specific criteria it was more likely to lead to some rationalisation of inaction, i.e. people tended to devalue this information, minimise their perceived risk, and use this as a reason for non-attendance [18].

The nature of mammography means that a decision about its personal relevance relies on a combination of physical and psychological considerations. As if to complicate matters, both of these sets of factors are subject to variations in the individual's perceptions too.

However the anecdotal themes of embarrassment, discomfort and pain [19] indicate that for a proportion of women the process itself is physically challenging, in a manner which may well be separate from any consideration about perceptions of the potential benefit of having a mammogram. Naturally any professional carrying out the screening will do their best to mentally prepare the individual and qualm any concerns, so it is not surprising that attendees are generally positive about the staff working in this field – it has even been noted that satisfaction with the practitioner can actually help to reduce reports of pain and embarrassment [20].

Nevertheless anyone experiencing serious discomfort or pain is likely to remember that feeling and hold that association with the experience of having a mammogram. It has been suggested that enhancing the levels of control clients have over the mammography procedure could further assist in countering discomfort [21]. Meanwhile research is ongoing to determine the compression forces required on the breast to obtain a viable image (see section "Perceptions of risk and pain" and Chaps. 20, 21 and 22) and clearly advances in practice are required to minimise the expectation and/or perception of pain or discomfort from the process of deciding whether or not to attend or re-attend.

Beyond the Health Beliefs Model

The Health Beliefs Model also highlights the cost-benefit analysis made by an individual which determines their next step after assessing their personal risk. For a positive decision to attend screening, it has been suggested that the benefits of the behaviour should outweigh the potential barriers to taking action. For example, this requires confidence in the ability of the mammogram to detect cancer, although painful, or otherwise off-putting, experience can over-ride this potential benefit [7].

The Theory of Planned Behaviour [22] goes further to consider judgements of what is the prevalent social expectation when deciding whether to attend or not – in other words do family members, friends and colleagues go for screening? However there are limitations in the ability of either approach to predict behaviour. For example studies conducted in different ethnic groups have pointed to the usefulness of the Health Beliefs Model; but additionally suggest the role of culturally distinct factors, in determining attendance for mammography [e.g. 23–25].

Previous research has documented that uptake in women in some groups may be negatively influenced by such factors as lack of knowledge, language barriers, reduced access to medical services and unhelpful attitudes of health professionals [26]. However the role of social support, including a close friendship, supportive relationships with family, or membership of a group (e.g. as a volunteer) can positively predict attendance for a mammogram, whereas isolation from peers – such as indicated by living alone or with children only – or through absence of social participation, significantly increases the likelihood of non-attendance [27].

Furthermore, it is important to consider that mammography is one of three ways in which women are encouraged to take preventative action with regard to breast cancer, along with self-examination and a clinical consultation with their doctor if a sign or symptom is noted. More recent comparisons of women's perceptions in relation to all three techniques suggest fewer ethnic-group differences in perceived threat or barriers associated with each, but instead differences in the perceptions of the benefits of mammography, along with varying scores for self-efficacy and health motivation [28]. Individual differences due to enduring personal characteristics, such as self-efficacy, have also been proposed as key factors predicting compliance with health-related behaviours [29].

Taken together these findings suggest individual perceptions of factors beyond the individual's control make the prospect of having a mammogram – and a preventative approach to ill health generally – harder to follow through. The Malmo Diet and Cancer Cohort Study in Sweden has identified perceptions of lower levels of control among non-attenders, who might answer positively to questions such as 'things do not turn out the way I had wished' [27]. However efforts to combat weak control beliefs through encouraging women across the English county of Kent to plan to attend have yielded positive results, by increasing attendance for mammography. Women who were required to plan their attendance had tended to report reduced confidence in their capacity to overcome difficulties in attending and the act of planning helped them to problem solve in a way that may well have influenced their motivation to take up the screening invitation [30]. Such a focus on implementation intentions, i.e. helping to link planning and then acting, holds particular promise for those who have intentions to attend but see difficulties in doing so [30].

Joffe [31] points out that 'people are motivated to represent the risks which they face in a way which protects them, and the groups with which they identify, from threat' (p. 10). Consistent with this, it is more likely that women consider mammograms in a manner which strengthens the ability to build psychological defences, i.e. safeguarding feelings at an individual and social level. This is clearly a phenomenon shared by anyone rationalising a particular course of action and can mean changing one's beliefs (e.g. It is a good idea to attend for a mammogram) to justify one's behaviour (e.g. I did not attend my mammogram appointment), so that one believes differently (e.g. My friends tend not to go for a mammogram and they're fine, so I will be fine too). This example of cognitive dissonance illustrates how the logic of decision making about attending for a mammogram can be altered and yet the theoretical approaches considered so far assume such decisions are based on a controlled process free from the influence of negative emotions and from beliefs which disagree with the health promotion literature [32].

It has been recognised that recent experiences of stress outside of work increase the chances of not attending for a mammogram [27], however previous research has suggested that psychosocial factors such as fear and fatalism can negatively influence whether a woman accepts an invitation to attend for routine screening [33].

The Role of Negative Psychological Factors

Fear and anxiety can be effective barriers to screening as they have the effect of impairing both judgement and behaviour. When a woman is worried about the possibility of having breast cancer, and agonises over its possible detection by screening, she may decide not to attend for screening [34]. 'Psycho-social fear has the effect of impairing one's cognitive behaviour, thus creating dissonance and confusion while reducing the person's logical decision – making' [33, p. 98]. Consequently, this state of mind can detrimentally affect a woman's logical reasoning and cause them to avoid their routine mammogram.

Avoidance, as a strategy for dealing with fear, is readily understandable, but coping – that may be perceived as cognitive dissonance by some – can also play a role in fostering potentially unhelpful psychological defences. Hence, there can be reluctance to discuss the topic of breast cancer for associated fear of raising the probability of it occurring [35], of tempting fate by looking for trouble [36] or of challenging belief in one's good health by participating in a medical procedure [37]. 'Cancer fatalism represents a surrender of the human spirit to perceptions of hopelessness, powerlessness, worthlessness and social despair' [38, p. 135]. Women who fear they may have breast cancer who adopt this way of thinking may view screening as pointless, i.e. the cancer was 'meant' to happen anyway and there is nothing to be done about it, or indeed that if mammography can detect it, then it is already too late. This sense of helplessness in contemplating mammography has echoes in how technology is viewed by some within the screening process. Whether this emanates from the critique of a medical culture prioritising the ideas of 'boys with toys' [39] or the perception of screening as a challenge to female modesty [40], the emotional impact of having a mammogram, at least in the short-term, is often palpable.

A number of research studies have assessed anxiety levels associated with various stages of the breast screening process. The ongoing overestimation of risk has been mentioned above [10] and so it is perhaps unsurprising that women may experience initial alarm at being invited for screening. It has been argued that this may itself facilitate uptake of a mammogram, unless such levels of anxiety are provoked as to lead an individual to avoid screening for reasons previously discussed [21]. Practical solutions such as increasing regularity of contact with prospective attendees – for example by pre-screening invitations and personalised contact – mean that as well as raising awareness of the screening programme, women can become more habituated to the idea that at some point a screening appointment will be offered [41].

A UK-wide evaluation of 2009–2010 data found that following initial screening, 3.9 % of women were recalled for a further mammogram. Of these 81 % were false positive cases, in which the query triggering recall was satisfied and the women were eventually given an all-clear result [42]. Naturally concerns are raised by receipt of a recall invitation and 40 % of those categorised as false-positive cases report extreme anxiety [43].

In a Norwegian study this increased anxiety state was found to be transient, such that 4 weeks after screening, levels matched those of the general population and initial increases in depressive symptoms had declined. Not surprisingly, for women who were diagnosed with cancer, both anxiety and depression levels exceeded the population norms [44]. Despite the psychological impact of being recalled, this Norwegian study found 98 % of all women stated they would re-attend [44].

However a major review of the impact of being recalled on psychological well-being found a small increase in generalised anxiety together with significant increases in breast cancer specific anxiety, depression, fear and distress [45]. It has been noted that such specific effects may be experienced by women classed as false-positives up to 3 years later [42], which is the point of usual recall in the UK screening programme. The experience of having a false positive result may impact on subsequent attendance, with one study noting an additional 3 % of women deterred from taking up their next mammogram appointment [46]. For women with a family history of breast cancer and who receive a false positive result no comparable increase in negative psychological outcomes has been found, which may reflect their differing level of expectation about the screening process and what it may entail [2].

Conclusions

The range of relevant psychological factors in attendance and non-attendance for mammography includes beliefs about breast cancer, self-perceptions of control and self-efficacy, social support systems, demography, communications from the mammography service, past physical and/or psychological experience of screening, as well as challenging emotions and symptoms of psychological ill-health. It is likely that psychological models will continue to adapt to take these into account, but the role of the practitioner in knowing their local population and considering which factors may affect them is paramount.

Given the influential role that a negative experience can play in future attendance [47] and the identified importance of ensuring some sense of control for clients in their involvement in screening, attention to the psychological aspects of the process warrants careful consideration. With this in mind the UK's National Institute for Health Research recommends, 'clear, carefully worded information about the reason for the assessment and process of the assessment (but not in such detail that they become distressed without the support of the screening staff being present),' [42, p. xv]. In response to an independent review of breast cancer screening [48], there is a growing emphasis on developing 'patient invitation support materials…[to] better support them as they make an informed choice about screening' [16, p. 5].

References

1. Health and Social Care Information Centre. Breast Screening Programme, England: Statistics for 2012–13. 27 Feb 2014.
2. Tyndel S, Austoker J, Henderson BJ, Brain K, Bankhead C, Clements A, Watson EK. What is the psychological impact of mammographic screening on younger women with a family history of breast cancer? Findings from a prospective cohort study by the PIMMS management group. J Clin Oncol. 2007;25(25):3823–30.
3. Breast cancer campaign; breast cancer statistics. http://www.breastcancercampaign.org/about-breast-cancer/breast-cancer-statistics#./breast-cancer-statistics?&_suid=140065027052507587201572451 88. Accessed 12 May 2014.
4. National Cancer Institute. Mammography. http://www.cancer.gov/cancertopics/factsheet/detection/mammograms. Accessed 12 May 2014.
5. Carpenter CJ. A meta-analysis of the effectiveness of health belief model variables in predicting behaviour. Health Commun. 2010;25(8):661–9.
6. Rosenstock IM. Why people use health services. Milbank Meml Fund Q. 1966;44:94–127.
7. Hyman RB, Baker S, Ephraim R, Moadel A, Philip J. Health beliefs model variables as predictors of screening mammography utilisation. J Behav Med. 1994;17(4):391–406.
8. Hopwood P. Breast cancer perception: what do we know and understand? Breast Cancer Res. 2000;2: 387–91.
9. Haas JS, Kaplan CP, Des Jarlais G, Gildengoin V, Pérez-Stable EJ, Kerlikowske K. Perceived risk of breast cancer among women at average and increased risk. J Womens Health. 2005;14(9):845–51.
10. Yavan T, Akyü A, Tosun N, Iyigün E. Women's breast cancer risk perception and attitudes towards screening tests. J Psychosoc Oncol. 2010;28(2):189–201.
11. Jones SC, Magee CA, Barrie LR, Iverson DC, Gregory P, Hanks EL, Nelson AE, Nehill CL, Zorbas HM. Australian women's perceptions of breast cancer risk factors and the risk of developing breast cancer. Womens Health Issues. 2011;21(5):353–60.
12. Cull A, Anderson EDC, Campbell S, Mackay J, Smyth E, Steel M. The impact of genetic counselling about breast cancer risk on women's risk perceptions and levels of distress. Br J Cancer. 1999;79:501–8.
13. Evans DGR, Blair V, Greenhalgh R, Hopwood P, Howell A. The impact of genetic counselling on risk perception in women with a family history of breast cancer. Br J Cancer. 1994;70:934–8.
14. Hopwood P, Long A, Keeling F, Poole C, Evans DGR, Howell A. Psychological support needs for women at high genetic risk of breast cancer: some preliminary indicators. Psychooncology. 1998;7:402–12.
15. Watson M, Lloyd S, Davidson J, Meyer L, Eeles R, Ebbs S, Murday V. The impact of genetic counselling on risk perception and mental health in women with a

family history of breast cancer. Br J Cancer. 1999;79: 868–74.
16. NHS Breast Screening Programme. Annual review. Sheffield: NHS; 2012.
17. Cameron D. Reviewing the evidence for breast screening, NHS Breast Screening Programme Annual Review. Sheffield: NHS; 2012.
18. Steckelberg A, Kasper J, Redegeld M, Muhlhauser I. Risk information – barrier to informed choice? A focus group study. Soz Preventivmed. 2004;49(6): 375–80.
19. Keefe RJ, Hauck ER, Egert J, Rimer B, Kornguth P. Mammography pain and discomfort: a cognitive behavioural perspective. Pain. 1994;56:247–60.
20. Hamilton EL, Wallis MG, Barlow J, Cullen L, Wright C. Women's views of a breast cancer service. Health Care Women Int. 2003;24:40–8.
21. Marks DF, Murray M, Evans B, Willig C, Woodall C, Sykes CM. Health psychology: theory, research and practice. 2nd ed. London: Sage; 2005.
22. Ajzen I. From intention to actions: a theory of planned behaviour. In: Kuhl J, Beckmann J, editors. Action-control: from cognition to behaviour. Heidelberg: Springer; 1985. p. 11–39.
23. Wu TY, West B, Chen YW, Hergert C. Health beliefs and practices related to breast cancer screening in Philippino, Chinese and Asian-Indian women. Cancer Detect Prev. 2006;30(1):58–66.
24. Vadaparampil ST, Champion VL, Miller TK, Menon U, Sugg-Skinner C. Using the health belief model to examine differences in adherence to mammography among African-American and Caucasian women. J Psychosoc Oncol. 2005;21:59–79.
25. Consedine NS, Magai C, Horton D, Neugut AI, Gillespie M. Health belief model factors in mammography screening: testing for interactions among subpopulations of Caribbean women. Ethn Dis. 2005;15(3):444–52.
26. Thomas VN, Saleem T, Abraham R. Barriers to effective uptake of cancer screening among black and minority ethnic groups. Int J Palliat Nurs. 2005;11(11): 562–71.
27. Lagerlund M, Sontrop JM, Zachrisson S. Psychosocial factors and attendance at a population-based mammography screening program in a cohort of Swedish women. BMC Women's Health. 2014;14:33. doi:10.1186/1472-6874/14/33.
28. Hajian-Tilaki K, Auladi S. Health belief model and practice of breast self-examination and breast cancer screening in Iranian women. Breast Cancer. 2012;21(4): 429–34.
29. Rosenstock IM, Strecher VJ, Becker MH. Social learning theory and the health belief model. Health Educ Q. 1988;15(2):175–83.
30. Rutter D, Quine L, Steadman L, Thompson, S. Increasing attendance at breast cancer screening: Field trial. Final report. University of Kent 2007.
31. Joffe H. Risk and the 'other'. New York: Cambridge University Press; 1999.
32. Sarafino EP. Health psychology: biopsychosocial interactions. 4th ed. New York: Wiley; 2002.
33. Talbert PV. The relationship of fear and fatalism with breast cancer screening among a selected target population of African American middle class women. J Soc Behav Health Sci. 2008;2(1):96–110.
34. Phillips JM, Cohen MZ, Moses G. Breast cancer screening and African American women: fear fatalism and silence. Oncol Nurs Forum. 1999;26(3):561–71.
35. Blaxter M. The causes of disease: women talking. Soc Sci Med. 1983;17:59–69.
36. Russell KM, Swenson MM, Skelton AM, Shedd-Steele R. The meaning of health in mammography screening for African American women. Health Care Women Int. 2003;24:27–39.
37. Borrayo EA, Jenkins SR. Feeling healthy: so why should Mexican-descent women screen for breast cancer? Qual Health Res. 2001;11:812–23.
38. Powe BD. Cancer fatalism – spiritual perspectives. J Relig Health. 1997;36(2):135–7.
39. Kearney AJ. Increasing our understanding of breast self-examination: women talk about cancer, the health care system and being women. Qual Health Res. 2006;16(6):802–20.
40. Borrayo EA, Jenkins SR. Feeling indecent: breast cancer screening resistance of Mexican-descent women. J Health Psychol. 2001;6:537–49.
41. Zelenyanszki C. Maximising screening attendance: a reference guide. NHS: North West London Cancer Network; 2009.
42. Bond M, Pavey T, Welch K, Cooper C, Garside R, Dean S, Hyde C. Systematic review of the psychological consequences of false-positive screening mammograms. Health Technol Assess. 2013;17(13):1–170.
43. Schwartz LM, Woloshin S, Fowler FJ, Welch HG. Enthusiasm for cancer screening in the United States. J Am Med Assoc. 2004;291:71–8.
44. Bredal S, Kåresen R, Skaane P, Engelstad KS, Ekeberg Ø. Recall mammography and psychological distress. Eur J Cancer. 2013;49(4):805–11.
45. Salz T, Richman AR, Brewer NT. Meta-analyses of the effect of false-positive mammograms on generic and specific psychosocial outcomes. Psychooncology. 2010;19:26–34.
46. McCann J, Stockton D, Godward S. Impact of false-positive mammography on subsequent screening attendance and risk of cancer. Breast Cancer Res. 2002;4. doi:10.1186/bcr455. Accessed 1 June 2014.
47. Marshall G. A comparative study of re-attenders and non re-attenders for second triennial National Breast Screening Programme appointments. J Public Health Med. 1994;16:79–86.
48. Marmot M. The benefits and harms of breast cancer screening: an independent review. The Lancet. 2012;380(9855):1778–86.

11 Emotional Intelligence

Stuart J. Mackay

Sue's story (see Chap. 9) is, as you might expect, full of emotion. She vividly describes her roller coaster experience in a series of powerful descriptions of what she is feeling. But, before we explore her emotions we need to define the term. This is problematic as it depends upon your view of the world, e.g. behaviourists might define the term differently to a philosopher. One useful and broad term used in psychology is that it is a complex state of feeling that results in physical and psychological changes that influence thought and behaviour [1]. The emotions demonstrated in Sue's story are indicated below:

The negative emotions/feelings demonstrated by Sue include

- "*..approached the machine with trepidation*"
- "*I was becoming frightened*"
- "*I felt the bottom fall out of my stomach*"
- "*I felt totally overwhelmed*"
- "*I was shocked*"
- "*I fell into a heap of uncontrollable sobbing, feeling that I was the main character in a nightmare*"
- "*I had to endure the colossal stress of waiting for results*"
- "*I was frankly terrified*"
- "*the treatment that filled me with the most fear*"
- "*I was so depressed. I had coped well up to this point*"

The positive emotions/feelings demonstrated by Sue include-

- "*She boosted me by stating….*"
- "*The joys of normal breathing*"
- "*My friends were caught up in my relief and positive spin*"
- "*Just talking to someone who had survived was so uplifting*"
- "*They made me feel confident and in caring hands*"

As well as emotion there is also a series of statements which show Sue's physical and emotional needs and expectations during this difficult time.

Reader Activity: Please re-read Sue's story and try to identify her expressed physical or emotional needs.

Sue needed to "*hold the nurses hand*" and felt there was value in "*the need to be distracted by small talk and reading waiting room notices*". She also recognised other distraction techniques, "*the staff were so chatty with me - which is exactly what I needed*". Sue states that "*The nurse merely watched the procedure*". This demonstrates Sue's expectation that the nurse should have engaged more in her care. Might the nurse have done more to help in some aspect of the procedure or maybe focus more on the patient and demonstrate some care?

Sue's story demonstrates the emotional intelligence (EI) of the patient and staff. Emotional

S.J. Mackay
Medical Imaging and Radiotherapy Directorate, School of Health Sciences, University of Liverpool, Brownlow Hill, Liverpool L69 3GB, UK
e-mail: s.mackay@liverpool.ac.uk

P. Hogg et al. (eds.), *Digital Mammography: A Holistic Approach*, DOI 10.1007/978-3-319-04831-4_11,

intelligence can be defined as the extent to which people can recognise, process and utilise emotional information [2]. People with high emotional intelligence are able to recognise emotions in themselves and in others, to understand what those emotions are and their consequences. They are able to implement a strategy designed to bring about a desired outcome. In the context of Sue's story, she describes searching on the internet and discovering information about her disease and prognosis. Discovering that "*40 % of women die within three years*" made her feel depressed and less able to cope. She mentioned this to the therapy radiography staff on her last day of radiotherapy treatment. The staff will have listened to this and recognised the strong negative emotion this invoked in Sue. They probably realised that this information was having, and would continue to have, a strong negative effect on Sue which might affect her perspective of her disease, treatment and quality of life. A strategy was implemented, to recruit the help of an oncologist, and for the therapy radiographer and oncologist to give some context to the information she had discovered. They explained that medical statistics are based on large groups of people but they are unable to predict at an individual level and she should consider the cancer cured. This clearly had a positive effect on Sue.

This broad EI definition is neatly applied to a real world situation here but to really understand EI we need to go further into the concept and explore the different models that have been described in the literature. There are essentially three models of EI – ability model, trait model and mixed model.

The ability model [3] states that emotions are useful sources of information and help in making sense of and navigating the social environment. In this model, EI is seen to comprise mental abilities, skills or capabilities and is therefore about the capacity to reason about emotions and of emotions to enhance thinking. The model is divided up into what they call Branches – namely Emotional Perception, Emotional Integration, Emotional Understanding and Emotional Management. These are then subdivided into emotional Tasks. This model – assessed using the oldest EI measurement tool called the Mayer, Salovey and Caruso Emotional intelligence test (MSCEIT) – is claimed by the authors as the only objective EI test.

The Trait EI model considers EI as a series of personality traits. Personality traits are often conceptualised as a hierarchical system with named traits (e.g. extroversion) at the top of the hierarchy. Traits are defined by a person's characteristics, the next level down in the hierarchy. The characteristics are derived from consistent aspects of an individual's behaviour. Petrides [4] describes the trait EI model as a constellation of emotional self-perceptions located at the lower levels of personality hierarchies. He uses the published and validated Trait Emotional Intelligence Questionnaire (TEIQue) to measure this model and describes the Global Trait EI which is made up of four factors called Well-being, Self Control, Emotionality, Sociability. Each factor is subdivided into several facets of which there are 15 in total (Table 11.1). Further information can be obtained from Petrides' website (www.psychometriclab.com).

The third model, called the mixed model, consists of social and emotional competencies. Key writers in this model are Goleman and Boyatzis; further information can be obtained from www.eiconsortium.org. They developed a theory [6] of work-based performance based on emotional intelligence. This consists of emotional competencies grouped into four clusters and twenty-two competencies. The clusters are self-awareness and self-management, social awareness and relationship management. The instrument (questionnaire) developed to measure this model is the Emotional Competence Inventory-University version (ECI-U).

Does EI Have Value in Healthcare?

The EI construct is only 20 years old and although research has already been undertaken over this time to explore the value of EI in healthcare, this work remains in its infancy. Nonetheless, there is evidence of the value of EI in medicine, nursing, radiography, physiotherapy and psychology.

Table 11.1 The trait emotional intelligence model demonstrating the 4 factors and 15 facets. NB the self-esteem facet is linked to both Sociability & Well-being

Factors	Facets	High scorers perceive themselves as …
Well-being	Trait happiness	Cheerful and satisfied with their lives
	Self-esteem	Successful and self-confident
	Trait optimism	Confident and likely to 'look on the bright side' of life
Self-control	Adaptability	Flexible and willing to adapt to new conditions
	Emotion regulation	Capable of controlling their emotions
	Impulsiveness (low)	Reflective and less likely to give in to their urges
	Self-motivation	Driven and unlikely to give up in the face of adversity
	Stress management	Capable of withstanding pressure and regulating stress
Emotionality	Emotion perception (self and others)	Clear about their own and other people's feelings
	Emotion expression	Capable of communicating their feelings to others
	Relationships	Capable of having fulfilling personal relationships
	Trait empathy	Capable of taking someone else's perspective
Sociability	Social awareness	Accomplished networkers with excellent social skills
	Self-esteem	Successful and self-confident
	Assertiveness	Forthright, frank and willing to stand up for their rights
	Emotion management (others)	Capable of influencing other people's feelings

Adapted from Petrides [5]

Arora [7] undertook a systematic review of the relationship between EI and doctors core competencies of the Accreditation Council for Graduate Medical Education. They found high EI positively contributed to the doctor-patient relationship, increased empathy, teamwork and communication skills, stress management, organisational commitment and leadership. It was noted that many of the studies were cross sectional in design and that more longitudinal research was needed to explore the long term impact of EI.

A key narrative review [8] of EI in nursing concluded that understanding and recognising emotion is a high order skill, vital to nursing practice. The authors also believed that understanding, detecting and conveying emotion is pivotal to a profession that requires sensitivity within relationships. Further evidence of its value came from Rankin [9] who explored the relationship between EI outcomes of a nursing degree programme and found positive correlations between practice performance of 1st years nursing students and EI. This was a small study of 1st year nurses only, so further research is required. The role of EI in care of dying among accident and emergency nurses was characterised in a qualitative study [10]. They found nurses were better able to manage the emotional labour of caring for the dying and their relatives through the development of EI.

The evidence in physiotherapy research has not demonstrated a positive relationship between EI and physiotherapy performance. Lewis [11] explored the relationship between EI and the clinical performance but found no significant correlations. Their study used the MSCEIT and a published clinical performance instrument for physiotherapy. Another study [12] also failed to show a relationship between EI and performance in physical therapy students. There were no statistically significant differences found in EI between physical therapy student scores at the start of the programme and after their first clinical block. This study used the Barr on EQi – a mixed model instrument. Both these studies were small and further research is needed to explore the role of EI in physical therapy performance.

Radiography

There have been no empirical studies identified in radiography, using science direct, Scopus and Google scholar, which provide evidence for a relationship between emotional intelligence and clinical performance. However there have been two benchmarking studies [13, 14] and three narrative reviews [15–17]. One study [13], which used the

Trait EI model, showed that radiographers are more emotionally intelligent than the general population, scoring more highly on Global EI along with three of the four factors, Well-being, Self control and Emotionality. Interestingly no differences were identified between diagnostic and therapeutic radiographers. The EI of different subspecialties of radiographer e.g. Mammographer, MR radiographer, nuclear medicine radiographer, were compared. Mammographers scored more highly than other subspecialties for well-being and emotionality. It can be seen from the descriptions in Table 11.1 that mammographers, as a group, perceive themselves, more so than other radiographer subspecialties, as cheerful, confident and with a positive outlook, plus they are able to perceive their own and others feelings, are able to communicate those feelings and are empathic. These are vitally important traits when managing clients/patients with possible breast cancer in what could often be described as an emotionally charged environment.

The narrative reviews discuss the theoretical value that EI might have in a radiography context. One paper [15] uses a case study approach with a real patient's experience and explains how emotional intelligence can be used to avoid the objectification or de-personalisation of the patient that can happen in healthcare particularly as a result of stress and fatigue [18]. With the increase in numbers of clients expected following the age extension for breast screening [19] and the short time period within which to image each patient it is likely that the busier environment in breast screening could be more stressful for staff. Development of EI skills which help staff to manage stress and promote wellbeing is a possible solution to this problem. Further research is needed to demonstrate whether there is a link between EI and patient care or clinical performance in radiography.

Can Emotional Intelligence Be Taught and Developed?

A growing body of evidence now exists to show that EI skills can be taught and developed. Two key papers demonstrated this in psychology students [20, 21]. A controlled experimental design was used in three separate experiments. They showed that emotional intelligence could be changed with an evidence-based training programme. These programmes lasted 18–20 h and were delivered over several weeks allowing participants to apply the taught theory to the real world. The syllabus covered holistic EI skills rather than focussing on one aspect of EI and results showed sustainable improvements in emotional functioning and long-term personality changes. There were also important positive implications in various other measures such as life satisfaction and proficiency in social relationships. A range of educational activities are available for improving one's EI. The Higher Education Academic website contains activities [22] that can improve self awareness, relieve stress and active listening.

A further excellent resource to improve EI in the area of facial and body language recognition is via the University of California at Berkley website called Greater Good [23]. This site presents a facial and body language recognition multiple choice quiz. A series of faces are presented with response options asking the participant to select the one corresponding to the emotion demonstrated by the face. It then marks your response and provides you with a detailed answer explaining the characteristics of the facial expression/body language which would indicate the emotion being felt by the individual.

Applied Emotional Intelligence in Mammographic Practice: The Anxious Patient/Client

Seminal work by Ekman and Friesen [24] concluded that six facial expressions are universal across cultures, these are happy, angry, sad, anxious, disgusted and surprised and that each of them is characterised by a particular facial muscular pattern. The ability to recognise these expressions of emotion is important to any healthcare practitioners including the mammographer. Recognising these facial expressions as being present in the patient will enable you to link them to the related emotion and thereby better understand what the patient is feeling. This is the essence of empathy, which is defined as an essential part of both emotional functioning and interpersonal cognition, making individuals particularly attentive to both the mental states and emotions of other people [25]. If we use the expression of anxiety as an example, how would a mammographer recognise that a patient would be feeling anxious? To help explain this I interviewed a mammography practitioner who is currently practising and examined the literature to identify how this might be done in practice.

Recognising Anxiety in Patients

Patients present with a wide range of features that might indicate they are anxious or fearful of their awaited procedure. This was described as worse for symptomatic patients who present with a possible pathology (following earlier interaction with the breast screening service) compared to screening patients who attend to have their perceived 'normality' confirmed. As described by the practising mammography practitioner, when the patient/client first arrives in the department it is the receptionist who meets them. At this stage the highly anxious state of some patients can be identified and passed on to the mammography practitioner, giving them early warning that a high level of EI may be required with this patient interaction.

The University of California [23] explains that when we are anxious or fearful our eyebrow muscles contract, pulling eyebrows up and in, lower eyelids contract and upper eyelids raise making our eyes open wider than usual. Lip corners pull sideways tightening and elongating the mouth, our jaw drops and the mouth hangs open. Plus our eyebrows are relatively flat when we're afraid. Mammography practice suggests that anxiety or fear of the procedure can be observed in the behaviour and body language. Some patients talk incessantly; others appear agitated or act as though they are very hot. Others appear distracted or disinterested or speak in a very quick or excited manner.

Recognising emotions of others in practice is not always a science. Occasionally intuition is used by the mammography practitioner to identify a woman's mood, or indeed occasionally that of a man seeking the service. Of course the other usual method of identifying emotion is to ask the patient/client how they are feeling. Sometimes women attending their first mammography screening have been exposed to frightening stories. Friends or family have told them how painful the examination is going to be and, as reported by the mammography practitioner interviewed, that they 'clamp you to the machine'. Alternatively they might have a family history of breast cancer and be very anxious about the result of their examination, a likely cause of high anxiety.

Having recognised that the patient is anxious or fearful the next action of the mammography practitioner would be to try and put in place some action or behaviour that would help to reduce the anxiety or fearfulness.

Reducing Patient Anxiety: Calm and Re-assure

The behaviour of the mammography practitioner towards the patient is crucial in helping to reduce anxiety, gain compliance and perform a high quality X-ray examination. Evidence has shown that the experience of women during a mammogram can have a detrimental effect on the response rate to a screening invitation [26].

The techniques used in practice to achieve the goals in the previous paragraph are many and varied and this is just a sample of current techniques that have been tried and found to be successful. There will be techniques that do not appear in this list and new techniques not yet conceived.

Distraction is one of the common techniques used where the mammography practitioner will chat to the women and encourage her to talk in an attempt to get her to think of something other than the situation she is in. In Sue's story she describes "*the need to be distracted by small talk and reading waiting room notices*". She appreciated chatting and found it was beneficial to her care. This chatting was often going on during the procedure so the mammography practitioner carried on positioning, setting exposures and applying compression force. Another distraction is making the women feel part of the procedure by asking them for their help in positioning. This makes them think about the present giving less time to focus on the worry.

Empathising was described as a way of helping reduce women's anxiety. Saying things like the following can help, "*yes this is a nerve wracking procedure*", "*no it is not a very nice procedure*", "*a lot of women get anxious about having a mammogram that's quite usual*". Explaining that the procedure will be over quite soon is also seen as a way of helping women to cope.

A lot of the worry was thought to be because women felt out of control and didn't know what was going to happen to them, so a response is to explain what is happening or going to happen at each stage of the procedure.

The scare stories can also be tackled by explaining that the procedure "*can be uncomfortable - but not for very long*", that "*you are in a good hospital as they are very thorough here*"; and you could tell the patient that "*they have done the right thing coming along and getting this sorted*". Some women might believe they are being overly fussy but you can explain that they are not and tell them that "*this is a normal response to this procedure*".

In short, talking to patients/clients can give them re-assurance about the examination or their response to it.

Finally, let us return to extracts from Sue's story to remind ourselves how comforting emotionally intelligent healthcare staff can be to patients: Sue describes "*The pleasant delightful registrar*" *and that* "*staff were as supportive as ever*". It is worthwhile concluding this chapter with Sue's words as they tell us how valuable healthcare staff are in supporting patients: She informs us "***how very important human beings are in supporting each other through the challenges of life. This is especially so in the caring professions- a small comment can have a massive impact for good or ill***".

Acknowledgements Many thanks to Mrs Suzanne Mckillop, Breast Screening Mammographer, Linda McCartney Centre, Royal Liverpool and Broad Green University Hospital Foundation Trust for offering her skills and experience in mammography.

References

1. Cherry K. Theories of Emotion. http://www.psychology.about.com. No date. Accessed 09 May 14.
2. Davey G, editor. Encyclopaedic dictionary of psychology. London: Hodder-Arnold; 2005. p. 306.
3. Mayer JD, Salovey P. What is emotional intelligence? In: Salovey P, Slyter D, editors. Emotional development and emotional intelligence: implications for educators. New York: Basic Books; 1997. p. 3–31.
4. Petrides KV, Pita R, Kokkinaki F. The location of trait emotional intelligence in personality factor space. Br J Psychol. 2007;98:273–89.
5. Petrides KV. Technical manual for the trait emotional intelligence questionnaires (TEIQue) (1st ed 4th Printing). London: London Psychometric Laboratory; 2009.
6. Goleman D, Boyatzis RE, McKee A. Primal leadership: realizing the power of emotional intelligence. Boston: Harvard Business School Press; 2002.
7. Arora S, Ashrafian H, Davis R, Athanasiou T, Darzi A, Sevdalis N. Emotional intelligence in medicine: a systematic review through the context of the ACGME competencies. Med Educ. 2010;44(8):749–64.
8. Bulmer Smith K, Profetto-McGrath J, Cummings G. Emotional intelligence and nursing: an integrative literature review. Int J Nurs Stud. 2009;46: 1624–36.
9. Rankin B. Emotional intelligence: enhancing values-based practice and compassionate care in nursing. J Adv Nurs. 2013;69(12):2717–25.
10. Bailey C, Murphy R, Porock D. Professional tears: developing emotional intelligence around death and dying in emergency work. J Clin Nurs. 2011;20: 3364–72.
11. Lewis E. Emotional intelligence as a predictor for clinical performance in professional physical therapy students. Internet J Allied Health Sci Pract. 2010; 8(4).
12. Larin HM, Benson G, Martin L, Wessel J, Williams R, Ploeg J. Examining change in emotional-social intelligence: caring, and leadership in health professions students. J Allied Health. 2011;40(2):96–102 (7).
13. Mackay SJ, Hogg P, Cooke G, Baker RD, Dawkes T. A UK-wide analysis of trait emotional intelligence within the radiography profession. Int J Radiogr. 2012;18(3):166–71.
14. Mackay SJ, Baker R, Collier D, Lewis S. A comparative analysis of emotional intelligence in the UK and Australian radiographer workforce. Int J Radiogr. 2013;19(2):151–5.

15. Mackay S, Reason J, Fawcett T, Mercer C. Are radiographers emotionally intelligent? Synergy. 2010;9:24–26, ISSN 1360-5518, http://synergy.sor.org/may2010/research.
16. Mackay SJ, Pearson J, Hogg P, Fawcett T, Mercer C. Does emotional intelligence make for good leaders? Synergy. 2010;22–24.
17. Faguy K. EI in health care. Radiol Technol. 2012; 83(3).
18. Rimmer RB, Bedwell SE, Bay R, Drachman D, Tory A, Foster KN, Caruso DM. Emotional intelligence in the burn centre and surgical intensive care unit-A possible solution for improving employee satisfaction and reducing turnover and burnout. Eur Burn Assoc Congr. 2009;Supp 1:S29–30.
19. Age Extension Project Group. Guide to implementing the breast screening age extension; NHSBSP good practice guide. Sheffield: NHS Cancer Screening Programmes; 2010.
20. Nelis D, Quoidbach J, Mikolajczak M, Hansenne M. Increasing emotional intelligence: (how) is it possible? Personal Individ Differ. 2009;47:36–41.
21. Nelis D, Kotsou I, Quoidbach J, Hansenne M, Weytens F, Dupuis P, Mikolajczak M. Increasing emotional competence improves psychological and physical well-being, social relationships, and employability. Emotion. 2011;11(2):354–66.
22. Dudiak H, Pope D, Qualter P, Gardner K. Emotional intelligence within personal development planning: teaching EI in universities. Higher education academy website. http://www.heacademy.ac.uk/resources/detail/subjects/psychology/Emotional_Intelligence_within_Personal_Development_Planning_Teaching_EI_in_Universities&utm_source=All_Academy&utm_medium=email&utm_campaign=STEM-psychology-june-2012&utm_content=content3?dm_i=12ZA,UYF0,5DN4DO,2JREG,1. Accessed 4 April 2014.
23. University of California, Berkeley, The Greater Good Body Language Quiz. http://greatergood.berkeley.edu/ei_quiz/. No date. Accessed 4 April 2014.
24. Ekman P, Friesen WV. Constants across cultures in the face and emotion. J Pers Soc Psychol. 1971;17:124–9.
25. Davis MH. The effects of dispositional empathy on emotional reactions and helping: a multidimensional approach. J Pers. 1983;51:167–84.
26. Brett J, Austoker J. Women who are recalled for further investigation for breast screening: psychological consequences 3 years after recall and factors affecting re-attendance. J Public Health. 2001;23(4):292–300.

Client-Practitioner Interactions within Breast Care Services

12

Julie M. Nightingale, Fred J. Murphy, and Rita M. Borgen

Introduction

United Kingdom (UK) breast care services are delivered within one of two models. Clients presenting with breast symptoms (*symptomatic*) are assessed within a 'one stop' (all done at one hospital attendance) out-patient setting whilst asymptomatic clients currently aged 50–70 (*screening*) are invited for 3 yearly breast screening by the National Health Service Breast Screening Programme (NHSBSP). A proportion of the latter are recalled for further assessment should a mammographic abnormality be suspected (*assessment clients*). Many other health care systems around the world also offer these three breast care approaches (symptomatic, screening and assessment services), though the timeframe between screening invitations and the age range of clients varies within the screening services (see Chap. 8).

These services are delivered by a multidisciplinary group of health professionals supported by other vital staff such as receptionists and support workers, and all require good communication skills. It is likely that the communication skills employed by staff within a breast service are well practised, yet it is important to remember that for an individual client each interaction is a unique experience which should leave them with a sense of value and recognition of their individuality.

The importance of the health care professional to recognise and acknowledge individual client needs in order to provide a satisfactory client experience has been highlighted in NHSBSP guidelines [1]. Within the UK screening environment the health care professional is likely to be a qualified radiographer with post-graduate mammography education and training (practitioner) or a mammography assistant practitioner. However clients attending either symptomatic or assessment clinics will meet a range of different health professionals within a single clinic attendance including mammography practitioners, breast care nurses, clinicians (radiologists or breast surgeons), health care assistants and receptionists. It is important that all of these staff groups are able to communicate effectively and compassionately, and in the UK the completion of advanced communication skills training is a requirement for those core members of the team who have direct contact with [suspected] cancer patients [2]. However concerns have been raised in several annual UK peer review exercises regarding poor compliance with this national requirement [3, 4], so it is important not to be

J.M. Nightingale (✉) • F.J. Murphy
School of Health Sciences, University of Salford, Frederick Road, Salford M6 6PU, UK
e-mail: j.nightingale@salford.ac.uk; f.j.murphy@salford.ac.uk

R.M. Borgen
Breast Screening Service, East Lancashire Hospitals NHS Trust, Casterton Avenue, Burnley BB10 2PQ, UK
e-mail: Rita.borgen@elht.nhs.uk

P. Hogg et al. (eds.), *Digital Mammography: A Holistic Approach*,
DOI 10.1007/978-3-319-04831-4_12, © Springer International Publishing Switzerland 2015

complacent. This chapter will now explore the nature and challenges of practitioner-client interactions within the routine screening setting and the assessment/symptomatic clinic.

The Breast Screening Experience

Research has shown that clients who participate in breast screening are generally positive about their experience [5]. Clark and Reeves identified in a recent literature review that women experienced diagnostic breast procedures in unique and diverse ways, and they identified five commonly reported themes that influenced the experience: fear, pain and discomfort, waiting, the physical environment and staff interactions [5]. In particular they argued that poor communication or interaction by the radiographer can have a negative influence on patient experience, a finding also supported by Davey [6]. It is important that the nature of any negative experiences are understood, including the impact they may have on the client and their wider social network (see also Chap. 7). A poor experience may be communicated to friends and family, heightening anxiety in those who may subsequently be invited for screening. Indeed Sharp et al. found that clients were influenced by accounts from others, often spread via social media (see also Chap. 11) [7]. Some may have been embellished, but they were nevertheless very 'real' to them at the time, possibly causing increased anxiety.

The client experience is likely to be influenced by the beliefs and values of the practitioner performing the examination [8], who is engaged in a complex decision making process that involves a range of human and technological facets (see Fig. 12.1) [9]. Screening mammograms are performed within a very tight time allocation, (typically six minutes), potentially influencing the client-practitioner interaction to be focussed to addressing technical considerations above care and compassion.

Clients may experience a range of emotions during the procedure and some degree of discomfort related to the application of compression force. Although the number of women

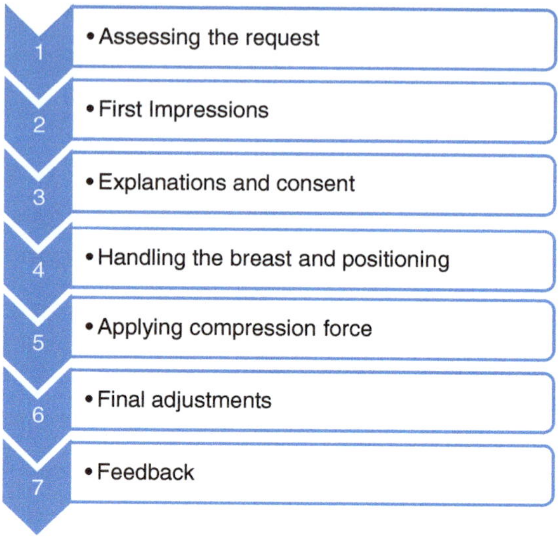

Fig. 12.1 Complex decision making and problem solving in mammography – the seven stages of the mammography examination (Taken from Nightingale et al. [8] reprinted with permission from Elsevier)

experiencing pain has been reported to be as low as 6 % [10], moderate pain may be experienced in up to 50 % of women [11]. While Poulos identified that discomfort rather than pain is a more appropriate descriptor of the mammography experience [12], one recent qualitative study noted that almost without exception mammography was described by women as painful [13]. Dibble et al. estimate that up to 8 % of women consider delaying or missing screening appointments due to the pain experienced at previous examinations [14].

Most interventions to reduce mammography pain or discomfort (e.g. pre-examination pain relief) have not been successful, however the provision of written and verbal information were identified within a systematic review to be the most helpful intervention in counteracting the 'experienced' discomfort. [15] However negative experiences are also associated with factors other than pain, such as a perceived lack of information, especially about benign breast conditions, and the demeanour and attitude of the practitioner [16].

Socio-demographic variables such as age, family history and breast size do not seem to be consistently associated with the amount of pain experienced during a mammogram [6].

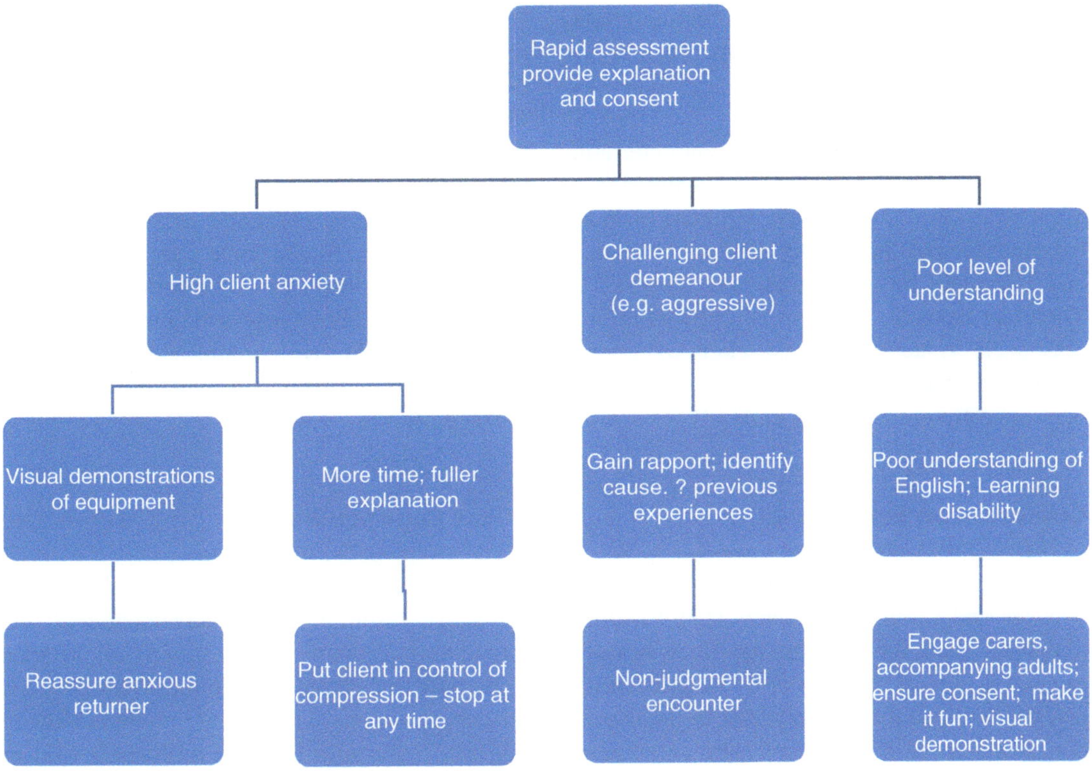

Fig. 12.2 Psychological approaches – rapid decision making upon first meeting the client (Adapted from Nightingale et al. [8] reprinted with permission from Elsevier)

Conversely, nervousness and anxiety have been found to be associated with painful mammograms [6], suggesting that there is an emotional component to the experience and/or tolerance of pain. This link offers practitioners a brief window of opportunity to potentially influence the degree of perceived discomfort, by initiating strategies to reduce nervousness and anxiety. For further information about pain see Chap. 14.

Practitioner Strategies

Nightingale et al. identified rapid practitioner decision-making on first meeting the client that enabled a range of anxiety-reducing strategies to be implemented (Fig. 12.2) [9]. Practitioners employ various strategies to produce quality diagnostic images whilst demonstrating empathy and professionalism. These include facilitating a degree of client empowerment by encouraging the clients to comment on the level of compression force themselves, or at least advising when the level is uncomfortable [8, 9].

Clarke and Iphofen offered an individual patient perspective which identified that being encouraged to say 'stop' during a procedure was very empowering [17], and indeed Bruyninckx et al. also stressed that this very act of speaking out could reduce perceived pain levels [18]. However some clients may insist on stopping the application of compression force when it is insufficient for acceptable image quality, thus giving the practitioner a dilemma. How the practitioner addresses this dilemma will have implications for either image quality, client experience, or both, and these difficult practitioner-client interactions are found to be influenced to some extent by the values and behaviours of the individual practitioner, and indeed the culture of the wider screening unit. Murphy et al. identified within some mammography screening units what they described as 'tribal' cultural influences upon mammography practitioners where [compression] practice was not necessarily supported by an evidence base but more associated with local social factors [8]. They recognised that the mammography practitioner-client interaction was a paradox of humanistic caring against the demands of imaging technologies, presenting difficult challenges and decisions for individual practitioners [8]. Therefore from the study of Murphy et al. it is reasonable to suggest that the client experience may differ from one practitioner to another, and between different screening units [8].

Compression Techniques

The application of compression force varies between and within practitioners [19]. Since the numerical scale for compression force is rarely referred to in some units but used as a guide in others, the look and feel of the breast tissue is often considered to be a better indicator of optimum compression force [8, 9]. Practitioners included in Murphy et al.'s study refer to subjective indicators such as gradual 'blanching' of the skin [8], but they also respond to verbal and non-verbal feedback from the client. Where clients appear to be struggling with the compression force, some practitioners use the 'fine tuning' of the hand compression, when available, (rather than relying solely on the foot pedal application) in order to apply force in a more controlled way [8].

Client Anxieties

Although the application of compression force appears to provoke anxiety in lots of women, several studies have identified other causes of anxieties as being very significant in the overall client experience. This includes issues associated with privacy, dignity, the process itself and understandably the implications of finding breast cancer [5, 6]. Murphy et al. found that practitioners identified overt differences in behaviour and anxiety levels between clients attending screening for the first time (*prevalent screen*) and those attending for follow up screening (*incident screen*), and this prompted different practitioner responses [8]. First attenders were often extremely anxious and a more detailed explanation was required, often including a demonstration of the equipment. Repeat attenders were often influenced by a prior 'poor' experience, requiring a degree of gentle persuasion by the practitioners [8, 9]. In some cases 'white lies' (harmless mistruths told in the belief it will benefit the client) about new and improved equipment were told to reassure clients that the discomfort they previously experienced will be reduced [8].

Client Engagement

Various client groups may have additional concerns that result in poor engagement with the screening programme. Such groups might arise from different ethnic and cultural backgrounds [20], those who have problems communicating in English, those with learning difficulties [21] or those with lack of mobility [22]. Engagement with such groups can be challenging [23], and interpersonal relationships between these clients and their social networks (family and close friends) influences breast screening behaviour [24, 25]. A need exists here for working closely with local group leaders and individual carers; there is likely to be a requirement to provide clear client information leaflets (including language translations and visual guides for learning disability), but there is no substitute on these occasions for an open and friendly approach to welcoming the client into the screening unit. However for some of these 'hard to reach' client groups, there may be a growing role for positive local, regional and national social media to encourage attendance for breast screening. Further information about social media can be found in Chap. 11.

The Breast Clinic Experience

Following breast screening a client may be recalled for a repeat mammography examination (*technical recall*) because the images are deemed to be non-diagnostic. UK practitioners should record no more than 3 % technical recalls with a target of 2 % [1]. Technical recalls use additional resources, result in additional radiation dose, and are inconvenient for the client, increasing their anxiety about the potential diagnosis.

Some clients, however, are referred to a breast clinic for additional investigations because an abnormality is suspected, and these include both symptomatic clients and screening assessment clients. There is inevitably a high degree of anxiety about potential findings for both client groups. Symptomatic clients will have identified a physical sign of breast disease (e.g. breast lump, nipple discharge) which their doctor considers requires urgent referral. While this will clearly be worrying for the symptomatic client, breast screening clients subsequently recalled to a breast assessment clinic are likely to experience an additional feeling of 'shock' (see also Chap. 7) [26]. Assessment clinic appointment letters which arrive unexpectedly have been criticised by low income ethnic minority women in one American study as being difficult to understand [27]. In the UK, there may be a delay of several days between informing the client of the need for their breast clinic appointment and the date of the actual appointment. In other countries the delay can be longer. These few days of delay may be filled with worry for the client, their friends and relatives; while some studies report that support from significant others is comforting, it does not diminish the women's anxiety [28]. The quality of the invitation letter and information leaflet are very significant in this pre-attendance period; personal contact by telephone from a health professional has also been found to be very beneficial in this early 'waiting' stage [28].

It is understandable that clients referred to a breast clinic will have anxiety related to the potential diagnosis of breast cancer. As this is the most common female cancer in Western civilisations, with a 1 in 8 lifetime risk of women developing the disease [29], it is highly likely that many women will have been in some way 'affected' by the disease, either through friends or relatives with the condition. Clients with a strong family history of the disease across several generations may experience heightened anxiety that is disproportionate to the actual risk factors [30] because they may be unaware of significant improvements in early diagnosis, treatment options and survival in recent years. Severe worry has been identified as a barrier to mammography use in higher risk women, but this is also found in normal risk populations [31]. There is once again a vital role for accurate verbal and written communication of appropriate information with clients. Nevertheless the degree of anxiety experienced by clients could be extremely high on entering the clinic, since they have had several days to consider the potential outcomes.

Client Interventions

Clients attending a screening assessment or symptomatic clinic are likely to have a combination of additional tests in a single visit, including: clinical consultations and breast assessment; standard mammography, additional mammographic projections, ultrasound scan; interventional procedures such as aspirations and biopsies. While the 'one-stop' visit may be resource efficient and give a more rapid diagnosis, inevitably the clients may feel they are on a diagnostic 'conveyor-belt', being passed from one room to another with little continuity. Similarly there is potential for the client to receive information very quickly which may not give them sufficient time to process and come to terms with the diagnosis, although in a survey by Hodgson et al. (n=46) all participants either agreed or strongly agreed that they had received sufficient information and enough time for discussion within their breast assessment clinic visit [32].

The assessment client journey could involve several individual staff-client interactions with a range of health care professions. While individual staff-client encounters are expected to be highly professional and empathetic, there is the potential for information overload and in some cases insufficient information being provided to the client. While staff are likely to make significant efforts to gauge the understanding and information needs of their clients, O'Connell et al. identified that many of the medical terms used in consultation with breast surgeons was not understood and this adversely affected the patient experience [33]. For this reason, the appointment of a named individual to act as a guide to escort the client through the clinic experience, where resources allowed, may be beneficial. Alternatively having the same person to 'open' the patient journey (initial greetings and explanations of the procedure) and to 'close' the journey at the end (summary of findings and next step), preferably in a pleasant and private environment, would facilitate personalised care.

Interventional Procedures

Clients where suspicion of cancer is high may require a biopsy, and these procedures may be associated with discomfort or even pain, although in one study the discomfort was categorised as only 'minimal' [34]. In most cases the biopsy results may take several days to be processed, requiring the client to return several days later. This additional wait can add to the client's anxiety, although in many centres the client will be placed under the care of a breast care nurse who will 'escort' them through the process and be a point of contact within the intervening period. They may also be their point of contact throughout their treatment should this be required.

Difficult Client Conversations

Difficult conversations with clients such as communicating bad news, is a necessary task within a breast clinic. The most senior staff will often be expected to engage in these conversations, which may leave a lasting impression on the client and any accompanying relatives. Sasson et al. found that radiology staff experienced stress explaining results to patients and responding to their emotions [35]. While educational courses exist to better prepare staff to engage in these difficult conversations, peer support and de-briefing is likely to be required to ensure the continuing well-being of the staff working regularly in this challenging environment.

Most clients attending a screening assessment clinic and a symptomatic clinic will be given a normal diagnosis and discharged. The screening clients will be invited to attend at the next routine screening interval.

Improving Re-attendance

While attendance at a screening assessment clinic is not the only factor to influence a clients' decision to participate in subsequent screening, the assessment clinic experience is intensely stressful, with increases in anxiety, worry and intrusive thoughts occurring in the short and medium term [36] One study also identified negative effects 6 months after the false positive result, but noted surprisingly that these were experienced at a similar level to women who had received a diagnosis of cancer [37]. Even after 3 years these women still reported greater negative psychosocial consequences compared to women with normal screening findings [37]. This 3 year timeframe coincides with an invitation for the next UK routine screen – just receiving such an invitation has been shown to increase negative thoughts [26].

Screening units should be proactive in encouraging re-attendance for false positive clients as well as those from client groups which are often under-represented in screening, using a variety of methods such as reminder letters and follow up phone calls [38]. However the most important predictor for encouraging re-attendance for breast screening is a good client experience, which, albeit constrained by time and resources, is within the gift of the practitioners working within the screening service.

References

1. NHS Breast Screening Programme. Quality assurance guidelines for mammography: Including radiographic quality control. April 2006. ISBN 1 84463 028 5. http://www.cancerscreening.nhs.uk/breastscreen/publications/nhsbsp63.html. Accessed 18 Aug 14.
2. National Cancer Peer Review Programme. Manual for cancer services: breast cancer measures version 1.1. 2014. http://www.cquins.nhs.uk/. Accessed 27 Aug 2014.

3. National Cancer Peer Review Programme. Report 2009/2010: Breast MDTs. http://www.cquins.nhs.uk/download.php?d=/resources/reports/NCAT_NCPR_Breast_Report_2010-11.pdf.
4. National Cancer Peer Review Programme. Report 2012/2013: Breast MDTs. http://www.cquins.nhs.uk/documents/resources/reports/2013/Breast%20NCPR%20Report%20September%202013.pdf.
5. Clark S, Reeves PJ. Women's experiences of the breast cancer diagnostic process: A thematic evaluation of the literature; Recall & biopsy. Radiography. 2015;21(1):89–92.
6. Davey B. Pain during mammography: possible risk factors and ways to alleviate pain. Radiography. 2007;13(3):229–34.
7. Sharp PC, Michielutte R, Freimanis R, Cunningham L, Spangler J, Burnette V. Reported pain following mammography screening. Arch Intern Med. 2003;163(7):833–6.
8. Murphy F, Nightingale J, Robinson L, Mackay S, Seddon D, Hogg P. Compression force behaviours: an exploration of the beliefs and values influencing the application of breast compression during screening mammography. Radiography. 2014. Accepted and in press. http://dx.doi.org/10.1016/j.radi.2014.05.009.
9. Nightingale J, Murphy F, Newton-Hughes A, Robinson L, Hogg P. Breast compression – an exploration of problem solving and decision making in mammography. Radiography. 2014. Ahead of print.
10. Poulos A, McLean D, Rickard M, Heard R. Breast compression in mammography; how much is enough? J Med Imaging Radiat Oncol. 2003;47(2):121–6.
11. Bai JY, He ZY, Dong JN, Yao GH, Chen HX, Li KA. Correlation of pain experience during mammography with factors of breast density and breast compressed thickness. J Shanghai Jiaotong Univ (Med Sci). 2010;30(9):1062–6.
12. Poulos A. Having a mammogram: how does it feel? The Radiogr. 2004;51:129–31.
13. Mathers SA, McKenzie GA, Robertson EM. 'It was daunting': experience of women with a diagnosis of breast cancer attending for breast imaging. Radiography. 2013;19(2):156–63.
14. Dibble SL, Israel J, Nussey B, Sayre JW, Brenner RJ, Sickles EA. Mammography with breast cushions. Womens Health Issues. 2005;15(2):55–63.
15. Miller D, Livingstone V, Herbison PG. Interventions for relieving the pain and discomfort of screening mammography. Database of Abstracts of Reviews and Effects (DARE). http://www.mrw.interscience.wiley.com/cochrane/clsysrev/articles/CD002942/frame.html. Accessed 26 July 2013.
16. Robinson L, Hogg P, Newton-Hughes A. The power and the pain: mammographic compression research from the service-users' perspective. Radiography. 2013;19:190–5.
17. Clarke KA, Iphofen R. Breast cancer: a personal reflective account. Synergy. 2006:12–16.
18. Bruyninckx E, Mortelmans D, Van Goethem M, Van Hove E. Risk factors of pain in mammographic screening. Soc Sci Med. 1999;49(7):933–41.
19. Mercer CE, Hogg P, Szczepura K, Denton ERE. Practitioner compression force variation in mammography: a 6-year study. Radiography. 2013;19(3):200–6.
20. Jafri NF, Ayyala RS, Ozonoff A, Jordan-Gray J, Slanetz PJ. Screening mammography: does ethnicity influence patient preferences for higher recall rates given the potential for earlier detection of breast cancer? Radiology. 2008;249(3):785–91.
21. Wilkinson JE, Deis CE, Bowen DJ, Bokhour BG. 'It's easier said than done': perspectives on mammography from women with intellectual disabilities. Ann Fam Med. 2011;9(2):142–7.
22. Liu SY, Clark MA. Breast and cervical cancer screening practices among disabled women aged 40–75: does quality of the experience matter? J Womens Health. 2008;17(8):1321–9.
23. Watson-Johnson LC, DeGroff A, Steele CB, Revels M, Smith JL, Justen E, Barron-Simpson R, Sanders L, Richardson LC. Mammography adherence: a qualitative study. J Womens Health. 2011;20(12):1887–94.
24. Kaltsa A, Holloway A, Cox K. Factors that influence mammography screening behaviour: a qualitative study of Greek women's experiences. Eur J Oncol Nurs. 2013;17(3):292–301.
25. Browne JL, Chan AYC. Using the theory of planned behaviour and implementation intentions to predict and facilitate upward family communication about mammography. Psychol Health. 2012;27(6):655–73.
26. Brett J, Bankhead C, Henderson B, Watson E, Austoker J. The psychological impact of mammographic screening. A systematic review. Psychooncology. 2005;14(11):917–38.
27. Marcus EN, Drummond D, Dietz N. Urban women's preferences for learning of their mammogram result: a qualitative study. J Cancer Educ. 2012;27(1):156–64.
28. Pineault P. Breast cancer screening: women's experiences of waiting for further testing. Oncol Nurs Forum. 2007;34(4):847–53.
29. Cancer Research UK. Cancer Statistics. http://info.cancerresearchuk.org/cancerstats/types/breast/. Accessed 02 Oct 2013.
30. Sauven P. Guidelines for the management of women at increased familial risk of breast cancer. Eur J Cancer. 2004;40(5):653–65.
31. Andersen MR, Smith R, Meischke H, Bowen D, Urban N. Breast cancer worry and mammography use by women with and without a family history in a population-based sample. Cancer Epidemiol Biomarkers Prev. 2003;12:314–20.
32. Hodgson L, Dixon A, Turley L. Vote of confidence. Imaging and Therapy Practice. 5–10 July 2013.
33. O'Connell RL, Hartridge-Lambert SK, Din N, St John ER, Hitchins C, Johnson T. Patients' understanding of medical terminology used in the breast clinic. Breast. 2013;22(5):836–8.

34. Brandon CJ, Mullan PB. Patients' perception of care during image-guided breast biopsy in a rural community breast center: communication matters. J Cancer Educ. 2011;26(1):156–60.
35. Sasson JP, Zand T, Lown BA. Communication in the diagnostic mammography suite: Implications for practice and training. Acad Radiol. 2008;15(4):417–24.
36. Rimer BK, Bluman LG. The psychosocial consequences of mammography. J Natl Cancer Inst Monogr. 1997;22:131–8.
37. Brodersen J, Siersma VD. Long-term psychosocial consequences of false-positive screening mammography. Ann Fam Med. 2013;11(2):106–15.
38. Costanza ME, Luckmann R, White MJ, Rosal MC, Cranos C, Reed G, Clark R, Sama S, Yood R. Design and methods for a randomized clinical trial comparing three outreach efforts to improve screening mammography adherence. BMC Health Serv Res. 2011; 11(145):1472–6963. Abstract only.

The Use of Digital Health Technology and Social Media to Support Breast Screening

13

Leslie Robinson, Marie Griffiths, Julie Wray, Cathy Ure, Julie R. Stein-Hodgins, and Geraldine Shires

Concept of Digital Health and Social Media for Promoting Health

'Digital health' is an overarching concept that currently lacks theoretical definition and common terminology. For instance, this broad and emerging field includes all of the following terms within its lexicon: mHealth, Wireless Health, Health 2.0, eHealth, e-Patient(s), Healthcare IT/Health IT, Big Data, Health Data, Cloud Computing, Quantified Self, Wearable Computing, Gamification, and Telehealth/Telemedicine [1]. However, whilst a definition is difficult to provide, in this overview it is considered that digital health is the use of digital media to transform the way healthcare provision is conceived and delivered. We consider it does this through three basic features.

Firstly, digital health provides individuals with easily accessible *information* in a range of formats to empower them to track, manage and improve their own and their family's health. Secondly, digital health refers to the technological developments that underpin its ability to provide *support at a personal level* including, the internet, social media, wireless devices and mobile networks as well as software sensing technologies and hardware sensors. Thirdly, digital health provision seeks to *improve access* to healthcare whilst improving the quality of service, reduce costs and deliver an increasingly personalised service.

The interest in digital health was driven by the proliferation of mobile devices, such as mobile phones and tablets, which in tandem with easily accessible mobile networks (mobile broadband and wi-fi) means the digital-enabled public has access to healthcare information at any time and almost anywhere. Significantly, in the United Kingdom (UK), over half of adults access the internet via their mobile phone, increasing to

L. Robinson (✉)
Department of Radiography, University of Salford, Frederick Road, Salford M6 6PU, UK
e-mail: l.robinson@salford.ac.uk

M. Griffiths
Salford Business School, University of Salford, The Crescent, Salford M5 4WT, UK
e-mail: m.griffiths@salford.ac.uk

J. Wray
School of Nursing, Midwifery, Social Work and Social Science, University of Salford, Mary Seacole Building, Frederick Road, Salford M6 6PU, UK
e-mail: j.wray@salford.ac.uk

C. Ure
Department of Media Psychology, University of Salford, Salford, UK
e-mail: c.m.ure@edu.salford.ac.uk

J.R. Stein-Hodgins
Breast Unit, Bolton Trust, Minerva Road, Bolton BL4 0JR, UK
e-mail: julieroxanne@gmail.com

G. Shires
Nightingale Centre, University Hospital of South Manchester (Wythenshawe Hospital), Southmoor Road, Manchester M23 9LT, UK
e-mail: geraldine.shires@uhsm.nhs.uk

P. Hogg et al. (eds.), *Digital Mammography: A Holistic Approach*,
DOI 10.1007/978-3-319-04831-4_13, © Springer International Publishing Switzerland 2015

86 % for smart phone users. Furthermore, 2 out of every 3 mobile devices is now driving a third of UK internet traffic. Importantly, it is not only younger people who make up these statistics. ComScore [2] reported that 55+ year old internet users are now accounting for 20.4 % of the online population.

But users are not just accessing information via the internet, they are increasingly turning to Mobile Applications or 'apps'. In 2012, more people used apps and browsed the web on their mobile devices [3]. In 2013, Apple reported there had been 50 billion app downloads and that customers were downloading around 800 apps every second amounting to around 2 billion apps per month. Consequently, apps are emerging as high demand sources of health information and patient self-management tools and there are approximately 1,000 new releases of health related apps every month with many existing health-related apps being updated. In order to introduce quality into this burgeoning market the US Food and Drug Administration (FDA) have introduced regulation for some types of medical apps and this is also being adopted by the UK National Health Service (NHS) [4].

The role *social media* can play in influencing individual health outcomes remains underexplored. Social media refers to a group of internet-based applications built on the ideological and technological foundations of Web 2.0, that allow the creation and exchange of user-generated content [5]. It is an umbrella term for a range of user-generated platforms including blogs and micro-blogs (Wordpress, Google Blog, Twitter); social networking sites (Facebook, Pinterest, LinkedIn); collaborative projects (Wikipedia); content communities (You Tube, Pinterest, Instagram); virtual social worlds (Second Life) and virtual gaming worlds (World of Warcraft). Utilising a range of these applications, patients can generate and use content related to health education, information, networking, research, support, goal setting and tracking personal progress [6]. It is estimated that in the UK 64 % of users use at least one social networking site [7]. Theoretically at least, extending patient participation beyond the physical space of the doctor's surgery and healthcare unit seems achievable if clinicians, academics and the general public can harness social media effectively. However whilst it would seem social media has the potential to be an effective addition to the armoury of digital patient support, currently health providers' use of social media to enhance patient services remains relatively limited [8].

The Use of Digital Social Media in Breast Screening and Symptomatic Contexts

This section relates the concept of digital health to breast imaging. For clarity, we refer to asymptomatic service-users, such as those of the breast screening service as clients. Symptomatic service-users are referred to as women. In the UK there is sparse evidence that digital health has been employed to its full potential within medical imaging and more specifically the asymptomatic breast imaging service. At the time of press, digital patient information, via the NHS Breast Screening Programme (NHSBSP) website, is still driven by web 1.0 technology. This provides useful information for helping women make decisions but does not enable user-generated content to be created. Women are therefore unable to engage with others via user forums or networks resulting in lack of support and a paternalistic approach to what information they can access. This is contrary to the empowerment agenda and ideology which underpins digital health. Outside the UK, and in particular in the United States of America (USA), web 2.0 technology has been used more widely to promote breast screening mammography. Pinky Swear is a Facebook site that was designed to remind women aged over 40 to attend scheduled mammography and has evolved as "a promise between friends to commit to annual mammogram screenings and promote breast cancer awareness". The fact that this was created and promoted by a private medical centre, may suggest women in the USA benefit from improved digital information because of their health service's imperative to attract business, an imperative which does not exist in the UK. Cancer charities are also prolific sources of digital health information and support through digital health approaches. For instance, in the UK, Breakthrough (etc) Breast Cancer has released a breast awareness app which promotes and advises on self-examination.

Access to digital information and support for symptomatic women in the UK is slightly better than that for asymptomatic women. However, again this is mainly as a result of externally provided resources (i.e. external to the imaging department). For example, a number of charity-run, digital health resources exist which are dedicated to patients with breast cancer, including approximately ten Facebook sites such as Breast Cancer Campaign and Breast Cancer Awareness. Many women share information in tweets about breast cancer on Twitter, and Breast Cancer Care has a strong Twitter presence.

A number of breast imaging centres have exploited digital health's potential for improving service access by trialling text messaging services for appointments and reminders, but the outcomes have yet to be published.

Currently there is still a long way to go in terms of imaging professionals becoming fully expert in ways of exploiting digital health for improving women's experiences within the breast screening service.

How Mammography Practitioners Can Enhance Their Communication with Patients Using Digital Technologies

The NHSBSP has national targets and one of the key performance indicators (KPIs) is to increase numbers of women attending for first and subsequent appointments. The innovative use of digital health technology by the BSP could enhance the woman's experience and therefore positively influence these KPIs. The following suggestions take the reader through the woman's NHSBSP journey, identifying potential points throughout this journey where the three benefits of digital health (information, personal support and improved access) might be realised.

Pre-examination

First, it is imperative that mammography practitioners identify their role in health promotion and should take an active involvement in breast cancer awareness campaigns. In this way, a digital social network (DSN) could be used to promote the value of attending breast screening mammography. Currently, the first contact with the woman is via the invitation letter. Information about digital resources such as a DSN could be included in the letter along with links to the client's breast screening unit's website. Information provided at this initial contact point means all women, attenders and non-attenders, would be made aware of the DSN and other sources of support.

Many women will have a similar set of Frequently Asked Questions (FAQs). The NHSBSP has a list of FAQs and the DSN could direct women to this. However, where a woman needs to speak to a mammography practitioner, for instance where their question has not been answered through the FAQs, digital technology provides more options and flexibility for communication. Presently, a woman has to find time during the day to telephone the breast screening unit and the mammography practitioner has to be available at that precise time to respond. With web 2.0 technology communication can be managed asynchronously and is therefore more efficient; texts and emails would be answered at the mammography practitioner's convenience without delaying the woman on the phone. Furthermore, discussion boards and forums could be used to respond through a wider audience thus dealing with the anxieties of several women simultaneously.

Appointment

Digital health technology could be used to enable women to manage their own appointments through access to an on-line booking and re-scheduling system. This is not only convenient for the woman but would also reduce calls to the unit office freeing up staff time to support those in attendance or to respond to emails, texts and forum queries. Smart phone technology might be used to support the service through SMS appointment reminders again linking to useful sources of support.

During the Examination

The environment has been criticised by women as being clinical and unwelcoming [9]. Digital screens displaying relaxing imagery in the waiting room and x-ray room may be effectively employed to address such criticisms. These have been found to have a positive impact on patient pain thresholds and to reduce anxiety in breast imaging contexts [10]. Others are using DVDs to help patients, whose first language is not English, to prepare for their examinations [11].

Post Examination

Post examination texts which provide details of results, follow-up assessment appointments and general breast awareness information could be sent. These functions would be automated and linked to the booking and patient records system. In this way when a woman's examination has been reported the relevant automated message would be sent.

Professional Social Networking

Breast imaging professionals would benefit from being digitally connected across a dedicated social and professional network. Such networks promote the sharing of best practice, learning, research and innovation, enabling practitioners to ensure the service they deliver is current and evidence-based.

Development of a Digital Social Network

Section three advocated a Digital Support Network (DSN) for women attending for breast screening. The following expands on this idea, providing a rationale and possible approach and then considers the complexities such an initiative might entail.

Whilst crucial for improving health outcomes, we know that mammography is associated with high levels of anxiety related to expectations of pain, positive diagnoses (i.e. that a cancer could be discovered) and the use of ionising radiation. Anxiety related to such fears can result in non-attendance [12]. Furthermore, research suggests that women who do attend can experience more discomfort if they are in heightened states of anxiety [9] which may lead to non-attendance at subsequent screening invitations.

Women attending for breast screening for the first time have said they are poorly informed about what to expect, that the NHSBSP patient leaflets are not memorable and that they preferred listening to the experiences of their friends and relatives instead. This is unsurprising given the earlier discussion within this chapter. Other studies supported this finding that women share stories about health via word-of-mouth spread through a range of social networks [13–15].

As discussed, the internet and web 2.0 technology has given rise to *digital* social networks. In 2012, Brenner [16] revealed that 73 % of women between 30 and 49 years of age used DSNs, reflecting the up-coming population of first-time attenders for breast screening.

A DSN dedicated to the asymptomatic breast screening population would therefore tap into women's preferences both for word-of-mouth approaches to gathering information about mammography and for on-line social networking. Such an initiative would also reflect NHS policy to improve patient access to on-line user-generated information, articulated in the UK government's 2010 NHS White Paper [17].

The creation of an effective DSN which is inclusive to the needs of all women would require their involvement at all stages; from inception and feasibility of the idea, design and testing of the prototype and evaluation of the final product. This is because the NHS breast screening population is not confined to one sector of society but includes women from the full gamut of communities that constitute multicultural Britain today. Furthermore, research has shown that what motivates women to attend or refuse breast screening may be differentiated on the grounds of ethnicity, education and socio-economic group [18–21]. For this reason, the content of a DSN would need to take into consideration the concerns of all such groups.

Not only content but also format and access would need to be inclusive. Ofcom data for 2013 [7] showed a difference between socio-economic groups (SEGs) in terms of access to the internet at home. Whilst 84 % of all those aged between 45 and 54 have access to the internet, this dropped to 62 % of those from the lower SEGs. However, with increasing proliferation of digital devices across all ages and all socio-economic groups this differentiation is quickly diminishing. Therefore, access to the relevant technology may not be an issue in the future, particularly for the future breast screening generations, as long as the DSN is structured to support access via mobile technology.

However, health behaviours are less easily addressed. According to Ofcom [7], searching the internet for health-related information and support is less likely by those from lower SEGs; only 7 % of C2DE groups declared weekly visits compared to 12 % of SEG ABC1 groups. This reflects research [22] showing that people from lower SEGs are less likely to seek out health-related communication and information at all (i.e. in any format, not just digitally). In designing a DSN which is of relevance to all members of society, there would need to be a better understanding of how the DSN might change health seeking information. Again, this would require user involvement in the design and development process and targeted promotion of the DSN might also be a requirement for some communities, because women who do not actively seek information are not likely to happen upon it by themselves.

Finally, it is essential that the role of the health professional or mammographic practitioner in the DSN is considered. Web 2.0 has not only provided a conduit for patients to network together but it has enabled them to access health professionals. It was suggested in 2007 that 18 % of the European population expected to be able to have consultations with health professionals online in the near future [23] and now many of the major on-line patient forums provide the user with access to discussion forums with a health professional.

The *level* of mammography practitioner involvement in a breast-screening network needs to be carefully considered. A site that is heavily managed will lose authenticity. However, lack of mammography practitioner involvement may result in negative stories being misunderstood and reinforced. An authentic DSN should not be censored to provide only 'happy' experiences. The stories women share should be 'real life' describing the reality of the mammogram. Stories from women who have not had such a good experience should be shared (although moderated to avoid exposing departments or naming staff) and other women encouraged to provide support to the person posting the narrative. It is important for women to know what to expect and maybe what they experienced was not the normal care women attending other places experience. The longitudinal impact of a DSN would be to influence repeat attendance, not provide inaccurate information that attracts women once to the service, who then drop out as their expectation did not match their experience.

These suggestions highlight the potential for digital technology, and in particular social networks to enhance a woman's experience but they are not without challenges. First, it is important to consider how a DSN would change working practices, in particular the way the practitioner communicates with the woman and more specifically their perceptions of social media. There is reticence on the part of imaging practitioners and health professionals more generally to engage in on-line discussion with patients perhaps because current systems of work make it difficult to imagine how such an approach could be integrated into working practice. However, digital technology allows non-synchronous communication which would allow practitioners to talk to women at a time convenient for all. Another possible barrier for staff is the fear of litigation and the potential threat of exposing their professional knowledge for judgement in the public domain. The discourse surrounding professionals using Facebook tends to be negative [24] and the reference to appropriate use of social media in professional codes of conduct also has the potential for establishing a culture of fear around the use of digital communication with clients. However, to ignore on-line comments can be more damaging.

Negative reviews through word-of-mouth are an inevitable feature of today's digital world [25–27]. The advantage of mammography practitioners responding to on-line comments through a dedicated breast screening platform is that they can respond to women with negative stories to tell, as well as reassure other women who may be affected by them. Thus the DSN becomes a rich source for open dialogue between women and mammography practitioners. This can be used to drive service improvements as mammography practitioners will be forced to reflect on how what they do influences the woman's experience. This benefit has recently been acknowledged in the production of a number of NHS 'essential guides' on social media for hospital executives and human resource managers encouraging people with strategic influence to become 'social media literate'. It is hoped that changes in attitude towards social media at the top of the institution will signal a shift in culture throughout the service.

Concern about access to digital health technology is also an issue if we are to ensure equal access to services across all communities. However, as we have seen, the proliferation of smart phones and other devices means access to the internet is increasing and technology inequality reducing [7]. Nevertheless, there is still some differential use of technology based on socio-economic grouping with D and E groups demonstrating lower usage. However, breast screening attendance rates in these communities are particularly low so more work needs to be done to discover the reasons. Digital health technologies are therefore not a panacea to address all causes of non-attendance however they can be used to improve a woman's experience in general and by offering an enhanced experience there is the possibility that it would improve second appointment attendance rates and the positive stories which spread by word-of-mouth; be these digital or otherwise.

References

1. Sonnier P. Story of digital health 2013. http://storyofdigitalhealth.com/definition/. Accessed 25 Feb 2014.
2. Comscore. Comscore releases '2013 UK digital future in focus' report'. 2013. https://www.comscore.com/Insights/Press_Releases/2013/2/comScore_Releases_2013_UK_Digital_Future_in_Focus_Report. Accessed 15 Mar 2014.
3. Handel MJ. mHealth (mobile health) – using Apps for health and wellness. Explore. 2011;7(4):256–61.
4. FDA. Mobile medical applications guidance for industry and Food and Drug Administration staff. 2013. http://www.fda.gov/downloads/MedicalDevices/DeviceRegulationandGuidance/GuidanceDocuments/UCM263366.pdf. Accessed 3 Mar 2014.
5. Kaplan AM, Haenlein M. Users of the world unite! The challenges and opportunities of social media. Bus Horiz. 2010;53:59–68. doi:10.1016/j.bush.2009.09.003.
6. Househ M, Borycki E, Kushniruk A. Empowering patients though social media: the benefits and challenges. Health Inform J. 2014;20(1):50–8. doi:10.1177/1460458213476969.
7. Ofcom. Adults media use and attitudes report. 2012. http://stakeholders.ofcom.org.uk/binaries/research/media-literacy/media-use-attitudes/adults-media-use-2012.pdf. Accessed 15 Mar 2013.
8. Sharma S, Reena K, Leung F-H. Health 2.0 – lessons learned. Social networking with patients for health promotion. J Prim Care Community Health. 2014. doi:10.1177/2150131914522061.
9. Robinson L, Hogg P, Newton-Hughes A. The power and the pain: mammographic compression research from the service-users' perspective. Radiography. 2013; 19(3):190–5.
10. Moving Essence. 2014. www.movingessence.net/ArtisticOverview.pdf.
11. BMA. When poverty and ethnicity combine. 2012. http://bma.org.uk/news-views-analysis/news/2012/february/when-poverty-and-ethnicity-combine. 4 Feb 2012.
12. Dibble SL, Israel J, Nussey B, Sayre JW, Brenner RJ, Sickles EA. Mammography with breast cushions. Women's Health Issues. 2005;15(2):55–63.
13. Maclean U, Sinfield D, Klein S, Harnden B. Women who decline breast screening. J Epidemiol Community Health. 1984;38:278–83.
14. Bilodeau BA, Degner LF. Information needs, sources of information and decisional roles in women with breast cancer. Oncol Nurs Forum. 1996;23:691–6.
15. Poulos A, Llewellyn G. Mammography discomfort: a holistic perspective derived from women's experiences. Radiography. 2005;11(1):17–25.
16. Brenner Joanna. Pew-internet: social networking. 2012. http://pewinternet.org/Commentary/2012/March/Pew-Internet-Social-Networking-full-detail.aspx. Accessed 5 Feb 2013.
17. DOH. Equity and excellence: Liberating the NHS. TSO. 2010.
18. Sokal R. A critical review of the literature on the uptake of cervical and breast screening in British South Asian women. Qual Prim Care. 2010;18:251–61.

19. Chiu LF, Moore J, et al. Communicating risk information about breast and cervical cancer and cancer screening to women from minority ethnic and low income groups. DOH, NHS Cancer Screening Programmes. 2009.
20. Edgar L, Glackin M, et al. Factors influencing participation in breast cancer screening. Br J Nurs Oncol Suppl. 2013;22(17):1021–6.
21. Rogers A. Factors influencing participation in breast cancer screening. Br J Nurs Oncol Suppl. 2013; 22(17):1021–6.
22. Ackerson LK, Viswanath K. The social context of interpersonal communication and health. J Health Commun. 2009;14:5–17.
23. Santana S, Lausen B, Bujnowska-Fedak M, Chronaki C, Kummervold PE, Rasmussen J, Sorensen T. Online communication between doctors and patients in Europe: status and perspectives. J Med Internet Res. 2010;12(2):e20. doi:10.2196/jmir.1281. http://www.jmir.org/2010/2/e20/. Accessed 14 Apr 14.
24. Levati S. Professional conduct among registered nurses in the use of online social networking sites. J Adv Nurs. 2014;70(10):2284–92. doi:10.1111/jan.12377. Epub 2014 Mar 12.
25. Bach SB, Kim S. Online consumer complaint behaviors: the dynamics of service failures, consumers' word of mouth, and organization-consumer relationships. Int J Strateg Commun. 2012;6:59–76.
26. Huang J-H, Hsiao T-T, et al. The effects of electronic word of mouth on product judgment and choice: the moderating role of the sense of virtual community. J Appl Soc Psychol. 2012;42(9):2326–47.
27. Wu PF. In search of negativity bias: an empirical study of perceived helpfulness of online reviews. Psychol Mark. 2013;30(11):971–84.

14 Pain in Mammography

Patsy Whelehan

Defining, Describing, and Measuring the Pain

What is pain? Since 1979, physical pain has been defined by the International Association for the Study of Pain (IASP) as "an unpleasant sensory and emotional experience associated with actual or potential tissue damage, or described in terms of such damage" [1]. So, even in the context of specifically *physical* pain, it is widely accepted that there are affective (emotional) dimensions alongside the sensory perceptions.

What, then, is discomfort, and what is the difference between pain and discomfort? This is difficult to answer with any degree of certainty. Physical discomfort is considered by some to be the same phenomenon as physical pain but simply less severe, and indeed the dictionary definition of discomfort is "slight pain". However, discomfort can be considered a separate and distinct phenomenon from pain, so it may not be wise to include both the terms pain and discomfort in a single measurement scale, as some authors on mammography pain have previously done.

For measuring pain, self-report is generally the preferred method because pain is essentially subjective and therefore best assessed by the person feeling it. While pain *can* be assessed by an observer, using behavioural indicators, this is generally a highly skilled process and only necessary for neonates, or patients with severe dementia [2].

When we set out to measure pain, we should avoid the mistake, sometimes made in the mammography literature, of formulating and using a measurement scale without first ensuring that we have good evidence of its validity and reliability. A *valid* scale is one that actually measures what it aims to measure and a *reliable* scale will produce the same or similar values for the same conditions on multiple occasions. There is no shortage of widely accepted, easy to use and well-validated pain scales. The three simplest and best known pain intensity scales are the 100 mm visual analogue scale (VAS), the numerical rating scale (NRS), and the verbal rating scale (VRS) (see Fig. 14.1) [3]. Although these scales are straightforward, the nomenclature can be a little confusing. For example, a VRS is not necessarily administered "verbally" or orally – in fact it is probably more commonly administered on paper. The NRS can also be administered either by someone asking the patient to state a number from 0 to 10, or by the patient making a mark against a number on paper or other medium. The VAS, as its name suggests, does need to be seen by the patient, who makes a mark on a line to indicate the pain level. The position of the mark is then measured in millimetres, giving a level on a scale of 0–100.

P. Whelehan
Medical Research Institute,
Ninewells Hospital and Medical School,
University of Dundee, Dundee DD1 9SY, UK
e-mail: p.j.whelehan@dundee.ac.uk

P. Hogg et al. (eds.), *Digital Mammography: A Holistic Approach*,
DOI 10.1007/978-3-319-04831-4_14, © Springer International Publishing Switzerland 2015

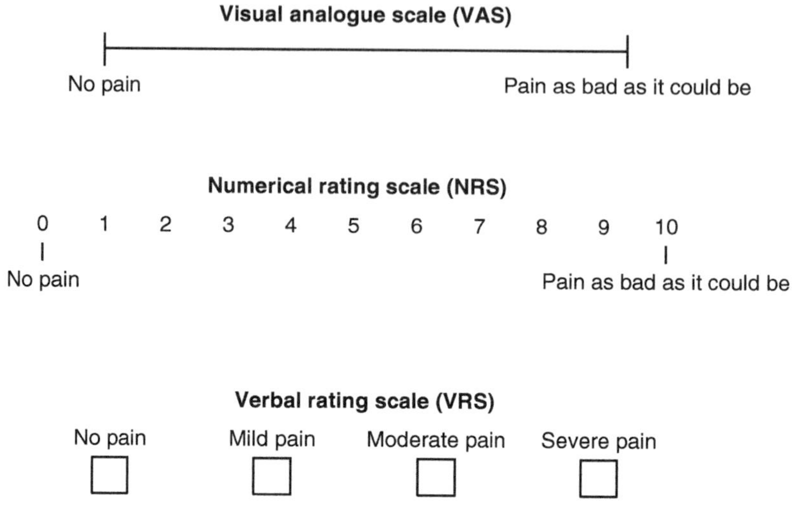

Fig. 14.1 Pain intensity measurement scales

A more sophisticated tool is the McGill Pain Questionnaire, which exists in long and shortened forms [4, 5]. This has the advantage of capturing richer data about the pain experience, including the affective dimension, but it is more difficult and time-consuming to complete. Finally, electronic devices are now becoming available to capture real-time pain data, for example using hand pressure exerted on a sensor to indicate pain intensity [6].

How Important Is the Problem of Pain in Mammography?

There are several ways in which we might assess the importance of pain in mammography as a problem. We could ask what proportion of women undergoing mammography experience any pain, or what proportion of women experience pain above a specified level. The literature in this area provides vastly variable findings, largely because of methodological limitations. Literature reviews have found that the proportion of women experiencing pain during their mammograms ranges from 1 to 92 % [7, 8], or from 6 to 76 % [9], so it is clearly difficult to use prevalence rates as a measure of the importance of the problem.

Perhaps a more appropriate measure of the importance of pain in mammography is whether, in the breast screening context, it affects behaviour; i.e. does it deter women from returning for future mammographic screening. Findings in the literature have varied on this question but a recent systematic literature review [10] has established that between 25 and 46 % of breast screening non-re-attenders give pain as a reason for not returning. This review also showed that when pain is measured at an index mammogram and compared with subsequent re-attendance rates, the risk of non-re-attendance is about a third higher in women who report pain than in those who do not (risk ratio: 1.34 [95 % CI: 0.94–1.91]). In the context of surveillance mammography for women previously treated for breast cancer, a study in 2012 [11] did not find an association between pain at mammography and annual mammography adherence. However, it was demonstrated that anxiety about the mammogram, and pain catastrophizing (e.g. “I became afraid that the pain would get worse”) were associated with non-adherence.

What Makes Mammography More Painful for Some Women Than Others?

This is another question which many authors have attempted to address. Numerous effects have been implicated as risk factors for pain in mammography but the evidence is inconclusive for many of them. This is partly because of weaknesses in the methodologies used in some studies, including the use of non-validated pain measurement instruments. In addition, it is difficult to separate the many potential co-variables and the complex interactions between them which are likely to exist.

An informal literature review published in 2007 [8] grouped the risk factors for mammography pain into biological, psychological and staff-related. Biological factors that have been linked with greater pain include breast tenderness; psychological factors include expectations of pain, and staff-related factors include clients' perceptions of staff attitude.

There is, perhaps, a fourth important category – technique-related. There is very little empirical evidence that the specific equipment model has an influence on mammographic pain, although many practitioners will suggest that it does. However, another obvious place to look for associations between technique and pain is the compression force exerted on the breast. This was investigated by Sullivan et al in 1991[12], whose findings suggested that pain *was* related to compression force. As it is recognised that applied force varies by practitioner [13], a strength of this study was that a single practitioner x-rayed all the participants. However, it is not stated that the cohort in the Sullivan study was asymptomatic (the age range would suggest not), nor was any differential presence of symptoms taken into account. Furthermore, the scale used to assess pain was non-standard and no evidence of validity or reliability was provided. A study by Poulos and Rickard later found no difference in discomfort between two cranio-caudal views when one was deliberately compressed less firmly than the other by the practitioner [14]. Clearly, a lack of robust empirical evidence for a relationship between compression force and pain does not necessarily mean that no relationship exists. The advent of digital mammography and tools for automated extraction of technique data may facilitate larger-scale and more definitive studies in this area.

Compression, and other aspects of technique, are discussed further in the next paragraph.

How Can We Reduce the Risk or the Level of Pain from Mammography?

Clearly, we should target those potentially modifiable factors which contribute most to the problem but, as described above, a surprising lack of clarity persists regarding what those factors are. A Cochrane systematic review, last updated in 2008 [15], found a shortage of effective interventions to reduce mammography pain. Interventions showing most promise in randomised controlled trials were: giving women sufficient information about the procedure prior to the mammogram; increasing women's control over the level of compression applied; and use of cushioning on the mammography machine. However, the latter two interventions both carried the risk of detriment to image quality, and the cushions, at least, involve additional cost.

An obvious potential pain reduction intervention is medication, and a number of studies have been conducted in this area. A well-conducted multi-arm, randomised, placebo controlled trial [16], which was published slightly too late to be included in the 2008 Cochrane review, evaluated the effects of lidocaine gel application and oral premedication with ibuprofen or paracetamol on mammography discomfort and satisfaction. The authors found a statistically significant but very small, and therefore probably clinically insignificant, difference in reported discomfort for lidocaine gel compared with placebo or no gel.

While researchers continue the quest for feasible, effective and cost-effective interventions to reduce pain in mammography, there are measures that all practitioners can take in their daily work which *may* reduce pain or discomfort and/or increase client satisfaction, without risk of causing harm or incurring additional costs. Provision of sufficient information and explanation should of course always be part of standard practice. In addition, it was demonstrated in one study that the risk of women reporting pain from mammography was reduced if they perceived that the radiographer told them that they could say "stop" if they became too uncomfortable, and if they perceived that they had had a conversation with the radiographer [17]. The method of assessing pain is not clearly described in this publication and there is no evidence of validity testing having been performed on the questionnaires. However, the finding of reduced pain risk if women are verbally offered some control over the level of compression is consistent with the randomised controlled trial evidence that pain can be reduced by giving more control to the women [18].

The 2008 premedication trial by Lambertz et al. [16] also produced important results from secondary analyses, showing that women who felt that the technologist (practitioner) had listened to them and made adjustments when asked to do so, had explained the procedure in understandable terms, and had seemed to care about them as people, reported lower discomfort and higher satisfaction. In turn, intention to re-attend for future screening was associated with satisfaction. This underscores the importance of excellent interpersonal skills and behaviours on the part of practitioners.

Deciding when the "right" amount of compression has been applied is challenging for the practitioner. Traditionally, we have been taught that the breast should feel taut, or the skin under the compression paddle should start to blanch [14, 19]. At the same time, it is inappropriate to apply more force than the woman finds acceptable. Here the practitioner's interpersonal skills are again important, in terms of being quick to notice non-verbal cues from the client which may indicate rising distress (see Chaps. 9, 10, 11, 12 and 13). Some departments prescribe a minimum compression force in an attempt to maximise image quality. This does not respect the holistic needs of the woman as an individual, nor the fact that breast tissue elasticity varies between women. Continuing to increase compression force when it is not resulting in further thickness reduction is futile and will only increase the risk or level of pain. It must be remembered that tissue elasticity (compressibility) varies between women and between different areas of the tissue in the field. Recent research has focussed on pressure (force per unit area) and how it is distributed across the compressed tissues in different women [20]. Work such as this has the potential to influence compression mechanism design [21] (see Chap. 22). However, it remains the task of the practitioner to make careful judgements about the appropriate level of compression force to apply, taking into account the look and feel of the breast tissue, the woman's responses, and the force readout.

Despite a shortage of published research evidence to show that positioning is crucial to minimising pain, experience and reasoning indicate that it is nonetheless the case. For example, centring too high for a medio-lateral oblique (MLO) view is likely to induce lengthwise tension in the pectoral muscle and breast, leading to more compression force being needed to hold the breast forward, and consequently a greater risk of pain. In addition to centring correctly, it is important to mobilise the breast maximally towards the medial direction for the MLO projection, to equalise tissue thickness as far as possible, thus reducing undue tissue pressure in localised areas. Full medial displacement will also reduce dragging on the skin as the paddle moves down. For the cranio-caudal projection, sufficient displacement of the breast in the superior direction will also minimise skin dragging (see Chaps. 15 and 21).

Summary

Pain in mammography is an important and somewhat intractable problem. However, excellence in mammographic practice can both minimise pain as far as possible and decrease the risk of women choosing not to re-attend for screening on account of poor experience.

References

1. IASP Subcommittee on Taxonomy. Editorial: the need of a taxonomy. Pain. 1979;6(3):247–52.
2. Curtiss C. Challenges in pain assessment in cognitively intact and cognitively impaired older adults with cancer. Oncol Nurs Forum. 2010;37:7–16.
3. Jensen M, Karoly P. Self-report scales and procedures for assessing pain in adults. In: Turk D, Melzack R, editors. Handbook of pain assessment. 3rd ed. New York: The Guildford Press; 2011. p. 19–44.

4. Melzack R. The McGill pain questionnaire: major properties and scoring methods. Pain. 1975;1(3): 277–99.
5. Melzack R. The short-form McGill pain questionnaire. Pain. 1987;30(2):191–7.
6. Schaffner N, Folkers G, Käppeli S, Musholt M, Hofbauer GFL, Candia V. A new tool for real-time pain assessment in experimental and clinical environments. PLoS One. 2012;7(11):e51014.
7. NHSBSP. Acceptability to women of full-field digital mammography (Equipment Report 0603). Sheffield: NHS Cancer Screening Programmes; 2006.
8. Davey B. Pain during mammography: possible risk factors and ways to alleviate pain. Radiography. 2007;13(3):229–34.
9. Armstrong K, Moye E, Williams S, Berlin JA, Reynolds EE. Screening mammography in women 40 to 49 years of age: a systematic review for the American College of Physicians. Ann Intern Med. 2007;146(7):516–26.
10. Whelehan P, Evans A, Wells M, MacGillivray S. The effect of mammography pain on repeat participation in breast cancer screening: a systematic review. Breast. 2013;22(4):383–94.
11. Shelby RA, Scipio CD, Somers TJ, Soo MS, Weinfurt KP, Keefe FJ. Prospective study of factors predicting adherence to surveillance mammography in women treated for breast cancer. J Clin Oncol. 2012;30(8): 813–9.
12. Sullivan DC, Beam CA, Goodman SM, Watt DL. Measurement of force applied during mammography. Radiology. 1991;181(2):355–7.
13. Mercer CE, Hogg P, Lawson R, Diffey J, Denton ERE. Practitioner compression force variability in mammography: a preliminary study. Br J Radiol. 2013;86(1022):20110596.
14. Poulos A, Rickard M. Compression in mammography and the perception of discomfort. Australas Radiol. 1997;41(3):247–52.
15. Miller D, Livingstone V, Herbison GP. Interventions for relieving the pain and discomfort of screening mammography. Cochrane Database Syst Rev. 2008; (1):CD002942.
16. Lambertz CK, Johnson CJ, Montgomery PG, Maxwell JR. Premedication to reduce discomfort during screening mammography. Radiology. 2008;248(3):765–72.
17. Van Goethem M, Mortelmans D, Bruyninckx E, Verslegers I, Biltjes I, Van Hove E, et al. Influence of the radiographer on the pain felt during mammography. Eur Radiol. 2003;13(10):2384–9.
18. Kornguth PJ, Rimer BK, Conaway MR, Sullivan DC, Catoe KE, Stout AL, et al. Impact of patient-controlled compression on the mammography experience. Radiology. 1993;186(1):99–102.
19. Bassett LW. Diagnosis of diseases of the breast. Philadelphia: Saunders; 2005.
20. Dustler M, Andersson I, Brorson H, Fröjd P, Mattsson S, Tingberg A, et al. Breast compression in mammography: pressure distribution patterns. Acta Radiol. 2012;53(9):973–80.
21. de Groot JE, Broeders MJM, Branderhorst W, den Heeten GJ, Grimbergen CA. Mammographic compression after breast conserving therapy: controlling pressure instead of force. Med Phys. 2014;41(2):023501.

Tissue Viability and Skin Tearing in Mammography

15

Melanie Stephens

Introduction

It has been acknowledged that some women are more sensitive to the handling and pressure exerted on their breasts during a mammogram than others [1]. This sensitivity can include heightened feelings of pain, skin reddening, tingling and bruising [2]; these are considered to be acceptable risks. A small proportion of women after mammography however, can go on to experience breast pain for days. Also they may develop pressure ulcers or skin tears. These pressure ulcers or skin tears are very rarely reported.

Within the UK, because of the advent of safer care for patients [3] and the reporting of avoidable harm through the NHS safety thermometer [4], the area of tissue viability needs to be addressed.

Risks of Mammography

To ensure a high quality mammogram image, that separates tissue components and reduces the dosage of radiation, compression of the breast is essential [5]. However applying compression force to the breast also increases the risk of tissue damage from pressure, shear and friction forces, resulting in iatrogenic injuries. The National Pressure Ulcer Advisory Panel (NPUAP) and the European Pressure Ulcer Advisory Panel (EPUAP) [6, 7] definitions of shear stress and friction clearly explain the risk mammography can cause from either applying forces to the breast, which causes two adjacent parts (the skin and underlying structures) to distort in the transverse plane or the rubbing of two surfaces together. The resultant damage can appear as a blister (friction), ulceration or tear of the epidermis or even skin breakdown that occurs days after the mammogram (pressure and shear).

The risks of skin breakdown are heightened when clients undergoing mammography are considered to be more at risk due to predisposing risk factors such as age, gender, dry and fragile skin or if the patient already has intertrigo, skin abrasions or lesions.

Defining Skin Tears and Pressure Ulcers

A pressure ulcer, according to the National Pressure Ulcer Advisory Panel [8], is a

> …localised injury to the skin and/or underlying tissue, usually over a bony prominence, as a result of pressure, or pressure in combination with shear. A number of contributing or confounding factors are also associated with pressure ulcers

M. Stephens
School of Nursing, Midwifery, Social Work and Social Sciences, University of Salford, Frederick Road, Salford M6 6PU, UK
e-mail: m.stephens@salford.ac.uk

P. Hogg et al. (eds.), *Digital Mammography: A Holistic Approach*,
DOI 10.1007/978-3-319-04831-4_15, © Springer International Publishing Switzerland 2015

Skin tears are considered to be traumatic injuries, varying from minor to complex wounds, which can result in the development of partial or full thickness injuries, where the epidermis has separated from the dermis or both layers of skin have separated from the underlying structures [9]. The problem arises when the damage has been caused through shear or friction forces as the type of wound that subsequently occurs can be categorised as both a pressure ulcer or skin tear. More research is needed to improve diagnosis of these types of wounds.

Where Do They Occur?

Pressure ulcers most commonly develop over bony prominences; however Fletcher [10] notes that device-related pressure ulcers can occur on other parts of the body, such as the breast. Skin tears can occur on any anatomical location, however in relation to mammography common places can be the inframammary fold or upper (inner or outer) aspects of the breast.

Predisposing Risk Factors

There are many predisposing risk factors that can contribute to the development of pressure ulcers and skin tears; they can either be intrinsically or extrinsically related. Extrinsic factors can be linked to direct pressure, shear and friction forces. Intrinsic factors are those that affect the physical, social and mental well being of clients. For mammography these factors can include:

Age: As aging occurs the skin thins and flattens. In conjunction, there is a loss in the number of blood vessels, nerve endings and collagen. This leads to a reduction in sensation, moisture balance, elasticity and temperature control. Atrophy and contraction of the dermis causes wrinkles and folds, whilst sebaceous glands reduce their level of activity causing the skin to dry out. The consequences of all these changes include skin fragility, furrowing and wrinkling of the skin [11–13]

History of previous skin damage, bruising, abrasions and intertrigo: Some clients may present with current bruising, skin abrasions, sores or tears and this increases the risk of further skin breakdown or worsening of their current skin condition [14]. For these cases breast imaging units should consider having local protocols in relation to informing the client of the risks of continuing with screening.

According to Wingfield [15] dry, fragile skin is frequently related to other skin diseases (eczema), illnesses (hypothyroidism) or environmental factors (central heating) and once the skin dries out it is more susceptible to cracks and splits. These may develop into infected wounds and sores.

Medication: Can affect skin structure and function and increase the risk of skin breakdown. For example, steroids can cause thinning of the skin; non steroidal anti-inflammatories can cause irritant dermatitis [16].

Diet and weight: A lack of adequate fats, carbohydrates, proteins, minerals, vitamins, fibre and water may predispose a client to increased risk of skin damage and delayed wound healing. Therefore clients who are either obese or emaciated are associated with a higher risk due to a lack of essential nutrition and hydration which promotes skin cell turgidity, elasticity and function [17].

Sensory impairment: Clients with altered cognitive or sensory impairment are at an increased risk of skin breakdown as they may not be able to perceive pain from pressure, shear and friction forces.

Co-morbidity: Many clients present with co-morbidities that affect skin status. These can include conditions such as cardiovascular, renal, endocrinology and respiratory diseases, which can alter the blood flow, oxygenation and nutrient levels and the removal of toxic waste from the skin.

Prevention of Tearing and Ulceration from Mammography

Preventing pressure ulcers and skin tears is complex in mammography as the device which potentially causes the damage forms the essential part of the diagnostic investigation. Nevertheless, assessment of the client's skin and risk factors when attending for mammography is vital. The mammography practitioner should note relevant factors which are reported by the client or observed through skin inspection before and after the mammogram. Findings should be documented in the client's notes. If required discussions of the risks of further skin damage should be carried out with the client if skin abrasions, tears or lesions are present.

As there is a lack of research in the prevention and management of pressure ulcers and skin tears current best practice includes consideration of:

- Reduction or elimination of pressure, shear and friction forces
- Correct positioning and alignment of breasts during the mammogram (see also Chap. 17)
- Obtaining pre-mammogram information in regards of skin care, nutrition and hydration, treatment of current lesions and skin tears
- Protection of susceptible skin areas during the mammography maybe be necessary

If a client develops a pressure ulcer or skin tear during or after the mammogram it is important to document accurately the wound and refer to the appropriate healthcare professional for advice and further management.

Pressure Ulcer and Skin Tear Classification Systems

Pressure Ulcers

In order to provide consensus across Europe in the care and management of pressure ulcers, EPUAP (2009) have developed a common classification system, as follows:

- Category/Stage I: Non-blanchable erythema
- Category/Stage II: Partial thickness, shallow open ulcer
- Category/Stage III: Full thickness skin loss, subcutaneous fat may be visible but bone, tendon or muscle are *not* exposed
- Category/Stage IV: Full thickness tissue loss with exposed bone, tendon or muscle

Additional Categories/Stages for the USA include Unstageable/Unclassified: Full thickness skin or tissue loss – depth unknown Suspected Deep Tissue Injury – depth unknown

Skin Tears

Payne and Martin [18] were the first practitioners to develop a classification system for skin tears and this is divided into categories and sub categories depending on the severity of the tear:

- **Category 1**: Skin tears without loss of tissue
- **Category 2**: Skin tears with partial tissue loss
- **Category 3**: Skin tears with complete tissue loss.

Since 1993 subsequent studies have explored the inter rate reliability of the classification system and general use in clinical practice) which has led to the development of a more universally acceptable classification Skin Tear Audit Research (STAR) Classification System [19, 20]. This system comprises three categories and two sub-categories of skin tears. The STAR Classification System is generally used in Australia, with early indications of implementation reported across the UK.

- **Category 1a**: a skin tear where the edges can be realigned to the normal anatomical position (without undue stretching) and the skin or flap colour is not pale, dusky or darkened.
- **Category 1b**: a skin tear where the edges can be realigned to the normal anatomical position (without undue stretching) and the skin or flap colour is pale, dusky or darkened.
- **Category 2a**: a skin tear where the edges cannot be realigned to the normal anatomical position and the skin or flap colour is not pale, dusky or darkened.
- **Category 2b**: a skin tear where the edges cannot be realigned to the normal anatomical position and the skin or flap colour is pale dusky or darkened.
- **Category 3**: a skin tear where the skin flap is completely absent.

Management and Other Considerations

If the mammography practitioner finds a pressure ulcer, skin tear, intertrigo or abrasion on the breast pre or post mammography procedure, it is imperative to discuss with the client subsequent management. This may include the practitioner carrying out some simple wound management and/or a referral to other services.

Simple steps to consider include:

1. Control of any bleeding and cleaning of the wound according to local policy
2. If the wound is a skin tear and it is feasible and viable, to realign any skin flap or tear
3. Assessment of the patient, their wound and the peri wound area adhering to local policy documents, in order to assess the degree of tissue damage or loss. This may include the use of either a pressure ulcer or skin tear classification tool, depending on the diagnosis
4. Apply appropriate dressings according to local policy dressing formulary
5. Referral to appropriate healthcare practitioner for follow up dressings
6. Discussion with the patient regards to findings and health education and promotion
7. Completion of any clinical incident or safety thermometer report forms

References

1. NHS Breast Screening Programme. Information and advice for health professionals in breast screening. Sheffield: NHS Cancer Screening Programme; 2002.
2. Cancerbackup. NHS breast screening: helping you decide. 2011. http://www.cancerscreening.nhs.uk/breastscreen/publications/nhsbsp.pdf.
3. Department of Health. NHS 2010–2015: from good to great. Preventative, people-centred, productive. London: DH; 2009.
4. NHS Quality Observatory. NHS safety thermometer. 2013. http://www.safetythermometer.nhs.uk/.
5. Dustler M, Andersson I, Brorson H, Fröjd P, Mattsson S, Tingberg A, Zackrisson S, Förnvik D. Breast compression in mammography: pressure distribution patterns. Acta Radiol. 2012;53(9):973–80.
6. National Pressure Ulcer Advisory Panel. Friction induced skin injuries – are they pressure ulcers? A National Pressure Ulcer Advisory Panel White Paper. 2012. https://www.npuap.org/wp-content/uploads/2012/01/NPUAP-Friction-White-Paper.pdf.
7. National Pressure Ulcer Advisory Panel. Shear Force Initiative Presentation. 2012b. http://www.npuap.org/wp-content/uploads/2012/03/Shear_slides.pdf.
8. National Pressure Ulcer Advisory Panel and European Pressure Ulcer Advisory panel. NPUAP Pressure Ulcer Stages/Categories. 2009. http://www.npuap.org/resources/educational-and-clinical-resources/npuap-pressure-ulcer-stagescategories/.
9. LeBlanc K, Baranoski S. Skin tears: state of the science: consensus statements for the prevention, prediction, assessment, and treatment of skin tears. 2011. http://www.skintears.org/pdf/SkinTearsConsensus-Statements.pdf.
10. Fletcher J. Device related pressure ulcers made easy. 2012. http://www.woundsinternational.com/pdf/content_10472.pdf.
11. Voegeli D. Factors that exacerbate skin breakdown and ulceration, Skin breakdown, the silent epidemic. Hull: Smith and Nephew Foundation; 2007.
12. Baranoski S, Ayello EA. Wound care essentials, practice principles. Springhouse: Lippincott, Williams and Wilkins; 2004.
13. Mistiaen P, van Halm-Walters M. Prevention and treatment of intertrigo in large skin folds of adults: a systematic review. BMC Nurs. 2010;9(12):1–9.
14. Stephen-Haynes J, Carville K. Skin tears made easy. Wounds Int. 2011;2(4):1–6.
15. Wingfield C. Managing dry skin conditions. Wound Essent. 2011;6:50–9.
16. British National Formulary. British National Formulary online. 2014. http://www.bnf.org/bnf/index.htm. Retrieved from 04 Apr 2014.
17. Johnston E. The role of nutrition in Tissue Viability. 2007. http://www.woundsinternational.com/pdf/content_182.pdf.
18. Payne RL, Martin ML. Defining and classifying skin tears: need for a common language. Ostomy Wound Manag. 1993;39(5):16–20, 2.
19. Carville K, Lewin G, Newall N, Haslehurst P, Michael R, Santamaria N, Roberts P. STAR: a consensus for skin tear classification. Prim Intention. 2007;15(1):18–28.
20. White W. Skin tears: a descriptive study of the opinions, clinical practice and knowledge base of RNs caring for the aged in high care residential facilities. Prim Intention. 2001;9(4):138–49.

Part III

Equipment

Mammography Equipment

16

C. John Kotre and Cláudia Sá dos Reis

Introduction

Mammography is one of the most technically demanding examinations in radiology, and it requires X-ray technology designed specifically for the task. The pathology to be imaged ranges from small (20–100 μm) high density microcalcifications to ill-defined low contrast masses. These must be imaged against a background of mixed densities. This makes demonstrating pathology challenging. Because of its use in asymptomatic screening, mammography must also employ as low a radiation dose as possible.

Background

In the past two decades technological developments in breast imaging have taken place [1, 2]. A milestone was the introduction of digital mammography systems in the 1990s. The main goal pursued by the mammography equipment industry has been to develop practical, inexpensive, harmless, equipment appealing to the patient and effective in identifying, localising and characterising abnormal tissues and signs of pathology within the breast [3–5].

Currently available technologies for breast imaging are used to identify structural or morphological differences in tumours, such as microcalcifications, tissue masses, angiogenesis, asymmetry and architectural distortion. Some of the more recently developed techniques can provide information about the biological or functional differences between tumours and normal tissues. However, until now there is not one single modality that can simultaneously achieve all these goals, that is, anatomy-physiology and pathology-related goals [1, 3].

Mammography is based on differential attenuation of X-ray photons in the breast tissues and this process is optimised when low energy photons are used. The varying composition and densities of the adipose and glandular tissues produce singular contrasts represented as dark and bright areas in the mammography image. However, the composition and density of glandular tissue and carcinoma are similar and their differentiation requires the use of low energy photons in the range 10–20 keV. For energies higher than 28 keV the linear X-ray attenuation coefficients of both tissues overlap, carcinoma and normal glandular tissue cannot be differentiated and diagnostic becomes compromised due to poor image contrast [6, 7].

C.J. Kotre (✉)
Christie Medical Physics and Engineering, The Christie NHS Foundation Trust, Wilmslow Road, Manchester M20 4BX, UK
e-mail: john.kotre@christie.nhs.uk

C.S. dos Reis
Escola Superior de Tecnologia da Saúde de Lisboa, Lisbon School of Health Technology, Av. D. João II, Lote 4.69.01, Lisbon 1990-096, Portugal
e-mail: claudia.reis@estesl.ipl.pt

P. Hogg et al. (eds.), *Digital Mammography: A Holistic Approach*, DOI 10.1007/978-3-319-04831-4_16, © Springer International Publishing Switzerland 2015

The subtle X-ray attenuation properties between normal and cancer tissues and the risks associated to ionising radiation demand imaging techniques that minimise dose and optimise image quality (IQ). This promotes the refinement of dedicated X-ray equipment for mammography (specialised X-ray tubes, adequate X-ray spectra systems) [6].

Technological advances over the last several decades have greatly improved the diagnostic sensitivity of mammography.

The Mammographic X-Ray Unit

Mammography is performed using dedicated equipment usually with a "C" shaped arm aimed at facilitating breast positioning. The C arm can be adjusted in height and angular orientation to adjust the compression plate and the breast support to the patient standing or sitting position.

The X-ray tube and digital receptor table assembly are mounted in opposition: the X-ray tube for the generation of the photon beam on the top head, a face protector, a compression paddle and the image receptor system on the lower arm (Fig. 16.1).

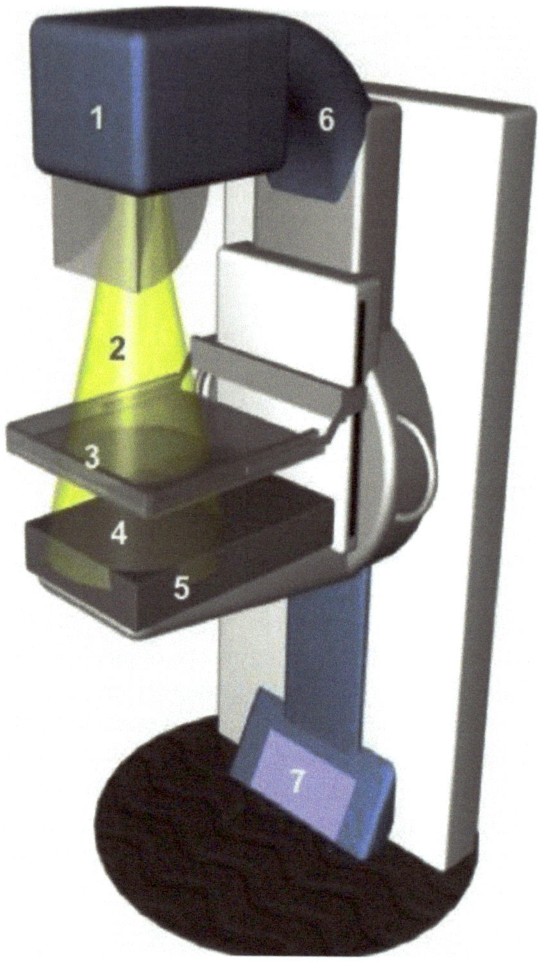

Fig. 16.1 Integrated direct digital mammography system. *1* X-ray tube, *2* X-ray beam, *3* compression paddle, *4* breast support, *5* detector, *6* C-arm, *7* monitor for angle, breast thickness and compression force (Image is courtesy of Mário Oliveira)

The stages for production of mammography images are acquisition, processing, display and post processing for interpretation and storage. In digital mammography each step is performed by an individual system that can be independently assessed and optimised. The image acquisition system is composed of an X-ray tube, breast compression plate and image receptor system.

The distance from the X-ray focus to the breast support platform is commonly around 60 cm. A moving anti-scatter grid is normally used which is situated just behind the low-attenuation (often carbon-fibre) table top and in front of the image receptor. Some designs work without an anti-scatter grid and make a software correction for the large-scale effects of scattered radiation in the image.

Due to the requirements for very high resolution, X-ray focal spot sizes must be small. Focal spots of approximately 0.3×0.3 mm are used for conventional mammography, with a size of 0.15×0.15 mm selectable for magnified views, where the breast is raised away from the image receptor on a special magnification table in order to produce a geometrically magnified view.

The X-ray tube is positioned within the unit so that the anode heel effect is employed to reduce X-ray intensity towards the nipple side of the field where the breast will be thinner. Heavy reliance is placed on the automatic exposure system of modern mammography units. These systems are capable of sensing the thickness and

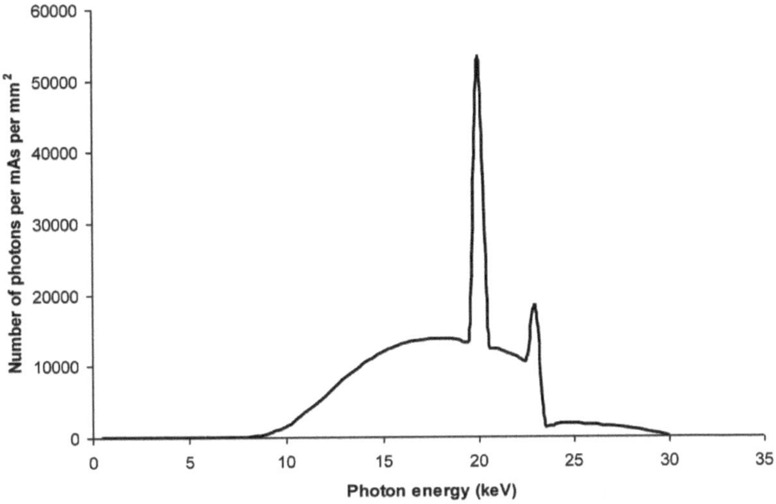

Fig. 16.2 X-ray spectrum for a typical rhodium target, rhodium filtered mammographic x-ray beam at 30 kV. The spectrum peaks around 20 keV due to the K-edge filtration produced by the rhodium filter. This spectrum is suitable for imaging moderate-sized breasts

composition of the compressed breast and then automatically selecting the tube potential, target and filter combination and exposure time required to give the optimal imaging exposure within the constraints of patient dose limitations.

The Mammographic X-Ray Spectrum

The X-ray spectrum from a conventional tungsten target, glass encapsulated, aluminium filtered X-ray tube is not optimal for mammography. The best subject contrast for between normal and malignant tissue is considered to be produced at a photon energy of around 20 keV, which is much lower than that used in normal radiography. Increasing photon energy will reduce contrast and reducing photon energy will lead to inadequate penetration of the breast and a large increase in patient dose, so the X-ray spectrum is critical. A range of mammographic spectra are used for digital mammography. The X-ray tube target may well be switchable (depending on the design) between molybdenum and rhodium, or rhodium and tungsten and the tube has a low attenuation beryllium output window. The beam is then filtered with either molybdenum, rhodium, silver or aluminium filters. The X-ray tube is operated at a voltage in the range 25–35 kV.

Figure 16.2 shows the spectrum of a rhodium target, rhodium filtered beam at a tube voltage of 30 kV. Rhodium has characteristic X-ray peaks at 20.2 and 22.7 keV, which contribute strongly to the limited range spectrum. Rhodium is again used as the filter because, due to the K-edge absorption, it strongly attenuates energies just above its own K-characteristic peaks as well as attenuating lower energies. The end result is a spectrum with most photons lying in a narrow band of energies.

Although the most common spectrum, this is not necessarily optimised for all breast thicknesses. For larger breasts, a more penetrating beam is optimal to avoid very long exposure times which bring the possibility of movement blur, tube overloading and high radiation doses. Figure 16.3 shows the spectrum of a tungsten target, aluminium filtered beam again at a tube voltage of 30 kV, with the X-ray tube again having a beryllium output window. Although the tungsten anode, aluminium filter combination was not used with film-screen mammography, it is well suited to the response of modern digital mammography receptors and is becoming a more common choice.

The shape of the spectrum is quite different from Fig. 16.2 and its peak is now at a higher energy, even though the tube voltage is the same. The tungsten target has no K-characteristic X-ray

Fig. 16.3 X-ray spectrum for a typical tungsten target, aluminium filtered mammographic x-ray beam at 30 kV

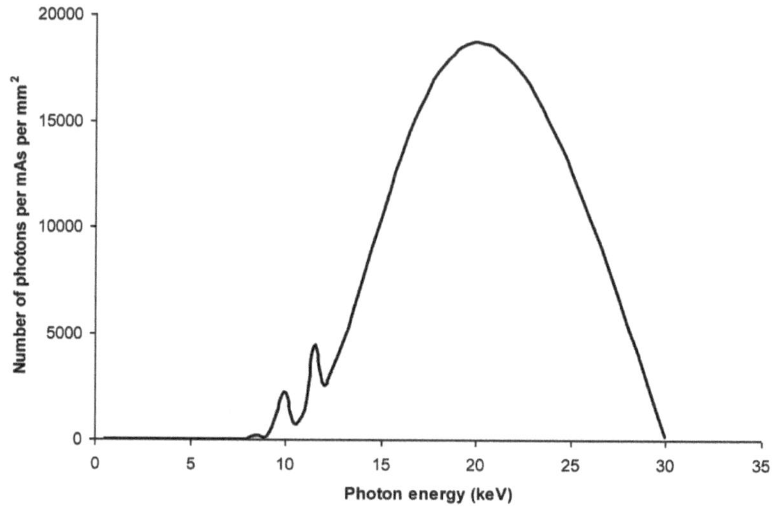

peaks in this energy range, and the aluminium filter, which similarly does not have a K-absorption edge in this energy range, does not preferentially attenuate the higher energy end of the spectrum.

Compression Paddle Design

In mammography the breast is compressed using a rigid transparent plastic compression plate which can be motor driven. The use of compression force reduces the thickness of the breast and holds it in place which gives a number of advantages:

- Better spatial resolution. The breast is brought closer to the imaging receptor so that magnification and focal spot blurring is reduced.
- Reduced movement blur, even at the relatively long exposure times (1 s typical) common in mammography.
- Less scattered radiation in the image. The beam path length through the breast is shorter, so there is less material to do the scattering. Reducing the proportion of scattered radiation in the image improves image contrast and reduces image noise.
- Improved image uniformity. Compression spreads the breast tissue out more evenly across the image and makes pathology easier to detect.
- Reducing the compressed breast thickness diminishes exposure time, decreasing the radiation dose delivered to the breast [8, 9].
- The reduced path length makes practicable the use of lower energy (less penetrating) X-ray spectra. This gives greater subject contrast.
- Small areas of pathology buried in glandular tissue can be better visualised, as malignant tissues tend to be firmer.

Compression in mammography is one of the few occasions in radiography where a technical advantage is gained without detriment to other aspects of the image; although there is a disadvantage in client discomfort. Modern mammography units can employ a system to measure the increasing amount of force resulting from a given small increase in compression to stop the motorised movement at a given compression. Many units use a motor driven assembly with more or less compression being applied by the practitioner; the practitioner has direct control over the amount of compression applied. It is suggested that the compression paddle must be controlled by hand during the final compression [8].The compression force maximum limit set on mammography systems is 200 Newtons. A range of compression paddles are normally supplied with a digital mammography unit to cover different types of projection. Some typical types are:

- Flat rigid paddle:
  This is the basic flat paddle that covers the whole of the area of the digital image receptor. The paddle maintains its shape parallel to the plane of the receptor and deforms only slightly when the compression force is applied. This is used for full-field MLO and CC views.
- Tilting flat paddle:
  This is a flat paddle that allows rotation against a spring resistance so that on compression the chest-wall edge of the plate will be higher than the nipple side. The advantages are claimed to be that the design holds the breast in place more firmly. This type of paddle is also used for full-field MLO and CC views.
- Sliding compression plate:
  This plate is suitable for imaging smaller breasts where the full area of the image receptor is not required. By sliding the plate to one side or the other, the MLO view can be achieved using the edge of the breast support table to improve positioning.
- Spot compression plate:
  This plate has a raised cylindrical area that applies extra compression force over a small area (Fig. 16.4). The advantages to spot compression are that better compression over the small area of interest is obtained, with all of the advantages above, but also that the spreading of surrounding parenchyma allows the outline of masses to be better visualised. Whereas features in superimposed tissue will spread out, mechanically harder malignant tissues will tend to retain their shape. Spot views are an additional examination often performed at assessment.
- Magnification compression plate:
  For magnification views, a different breast support table is used that raises the breast away from the plane of the image receptor by some 30 cm (depending on the magnification factor and focus-to-receptor distance), so that the image is geometrically magnified. The compression plate for this is smaller, as the X-ray field is smaller close to the focus, and often has a step in the support arm to allow it to fix to the compression system at a point lower than the magnification support table (Fig. 16.5). See also Chap. 25.

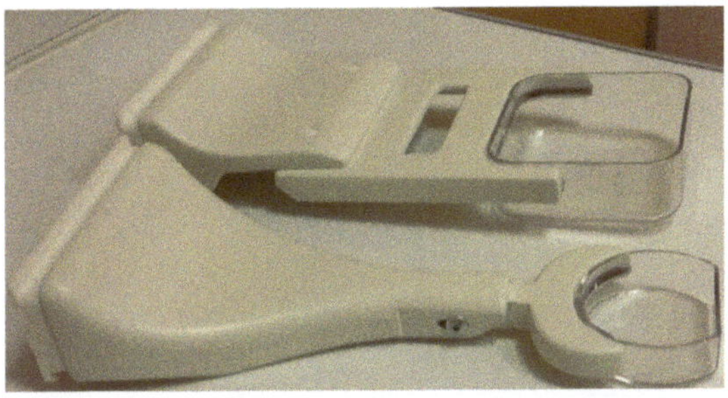

Fig. 16.4 Spot compression plate: this plate has a raised cylindrical area that applies extra compression force over a small area

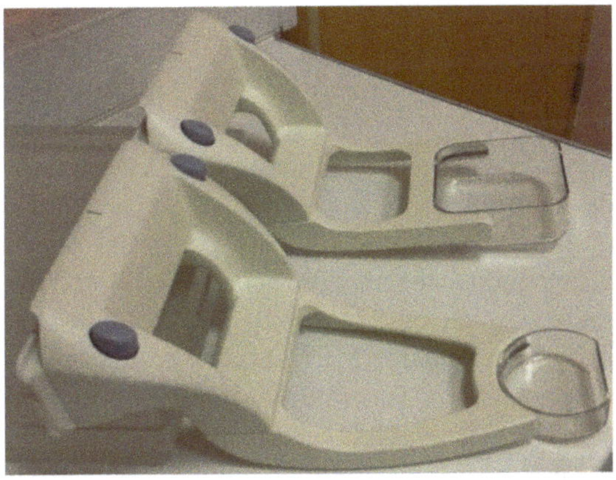

Fig. 16.5 Magnification compression plate: the compression plate for this is smaller, as the x-ray field is smaller close to the focus, and it often has a step in the support arm to allow it to fix to the compression system

- Biopsy compression plate:
  Various specialist compression plates may be required for biopsy systems where the plate has an aperture to accommodate the biopsy needle or device – Fig. 16.6. See also Chap. 33.

Further Advances

Recently American Mammographic has developed a paddle for screening mammography called S.O.F.T. This new paddle is used as an alternative to the conventional flat compression

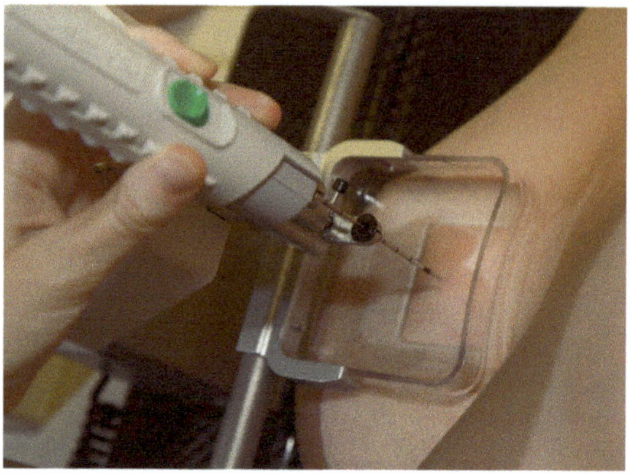

Fig.16.6 Specialist biopsy compression plate in use

paddle allowing a tilt for superior compression of the mid and anterior-breast with less patient discomfort.

Another compression paddle was developed also to reduce the pressure and discomfort on the thickest parts of the breasts. The compression paddle bends along the breasts when the paddle touches them. Also, with three slits on the front side and right and left lateral sides of the paddle, the pressure is dispersed.

The discomfort to the patient is the negative aspect of the compression although the tolerance to compression is variable among women (see Chap. 14). No recommendation is provided regarding the suitable compression force to take into account the characteristics of the breast, namely compressibility, composition and thickness. Several studies [10–15] investigated the best compression force in terms of dose, IQ and patient tolerance. One of these studies concluded that the amount of compression force has noticeable effects on IQ. Moreover, higher IQ rates were consistently associated with higher compression forces. The mean compression force required to produce a "perfect" image in digital systems was 121.3 N for CC and 134.2 N for MLO, whereas for analogue systems the compression force was 112.2 N and 129.7 N for CC and MLO, respectively. In this group of 1,200 patients, 2 % expressed dissatisfaction with the endured compression force [10].

Chapter 22 gives details on a new approach to breast compression, employing a system that uses pressure instead of force.

Digital Mammographic Image Receptors

Digital image capture was first introduced into mammography as 'small-field digital mammography' for needle and core biopsy guidance using detectors typically approximately 15 cm in size. Full-field digital mammography, with detector sizes up to the equivalent of the 24 × 30 cm was developed later.

The imaging advantages of digital mammography include a wide dynamic range and the separation of the image capture and image display functions, so that the image display can be varied to optimally show the full range of recorded X-ray intensities. This provides good visualisation of the skin line and nipple and has advantages when imaging dense breasts and younger women. There are a range of competing image capture technologies for digital mammography, and the choice of technology depends to some extent on the imaging task, be it screening or symptomatic, and the size and format of the hospital or clinic environment in which it will be operated. The range of technologies described below fit the state of the market at the time of writing, but this is an area where progress is still rapid.

General Features of Digital Mammographic Images

A digital image is not a continuous distribution of bright and dark, but is composed of a finite number of points (or 'pixels'), where each pixel has a value of brightness dictated by a stored numerical value. Digital images have the advantage that they can be enhanced and manipulated by computer to extract the maximum amount of diagnostic information. Digital images can be stored, transferred, copied without detriment and retrieved in a very efficient manner using computer mass data storage techniques. They have the disadvantage of a limit to spatial resolution caused by the finite pixel size. Digital mammography receptors usually have a linear response between pixel value and the radiation dose incident on the pixel over a very wide dynamic range, typically a factor of some 10,000:1. The choice of what patient dose is required for digital mammography is therefore driven by the signal-to-noise ratio required for a diagnostic image rather than a specific radiation dose to the receptor.

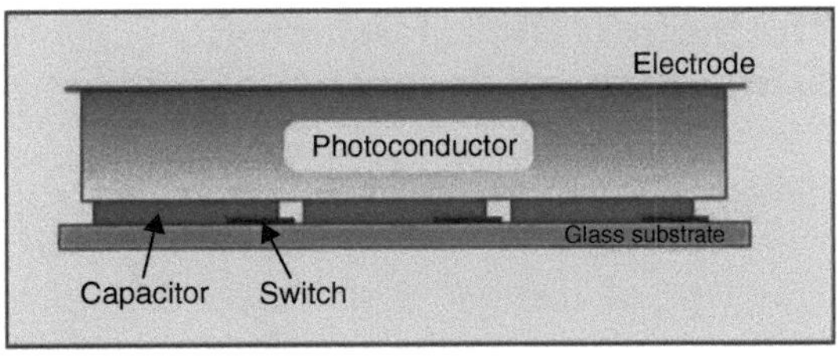

Fig. 16.7 Cross-section through a direct digital mammography image receptor. The photoconductor is a layer of amorphous selenium that allows electrons to flow across it when exposed to x-ray photons. The capacitor builds up a charge, proportional to the x-ray exposure for that pixel. The charge is transferred out of the device via the switch at the end of the exposure and converted to a numerical pixel value

The Direct Digital Detector: Amorphous Selenium

In direct conversion detectors the X-ray interaction is converted directly to an electrical signal using an amorphous selenium (a-Se) layer, behind which lies an amorphous silicon microcircuit layer which in turn is supported by a rigid substrate (Fig. 16.7). Selenium is a photoconductor, so is an electrical insulator in the dark, and a conductor when exposed to light or X-rays. The amorphous selenium is employed as a mammographic image receptor in the form of a thin layer (0.5 mm) with a voltage applied between a large area electrode across the front surface, and an array of charge collection electrodes, one per pixel, on the back surface. These are linked to capacitors to accumulate the charge released during the exposure. These are linked in turn to thin-film-transistor switches to provide a line-by-line read out arrangement in which the charge stored for an individual pixel is passed pixel-by-pixel along the line until it can be measured by electronics external to the imaging sensor. Incoming X-ray photons interact photo-electrically in the a-Se layer producing electrons and 'holes' (the vacancy where an electron should be). Because of the high voltage gradient across the thin a-Se layer, the electrons move towards the positive surface electrode and the holes towards the negative charge collection electrodes. The electrons and holes do not move sideways as they have to follow the direction of the electric field gradient, so image blurring from this source is minimal and the spatial resolution of the detector is good. At the end of the exposure, the charge signals (proportional to the radiation detected) from each pixel are read out via the thin-film-transistor switches and data lines. The charge signals are converted to digital values via charge amplifiers and with a digital-to-analogue converter and sent to the computer for assembly into an image.

The a-Se layer has good photon capture characteristics in the mammographic energy range, and the lack of sideways spread of the electrons and holes carrying the image information allow the a-Se layer to be made relatively thick, resulting in an efficient detector. As the receptor is mounted rigidly in the breast support table of the mammography unit, it is always in the same position with respect to the X-ray beam, allowing the use of 'flat-fielding'. This is an important image calibration in which the receptor is exposed to the unattenuated X-ray beam under test conditions, so that variation in the X-ray intensity across the field and variations in pixel-to-pixel sensitivity can be removed from subsequent images. The removal of these fixed noise sources further improves the efficiency of the receptor.

The Indirect Digital Detector: Scintillator and Amorphous Silicon

Indirect digital mammography detectors use a two-step process for X-ray detection [6, 16, 17]. This type of receptor is similar to that commonly employed in digital radiography, and consists of a thin crystalline scintillator layer closely coupled to amorphous silicon micro-circuit layer which is supported by a rigid substrate. Indirect conversion detectors work by first converting the incident X-ray distribution into a light image, then converting the light distribution into electrical signals addressable to a pixel location on the detector, see Fig. 16.8. The most successful scintillator is Thallium activated Caesium Iodide. This has excellent X-ray absorption characteristics and can be grown in a channelled crystal structure that acts like a fibre optic guide to prevent light spreading sideways giving to the detector improved spatial resolution. It is similar to the input phosphor material of X-ray image intensifiers. The scintillator layer is deposited onto an amorphous silicon micro-circuit array of light sensitive photo-diodes and associated electronics to measure the signal from each photo-diode. After the X-ray exposure is completed, a switching array of thin-film transistors and associated data lines allow the signals from the photodiodes to be fed out of the receptor array in sequence. These signals are then digitised and transferred to the computer to be assembled into an image.

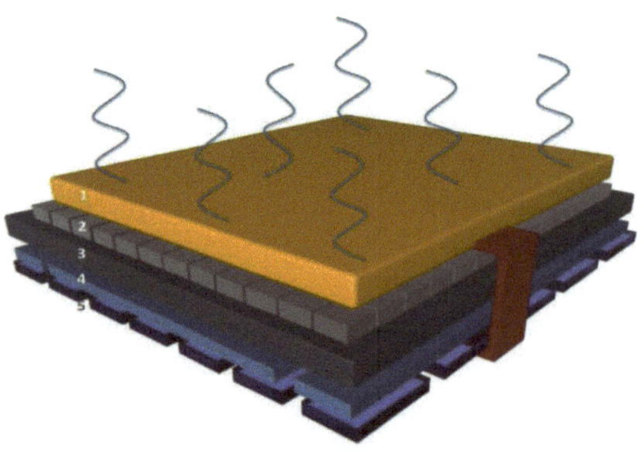

Fig. 16.8 Basic structure of detectors for digital mammography in integrated systems. *Layer 1* – detector material: CsI scintillator + transparent electrode or a-Se (amorphous selenium), *Layer 2* – a-Si array (amorphous silicon), *Layer 3* – base plate, *Layer 4* – driver board – readout board – driver board and *Layer 5* – glass substrate (Courtesy of Mário Oliveira)

This type of receptor is also mounted rigidly in the breast support table of the mammography unit, so the important flat-fielding correction described above can also be used, with the same removal of fixed pattern noise and resulting efficiency improvement.

Computed Radiography

Computed Radiography (CR) is based on the phenomenon of photo-stimulable luminescence. When X-rays are incident on a material such as europium doped barium fluorohalide, they produce high-energy photoelectrons which in turn produce ionisation that results in large number of lower energy electron–hole pairs. In conventional screen-film mammography this happens in a screen in close contact with the film where the electron–hole pairs recombine to emit light that then exposes the film. In photo-stimulable luminescence, however, less than 50 % of the electron–hole pairs recombine, the others are trapped apart due to the presence of the doped sites in the phosphor. These electron traps are crystal lattice defects where halogen ion vacancies occur in the otherwise regular ionic lattice. These so-called 'F' or 'Colour' centres are created during manufacture by prolonged irradiation of the imaging plate with high intensity X-rays and ultra-violet light. Following exposure, electrons can remain trapped at these defects for many hours or days, although the stored image gradually fades with time. The concentration of trapped electrons is proportional to the locally incident X-ray exposure. The electrons are trapped in this state until they are stimulated by light of a suitable wavelength in a CR plate reader, whereupon they are free to travel to the holes, recombine and emit light. The emitted light, which is linearly proportional to the locally incident X-ray intensity is then detected by a photomultiplier and digitised to form an image.

The CR cassette housing the image plate looks much like a screen-film cassette and can be used in substantially the same way. The readout is performed in a plate reader, which works by scanning an intense laser beam across the image plate on a line-by-line basis while the plate is slowly drawn through. A red laser is used to add enough energy to the trapped electrons to get them out of their traps and into the conduction band of the material. They can then move and recombine with a positive ion, dropping back to the ground energy state and in doing so emit their excess energy as a photon of blue light. This weak light signal is picked up by a light guide and sent via a blue filter (to keep out the red light of the stimulating laser) to a photo-multiplier tube that measures the amount of light. This signal is then digitised to produce the raw 'pixel value' associated with that particular location on the image plate.

The scanning laser is focused to a diameter of approximately 0.1 mm to define the pixel of the image (although note that the imaging plate is continuous and not divided into physical pixels). Following read-out, the image plate is exposed to high intensity light to completely erase any traces of the previous image, then reloaded into the cassette and ejected from the reader ready for reuse.

Because the CR cassette is not mounted rigidly in position, and a number of cassettes will normally be used in rotation, it is not possible to apply flat-fielding corrections in CR mammography, and the efficiency of the detector is reduced by the fixed pattern noise in the image arising from non-uniformity of the crystalline photostimulable phosphor. There is also an element of light spread in the phosphor from the read-out laser that leads to some blurring. New developments in 'needle plate' (caesium bromide) phosphors that have a channelled crystalline structure similar to that of caesium iodide (above) promise to improve the efficiency of CR mammography provided these delicate phosphors can be made robust enough for routine use.

Scanned Slit Linear Detectors

A quite different type of digital mammography unit that is rapidly increasing its share of the market is that employing a scanning fan beam of X-rays coupled to a moving one-dimensional detector. This geometry is attractive in terms of its ability to reject scattered photons using a slit collimator at the detector, so no anti-scatter grid is required. Also the one-dimensional detector can be made relatively complex and its signal transfer to the external electronics more direct than with a thin-film two-dimensional array. One commercial design employs a photon-counting detector based on those used in high-energy experimental physics. Using this approach, individual photons are counted in each pixel of the image and the pixel brightness is dictated by the total photons counted during the time the X-ray beam was swept over the pixel position. This has the advantage that low-level fluctuations caused by thermal excitation in the amplifiers and electronics can be rejected leaving only the higher energy photon counts, so a source of image noise can be negated. The motorised movements of the scanning beam are complex, the X-ray tube loading tends to be high and the scan time is generally longer than the exposure time for a two-dimensional receptor, but the overall performance of this technology is directly competitive with the more common amorphous selenium detectors.

Charge-Coupled Devices

Charge-coupled devices (CCD) are rarely used in full-field digital mammography due to the size limitations on the image receptor array, which is fabricated on a conventional silicon wafer. These are, however, common in devices designed for 'small field mammography' where the application is primarily to provide image guidance for biopsy procedures. A layer of scintillator, such as Caesium Iodide, is directly coupled to the light sensing CCD array in the small field device. Designs giving larger field sizes by coupling a larger area scintillator layer to the CCD using fibre-optic bundles or systems of mirrors and lenses have been produced, but the efficiency is generally reduced by light losses in these coupling systems.

The Automatic Exposure Control System

In the 1980s the automatic exposure control (AEC) system was implemented in mammography equipment [18] with the aim to provide uniform and reproducible exposure and penetration of the breast tissues, regardless of their thickness or composition.

Modern mammographic units make heavy use of the AEC to time the length of the exposure. The tube current is often fixed or varied in broad bands. Mammographic AECs can be very sophisticated, making allowance for the attenuation of the breast, the energy of the beam, and able to automatically select the best target/filter combination and kV on the most sophisticated designs.

AEC devices operate by measuring the amount of radiation that reaches the image receptor and terminating the X-ray production when an adequate level of exposure in detector is obtained. This system is composed of one (or more) radiation detectors, signal amplifier, density selector, comparator circuit, termination switch and a backup timer. AEC systems are also known as photo-timers. Considering the most typical configuration in mammography systems, the X-rays transmitted through the patient generate instantaneously a small signal in the AEC sensors located behind the image receptor. An amplifier boosts the signal, which is fed to a voltage comparator and integration circuit. When the accumulated signal equals a preselected reference value, an output pulse ends the exposure. If the detector or circuit fails a "backup timer" safety device terminates the X-ray after a pre-set time. AEC devices require calibration to set the adequate reference detector level for various X-ray exposure conditions.

In modern digital units the automatic exposure control can be set up to provide a constant contrast-to-noise ratio with increasing compressed breast thickness, or a compromise 'low dose' configuration in which the contrast-to-noise ratio is allowed to decrease slowly with increasing compressed breast thickness in return for a dose saving for the largest breasts. These functions are achieved using a complex set of relationships between kVp, target/filter combination and phototiming, which use inputs from the compression paddle position as well as energy-sensitive measurements of radiation transmission through the breast. Some designs use the output from the image receptor itself to provide a signal to the automatic exposure control, and this can be configured in a number of ways using software to provide a range of sensor patterns, or automatically locate the densest area of the breast to provide a reference signal.

In digital mammography systems the grey scale values are not dependent on the incident exposure but on image processing and display. The AEC calibration in digital mammography does not use the optical density as it is used in screen-film mammography systems. Nowadays, AEC devices are calibrated to suit the energy response of the image receptor [19]. The AEC is set up with a generic calibration curve adapted to each image receptor which gives adequate image quality, considering the potential and ensuring the lowest dose [7, 8].

In integrated digital systems, the AEC sensor is the detector itself or a region of it. The image acquisition starts with a short low dose exposure called pre-exposure of the breast and the resulting signal is sampled automatically to identify the densest areas of the breast. This information is used to select the optimised settings (e.g. T/F, kVp, mAs, e.g. tube/filter combination, tube potential, exposure time) [7].

Optimisation of Digital Mammography

The linear response and wide dynamic range of digital mammographic receptors means that images can be successfully acquired over a large range of doses. This provides a number of possibilities for optimisation and dose reduction, but equally also allows sub-optimal systems to acquire images at higher patient doses than are necessary. The phenomenon of 'exposure creep' has been identified in general digital radiography, where average patient doses can rise due to the natural human inclination to make the images look better, and the fact that images are not rejected for being 'too good'. In digital mammography a universal approach to dose optimisation is a still distant goal (although much research is in progress), but initial findings in well-controlled programmes with properly calibrated automatic exposure devices are that average patient doses with new digital units are lower than those for the screen-film systems they replaced. Modern automatic exposure control software may offer alternative combinations of automatic exposure factors that either optimise for contrast (at the expense of dose) or dose (at the expense of poorer contrast-to-noise ratio).

Display Devices

With a pixel size of 0.05–0.1 mm, and a typical field size for full-field digital mammography of 24×30 cm, a digital mammography image may well be composed of over 10 million pixels. Specialist medical-grade display monitors are required to provide an adequate display for primary reporting. Lower specification displays may be used as 'review' monitors in the mammography room for the practitioner to confirm the quality of image acquisition, but these should not be used for primary reporting. Most digital mammography monitors are now LCD flat-panel displays although some legacy equipment based on cathode-ray-tubes is also in use.

Although there can be some flexibility in the format of simultaneous image display for reporting, in general two high resolution monitors in portrait orientation will be required for a reporting workstation as usually two images need to be compared, but other monitors may be added to allow simultaneous comparison of prior screening mammograms. An additional low resolution monitor may be required to display patient information, work-lists and other textual diagnostic reports.

It is not generally expected that the display monitor will be capable of displaying the full resolution of the recorded image as a complete frame, but that magnification, pan and zoom within the image will be used to display all of the pixels when this is needed. Presently 5 megapixel monitors are recommended (approximately 2,000×2,500 pixels), so that only a proportion of the breast image can be displayed at full resolution.

An important distinguishing feature of medical-grade displays is their maximum luminance. Ideally this should be 450 cd/m^2 or higher (much brighter than standard computer displays) so that a large ratio between maximum and minimum can be maintained, and susceptibility to the effects of ambient lighting is reduced. Careful consideration to the design of the viewing room is still required, however, as the brightness of the monitor itself will light up the room (as well as more obvious light sources such as open doors and windows) and structured reflections of room surroundings and indeed the observer superimposed on the viewed image will reduce its contrast and may introduce distracting features.

The DICOM Greyscale Standard Display Function

DICOM is a medical image interchange standard that allows vendors to transmit images between their imaging systems and PACS, the Picture Archiving and Communication System. One element to DICOM that is particularly important from the radiological reporting standpoint is the Greyscale Standard Display Function (GSDF). This is based on a psychophysical model of the human visual system and is designed to maximise the number of 'just noticeable differences' that a given display can reproduce, and to give a perceptually linear greyscale, with the same small change in contrast visible in a dark part of the image as in a light part. Usually the GSDF boosts the signal in the white, but it will be different for CRT, flat screen displays and (if this is used) hardcopy film. If the GSDF is correctly implemented for a given monitor, it should give the best display that monitor is capable of in the viewing conditions where it is used. The GSDF attempts to make the best of the display's capabilities but cannot make a cheap display in poor viewing conditions as good as an expensive megapixel grey-scale monitor in good viewing conditions.

Display Tools

Display workstations would be expected to provide a user interface providing an efficient throughput of images and a range of display tools typically including

- magnification, zoom and pan (roam)
- contrast and brightness adjustment (windowing)
- image flip and rotation
- black/white inversion
- spatial measurement
- edge enhancement and noise reduction (spatial frequency filtering)

Some of these features are further explained below.

Windowing

Post processing of digital images by windowing is a very powerful feature of digital imaging that also applies to CT, MR and radioisotope imaging. Because in a digital image the brightness of a pixel is dictated by an integer number (the 'pixel number'), there are a finite number of values that the brightness level can take. Digital mammography systems might typically digitise to 12 bits (4,096 grey levels), whereas the display monitor will probably only have a capability of displaying 256 levels of luminance (8 bits). In addition, the human visual system is only capable of distinguishing about 100 grey levels in an image, even under ideal viewing conditions, so it follows that if all the information present in a digital image was displayed on the monitor at once, small differences in contrast, although recorded successfully, would not be distinguishable. The solution

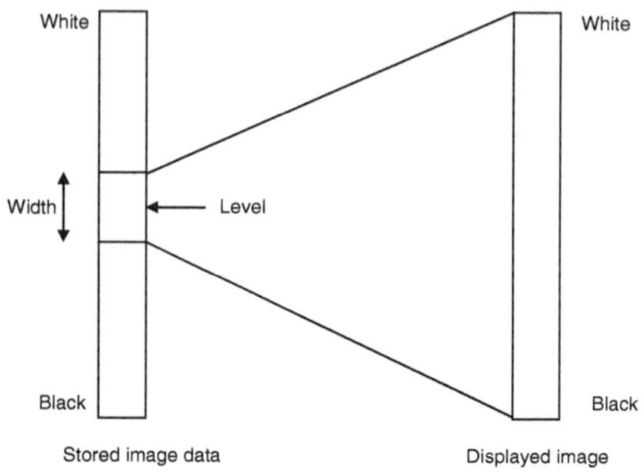

Fig. 16.9 Diagrammatic representation of image display windowing. The display width and level define a subset of the stored image grey levels which is expanded to fit the full luminance range of the display device

to this problem is to display only a selected range of pixel values, thus increasing the displayed contrast for that subset of levels. This 'window' of pixel number values is defined by a window 'width' and window 'level' (Fig. 16.9). By altering the display window width and level settings, the observer can optimise the display of the range of grey levels for the diagnostic task being undertaken, and any contrast recorded in the image can be displayed, but the time taken to make many such adjustments can become a factor in reporting high volumes of images. The user interface for window width and level adjustment is usually quite intuitive, using computer mouse or trackball, and preset window preferences can also save time.

Spatial Frequency Filtering

Images can be thought of and analysed as sets of spatial frequencies. In general, low spatial frequencies are associated with uniform greyness or slowly changing gradients, whilst high spatial frequencies are associated with sudden changes in brightness such as at sharp edges or patterns of dots or lines. By applying a spatial frequency filter, ranges of spatial frequencies can be enhanced or attenuated. Enhancing high spatial frequencies enhances the contrast of sharp edges e.g. microcalcifications and linear structures, and generally 'sharpens' the image. Unfortunately, high

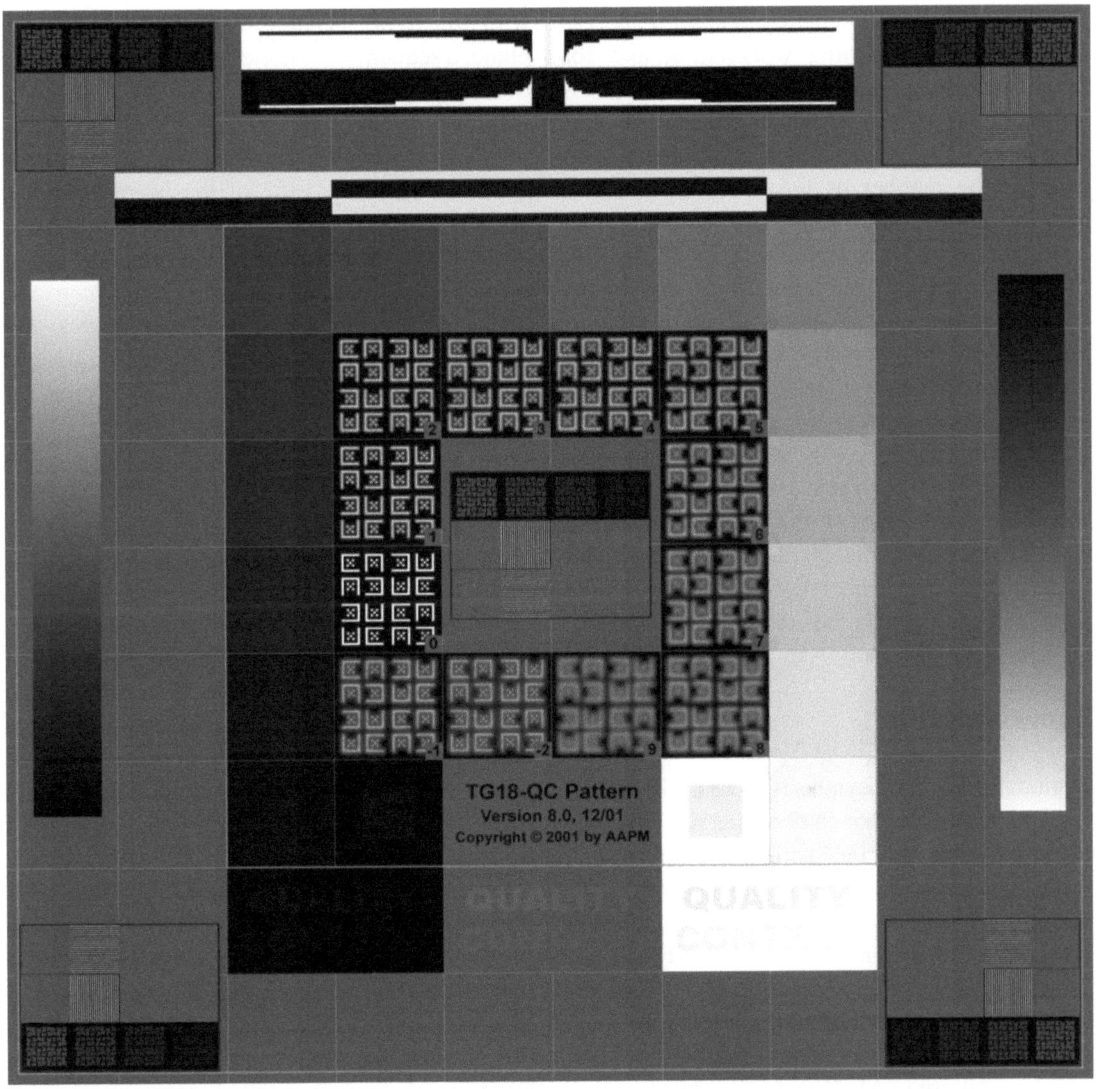

Fig. 16.10 A common quality control test object for display monitor testing. This is the AAPM Topic Group 18 (TG18) test pattern. The pattern features grey scale, image alignment, high spatial resolution and low contrast tests

frequency enhancement comes at the price of also boosting the noise that lies in this frequency band, so subtle enhancement is the most effective. Attenuating high frequencies effectively blurs the image, and this can be used to reduce the appearance quantum noise in some situations. Various layers of image processing, including spatial frequency filtering, are routinely used in digital mammography. Whilst this processing can make improvements to clinical images, it can also cause problems with quality control phantom images, for which the image processing often has to be deselected.

Quality Control of Display Devices

Monitor performance reduces with age, and regular quality control checks are required. Regular user checks should include the systematic visual checking of a test pattern, such as the SMPTE pattern or the AAPM TG-18 pattern (Fig. 16.10).

Images of a suitable pattern should be accessible from the reporting workstation and for review monitors. Quantitative tests of the monitor performance, which include measurements of luminance over a range of grey levels and assessment of the number of 'just noticeable differences' that the monitor can deliver in the lighting conditions where it is used. Some medical-grade monitors support self-calibration, where the monitor makes measurements of its own luminance output, and adjusts its calibration accordingly. The calibration again takes account of room lighting conditions so problems can arise if the lighting in the room at the time of self-calibration is not the same as when it is used for reporting. An element of monitor quality control is cleaning of the display screen, as dust and finger-marks etc. reflect light from within the room and can degrade the contrast of the image.

Tomosynthesis

Digital breast tomosynthesis (DBT) is a 3-D imaging technique that can be used to help overcome the main problem with conventional 2-D imaging, namely that a three-dimensional distribution of X-ray attenuation is being collapsed into a two-dimensional image plane. The result of that collapse is that it is not possible to distinguish between overlying and underlying features, or to visualise the depth relationship between objects. The use of MLO and CC views together helps to some extent, but the ideal would be a 3-D array of X-ray attenuation, from which to display any desired image plane. DBT falls some way short of that ideal, but does provide useful depth information. Further information on tomosynthesis is available in Chap. 30.

Image Acquisition

DBT can be carried out on suitably adapted conventional digital mammography units, making the technique an add-on to most modern designs. The breast is held compressed against the image receptor as normal, but instead of one exposure with the X-ray beam orthogonal to the image plane, a sequence of shorter exposures is made as the tube gantry moves through an angle. The result is a series of images, taken with the source of X-rays stepping through the swing angle which is typically ±15° of the normal vertical position. The projections will be subtly different, as the X-ray shadow of objects close to the top of the breast will appear to move relative to the image frame as the X-ray focus moves, but objects close to the support table will be imaged in the same place (Fig. 16.11).

Reconstruction

In order to produce the tomographic image, the series of projections must be reconstructed into a single image that emphasises features at a particular depth within the breast. In the simplest form of tomosynthesis, this is done by shifting the projection images with respect to the image frame, so that the features at a selected depth all appear in the same place within the frame. These shifted images are then added together. The addition reinforces the contrast of features in the selected plane, where they are in the same position, but tends to blur out objects in other planes.

The degree of blurring (or technically streaking, as the blur occurs in the direction of X-ray tube movement) increases with distance from the selected plane (Fig. 16.12). The result of image reconstruction is therefore an image reminiscent of film-screen tomography, where the observer can focus on objects in the intended image plane, but tends to 'see through' the blurred features in other planes. This is distinct from true tomography (e.g. CT), where each image is a true cross-sectional cut through the object with no overlying or underlying structure. More sophisticated DBT image reconstruction methods based on filtered back projection (a variant of CT reconstruction) or iterative techniques are used in commercial DBT designs, but because of the very limited range of angles at which the projections in DBT are recorded, these still cannot recover enough information to produce pure tomographic slices.

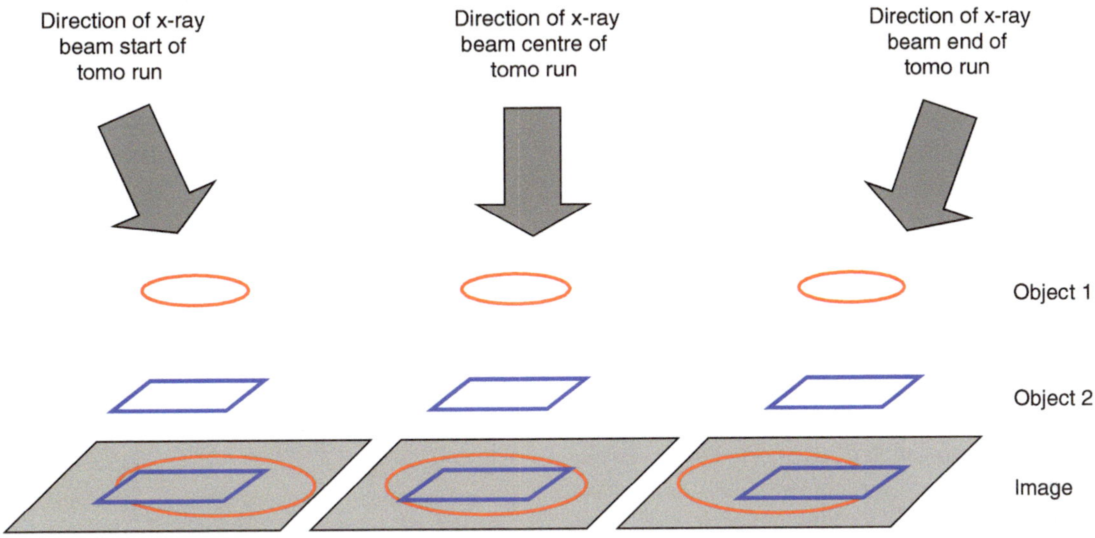

Fig. 16.11 Tomosynthesis image acquisition: the breast is held compressed against the stationary support table, and a sequence of small exposures is made as the tube gantry moves through an angle

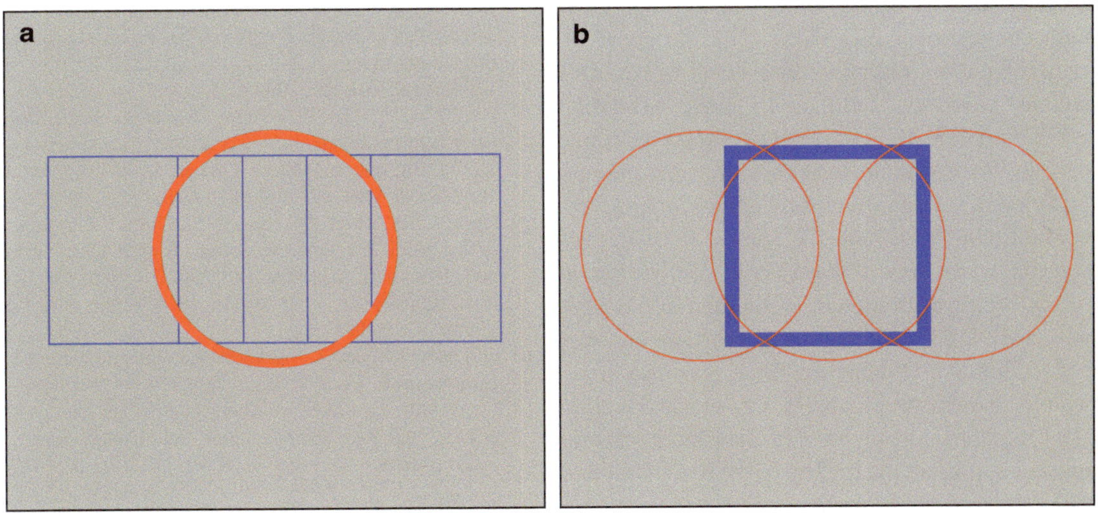

Fig. 16.12 In image (**a**) the individual projection images have been shifted and summed to reinforce the shadow of the circle, close to the top of the breast, leaving the square blurred out. In image (**b**) the images have been shifted less before summation, resulting in reinforcement of the shadow of the square, close to the support table, and blurring of the circle

Image Interpretation

To create a 3-D image stack suitable for mammographic reporting, the tomosynthesis reconstruction process must be repeated with the calculated in-focus plane shifted a few millimetres down from the previous one, and this cycle is repeated to eventually produce an image stack of perhaps 50 or 60 tomosynthesis images. The entire stack of tomosynthesis images can be reconstructed from just the one set of projections.

To report the images, the viewer controls the selected in-focus plane shown on the display screen, and this can be rapidly swept up and down through the image stack. The act of stepping through the images on the display allows the observer to build up a 3-D impression of the relative positions of features within the volume of the breast. For example, a small detail feature, such as a cluster of microcalcifications, will gradually come into sharp focus as the displayed in-focus plane approaches its true depth, then will fade out of focus as displayed image moves beyond it.

Radiation Dose for Tomosynthesis

The radiation dose to the patient from tomographic imaging would be expected to be marginally higher than for conventional 2-D views, because the X-rays forming the projection views at the extremes of the angular swing have to traverse a greater thickness within the compressed breast. Most commercial implementations aim to keep the dose for tomographic views comparable with conventional 2-D views. One proposal to keep the patient radiation dose down for examinations based on DBT is to make available another method of reconstructing the projections, but now to use them to reconstruct a synthetic 2-D view, i.e. an image closely approximating the conventional MLO and CC views. It is argued that the availability of these views could allow a whole breast examination to be carried out just with two DBT acquisitions per breast and no conventional 2-D imaging. This proposal may well in due course provide a way of introducing DBT into the mainstream of breast cancer screening, but at present the quality of the reconstructed 2-D view may not be quite as good as the conventional mammogram due to the approximations involved in its reconstruction.

References

1. Thierry-Chef I, Simonb SL, Weinstockc RM, Kwonb D, Linetb MS. Reconstruction of absorbed doses to fibroglandular tissue of the breast of women undergoing mammography (1960 to the present). Radiat Res [Internet]. 2012;177:92–108. http://dx.doi.org/10.1667/RR2241.1.
2. Gold H, Bassett W, Widoff E. Highlights from the history of mammography. Radiographics. 1990;10:1111–31.
3. Institute of Medicine – National Research Council. In: Nass SJ, Henderson IC, Lashof J, editors. Mammography and beyond: developing technologies for the early detection of breast cancer. 1st ed. Washington, DC: National Cancer Policy Board – Institute of Medicine; 2001. p. 1–311.
4. Joy JE, Penhoet EE, Petitti DB. Saving women's lives – strategies for improving breast cancer detection and diagnosis [Internet]. In: The National Academies, editor. Econ Policy. The National Academies; 2005. p. 1–385. http://www.ncbi.nlm.nih.gov/books/NBK22315/pdf/TOC.pdf.
5. Fass L. Imaging and cancer: a review. Mol Oncol [Internet]. 2008 [cited 25 Jul 2011];2:115–52. http://www.ncbi.nlm.nih.gov/pubmed/19383333.
6. National Breast Screening Quality Assurance. In: Moore AC, Dance DR, Evans DS, Lawinski CP, Pitcher EM, Rust A, et al., editors. The commissioning and routine testing of mammographic X-ray systems. York: Institute of Physics and Engineering in Medicine; 2005. p. 1–146.
7. Bushberg J, Seibert JA, Leidholdt Jr E, Boone J. In: Snyder A, DeGeorge T, editors. The essential physics of medical imaging. 2nd ed. Philadelphia: Lippincott Williams & Wilkins; 2002. p. 1–956.
8. Andolina V, Lyllé S. In: Sabatini P, editor. Mammographic imaging – a practical guide [Internet]. 3rd ed. Baltimore: Wolters Kluwer Health-Lippincott Williams & Wilkins; 2011. p. 1–610.
9. Bassett LW, Hoyt AC, Oshiro T. Digital mammography: clinical image evaluation. Radiol Clin North Am [Internet]. Elsevier Ltd; 2010 [cited 19 Jan 2012];48:903–15. http://www.ncbi.nlm.nih.gov/pubmed/20868893.
10. O' Leary D, Teape A, Hammond J, Rainford L, Grant T. Compression force recommendations in mammography must be linked to image quality. In: European Society of Radiology, editor. Eur Congr Radiol. 2011 [Internet]. Vienna: ECR 2011; 2011. p. 1–19. www.myESR.org4.
11. Poulos A, McLean D. The application of breast compression in mammography: a new perspective. Radiography [Internet]. 2004 [cited 2011 May 16];10:131–7. http://linkinghub.elsevier.com/retrieve/pii/S1078817404000434.
12. Poulos A, Llewellyn G. Mammography discomfort: a holistic perspective derived from women's experiences. Radiography [Internet]. 2005 [cited 5 Aug 2011];11:17–25. http://linkinghub.elsevier.com/retrieve/pii/S1078817404001002.
13. Spuur K, Poulos A, Currie G, Rickard M. Mammography: correlation of pectoral muscle width and the length in the mediolateral oblique view of the breast. Radiography [Internet]. Elsevier Ltd;

2010 [cited 19 Jan 2012];16:286–91. http://linkinghub.elsevier.com/retrieve/pii/S1078817410000581.
14. Bentley K, Poulos A, Rickard M. Mammography image quality: analysis of evaluation criteria using pectoral muscle presentation. Radiography [Internet]. 2008 [cited 29 Apr 2011];14:189–94. http://linkinghub.elsevier.com/retrieve/pii/S1078817407000090.
15. Spuur K, Hung WT, Poulos A, Rickard M. Mammography image quality: model for predicting compliance with posterior nipple line criterion. Eur J Radiol [Internet]. Elsevier Ireland Ltd; 2011 [cited 19 Jan 2012];80:713–8. http://www.ncbi.nlm.nih.gov/pubmed/20621431.
16. Smith A. Fundamentals of digital mammography: physics, technology and practical considerations. Hologic [Internet]. 2005; R-BI-016:1–12. http://www.ncbi.nlm.nih.gov/pubmed/14603590.
17. Yaffe MJ, Rowlands JA. X-ray detectors for digital radiography. Phys Med Biol [Internet]. 1997;42:1–39. http://www.ncbi.nlm.nih.gov/pubmed/9015806.
18. Thierry-Chef I, Simon SL, Weinstock RM, Kwon D, Linet MS. Reconstruction of absorbed doses to fibroglandular tissue of the breast of women undergoing mammography (1960 to the present). Radiat Res [Internet]. 2012 [cited 29 July 2012];177:92–108. http://www.ncbi.nlm.nih.gov/pubmed/21988547.
19. Mackenzie A, Doylo P, Honey I, Marshall N, O'Neil J, Smail M. Measurements of the performance characteristics of diagnostic X-ray system: digital imaging system – IPEM report 32 Part VII. York; 2010. p. 1–125.

17 Equipment Quality Control

Cláudia Sá dos Reis

Introduction

Mammography equipment must be evaluated to ensure that images will be of acceptable diagnostic quality with lowest radiation dose. Quality Assurance (QA) aims to provide systematic and constant improvement through a feedback mechanism to address the technical, clinical and training aspects [1, 2]; Quality Control (QC), in relation to mammography equipment, comprises a series of tests to determine equipment performance characteristics. The introduction of digital technologies promoted changes in QC tests and protocols and there are some tests that are specific for each manufacturer [2]. Within each country specific QC tests should be compliant with regulatory requirements and guidance [1]. Ideally, one mammography practitioner should take overarching responsibility for QC within a service, with all practitioners having responsibility for actual QC testing. All QC results must be documented to facilitate troubleshooting, internal audit and external assessment [3, 4].

Generally speaking, the practitioner's role includes performing, interpreting and recording the QC tests as well as reporting any out of action limits to their service lead. They must undertake additional continuous professional development to maintain their QC competencies [3]. They are usually supported by technicians and medical physicists; in some countries the latter are mandatory. Technicians and/or medical physicists often perform many of the tests indicated within this chapter.

It is important to recognise that this chapter is an attempt to encompass the main tests performed within European countries. Specific tests related to the service that you work within must be familiarised with and adhered too.

Tests for Quality Control

The QC tests in this chapter are based on recommendations from various organisations and documents, specifically: Institute of Physics and Engineering in Medicine (IPEM); National Health Service Breast Screening Programme (NHSBSP) [5, 6]; European Protocol (EP) (EUREF [4, 7, 8]); European Federation of Organisations in Medical Physics (EFOMP) [9]; and International Atomic Energy Agency (IAEA).

EP and EFOMP guidelines have been included because they aim to promote harmonisation of mammography practices within EU countries. EP guidance is disseminated within Europe and to date is adopted in more than 15 countries [10–17]. The NHSBSP guidance (United Kingdom) is used by various countries worldwide [1, 18].

C.S. dos Reis
Escola Superior de Tecnologia da Saúde de Lisboa (ESTeSL), Lisbon School of Health Technology, Lisbon, Portugal
e-mail: claudia.reis@estesl.ipl.pt

P. Hogg et al. (eds.), *Digital Mammography: A Holistic Approach*,
DOI 10.1007/978-3-319-04831-4_17,

IAEA and EFOMP guidelines are the most up-to-date documents for digital mammography QC [3]. For general QC tests, all the above documents provide guidance on periodic testing, to address image acquisition, detection systems, image processing, image display and others tests (e.g. electrical and mechanical tests) [3–6, 19–21].

The tests that are commonly recommended in all the guidance documents are presented in this chapter.

Tests for Acquisition Systems

X-Ray Tube and Generator

Various tests (reproducibility and accuracy, focal spot size, tube output, HVL, etc.) can be performed to assess this part of the equipment. However, with the introduction of digital technologies the majority are no longer done by mammography practitioners due to the stability of the X-ray generators that are currently in use. The QC tests that are in use are those related to dosimetry – tube output and Half Value Layer (HVL) [9].

Procedure and Materials

The performance of the X-ray system is assessed through measurements of the X-ray tube output (in air). Measurements should be undertaken with a calibrated dosimeter [9].

The dosimeter should be positioned at 4 cm from the chest wall edge laterally centred on the image receptor (the perspex it is not positioned on the image receptor but on top of breast support platform) and irradiated using a collimated radiation beam. The compression paddle should be removed for the measurements [4]. Tube output should be measured for all target-filter combinations used in clinical practice (e.g. Mo/Mo, Mo/Rh, Rh/Rh, W/Rh, W/Ag). Repeating this test with the paddle on can be done if you want to ascertain the attenuation of the paddle for dosimetry purposes.

Output measurements need to be repeated using 2 mm aluminium filtration (or 4.5 cm PMMA) attached to the tube port using a broad X-ray beam geometry to mimic the attenuation and scatter of the breast. The output should be measured across a range of mAs values (10, 20, 40, 80, 120 and 180). This data is required to characterise the detector response function (signal transfer function – STP).

Frequency

At equipment acceptance and annual checks. Within the UK this is every 6 months.

Expected Results

Output at 28 kVp for target filter Mo/Mo – the reference acceptable and achievable X-ray tube output values recommended by EUREF are >30 μGy/mAs and >40 μGy/mAs, respectively.

Tests for Detection Systems

Alignment of X-Ray Field to Optical Field

The aim of this test is to evaluate coincidence of X-ray and light fields. The chest wall edge is most important. Misalignment may result in breast tissue being missed or non-breast tissue being imaged: the latter increases dose for no benefit; the former could mean pathology is missed.

Procedure and Materials

The light field edges must be identified using radio-opaque markers, an X-ray image is then produced and evaluated. Difference between X-ray and light fields is assessed.

Frequency

At equipment acceptance and annual checks. Within the UK this is every 6 months.

Expected Results

Misalignment should be less than 5 mm along any edge [4, 6].

Compression Force and Thickness Accuracy

Some systems use compressed breast thickness to auto-select kVp and T/F, consequently it is important to assess the thickness indicator accuracy; thickness reduction is achieved by the application of compression force [3].

Procedures and Materials

Prior to testing compression force, the compression paddle should be inspected to identify physical damage (e.g. cracks). Compression force can be evaluated by placing weighing scales on the breast platform and centred under the compression paddle. The compression paddle should be moved up to the maximum compression force supported by the system (generally 180 or 200 N). Care must be exercised so as not to damage the mammography equipment. Results from the mammography machine and weighing scales should be compared. The next test considers compression force maintenance over 30 s or 1 min – to identify if there is any compression force drop over time [3, 4].

To verify breast thickness readout accuracy display, a rectangular poly-methyl methacrylate (PMMA) phantom with three different thickness (20, 45 and 70 mm) is used. This is aligned with the chest wall and centred on breast platform. Typically 80 N is applied and the machine given thickness readout is recorded. Phantom and machine given readout thickness are then compared.

Frequency

Monthly, or more frequently as required by guidance.

Expected Results

The display value for compression force readout on the mammography machine should be within ±20 N of the display on the weighing scales; if the display on the weighing scales is higher than 200 N the machine should be taken out of action and reported immediately. For breast thickness indicator should be ±5 mm [3, 4].

Signal Transfer Function

Procedures and Materials

The signal transfer property (STP) establishes the relationship between the entrance air kerma at the detector and the pixel value in pre-processed images. It is useful to understand how the detector transforms the input into an output signal.

Measurement of STP can be performed using images produced with an attenuated beam by having 2 mm thick aluminium plate attached to the tube port to mimic the attenuation of a standard breast. The compression paddle (optional) and the grid are removed for the image acquisition. Non-processed (raw) images can be acquired either (a) a standard tube voltage (28 kVp) across a wide range of entrance air kerma values (nominal 12.5, 25, 50, 100, 200 and 400 μGy) or (b) in the UK factors selected by the AEC when exposing a standard breast. The mAs values required to produce the aimed receptor air kerma values are determined from the output measurements previously performed [22].

For each image, measurements of the mean pixel value and standard deviation must be undertaken in the Region of Interest (ROI) of 1 cm^2 at 6 cm from the image chest wall edge [4].

For mammography systems with a linear STP response (DR systems) the mean pixel value should be plotted against the entrance air kerma; linearity is assessed using software [22].

Frequency

For equipment acceptance and 6 monthly checks.

Expected Results

Correlation coefficient should be $R^2 > 0.99$ [4, 22].

Automatic Exposure Control System (AEC)

The AEC controls the exposure to the detector; its performance testing is crucial as it has a direct impact on image quality and patient dose (see also Chap. 15). This test is recommended because it provides information regarding the global performance of mammography equipment [1].

Various methods have been proposed and metrics have been developed, e.g. detector air kerma, detector dose index, pixel value, Signal to noise Ratio (SNR) and Signal difference to Noise Ratio (SdNR) equivalent to Contrast to Noise Ratio (CNR).

Procedures and Materials

Here the SdNR method is explained. SdNR is measured from images produced with a PMMA phantom and a low contrast object (aluminium 0.2 mm thick, >99.9 % purity), see Fig. 17.1 [22].

SdNR and dose should be measured in at least three different thicknesses (20, 45 and 70 mm) which are considered to mimic attenuation and scatter provided by a thin, average and large breast. The PMMA breast phantom is composed of various 0.5 or 1 cm slabs piled up on top of each other to produce the necessary thickness. A small aluminium square (1 cm × 1 cm and 0.2 mm thickness) must be positioned below the top slab at 6 cm from the chest wall edge. In the UK it is placed on top of the bottom slab and then built up with additional PMMA on top.

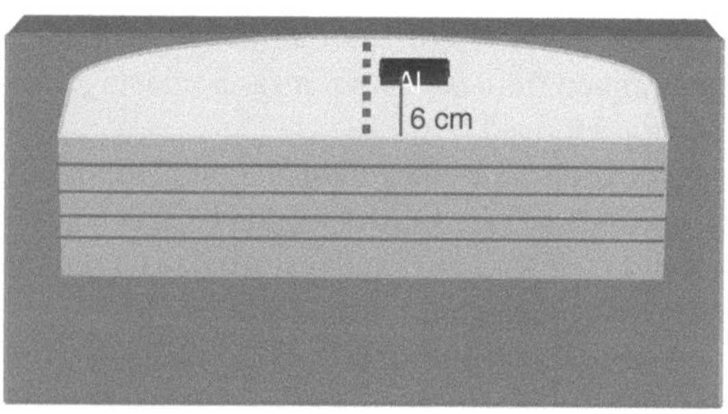

Fig. 17.1 PMMA phantom used to perform the AEC testing

The PMMA phantom is placed on the perspex it is not positioned on the image receptor but on top of breast support platform with an overhang of 5 mm out from the chest wall edge and laterally centred in the image field. The radiation field size should be collimated to cover the complete phantom.

The compression paddle must be positioned in contact with the PMMA slabs and a consistent compression force is recommended e.g. 60 N. For AEC systems with options for positioning the AEC (X-ray sets associated with CR systems and some DR e.g. Hologic Dimensions) the midline position is selected and a region that would not be affected by the Aluminium square.

Images should be acquired using AEC and associated exposure settings typically used in clinical practice. Images are acquired for the three PMMA thicknesses. For the standard thickness (45 mm PMMA) the procedure should be repeated three times.

For thicknesses ≥40 mm, low attenuation material spacers can be positioned at the edges of the phantom to achieve the intended equivalent [breast] thickness. This is important because some mammography systems adjust the X-ray settings according to the detected breast thickness or compression force.

Only raw images with the processing algorithm turned off are used, acquired in a "raw", "unprocessed" or DICOM "for processing" format depending on the system used.

For each image, measurements of the mean pixel value and its standard deviation are performed in ROIs (1 cm^2) in aluminium and the surrounding background. Pixel values are corrected using STP data and SdNR is calculated:

$$SdNR = \frac{\text{mean pixel value}(\text{signal}) - \text{mean pixel value}(\text{background})}{\text{background standard deviation}} \tag{17.1}$$

Table 17.1 Acceptable (Accep.) and Achievable (Achiev.) reference levels for SdNR in mammography proposed by IAEA for thicknesses of 20, 45 and 70 mm [3]

	Compressed breast thickness [mm]					
	20		45		70	
Mammography system	Accep.	Achiev.	Accep.	Achiev.	Accep.	Achiev.
GE 2000D – DR	8.9	12.9	7.9	11.5	6.9	10.0
GE DS – DR	8.9	12.9	7.9	11.5	6.9	10.0
GE Essential – DR	12.7	18.4	11.3	16.5	9.9	14.4
Fuji Amulet – DR	6.1	8.7	5.5	7.8	4.8	6.8
Siemens Inspiration – DR	4.4	6.3	3.9	5.7	3.4	5.0

Frequency

Every 6 months, or more frequently as required within the UK: Daily for Radiographers at 4 cm and monthly for 2 and 6/7 cm.

Expected Results

Using the SdNR method, the IAEA reference values can be used (Table 17.1).

Detector Uniformity and Artefacts

Image receptor uniformity is essential and uniformity testing should be performed regularly. Uniformity problems in digital systems can be caused by inappropriate calibrations of the image field or due to artefacts caused by defects on the detector [9, 23]. There are also noted problems with the target, filters, grid and paddle if looking at the system rather than just detector.

Procedures and Materials

Uniformity can be assessed using flat field uniform images produced with an attenuated X-ray beam with a 2 mm Al foil attached to the tube port. Most manufacturers supply a large area block of PMMA which can sit over the breast support platform as an alternative to Al over the tube. The image receptor can be imaged using clinical exposure parameters to achieve an air kerma of approximately 100 μGy at the image detector. The images can be acquired either (a) without grid and without compression paddle and also without processing (raw images) or (b) with the grid to asess the system clinically. A large radiation field should be used (broad beam), typical for clinical use.

Pixel values should be corrected using STP data before making ROI measurements. The mean pixel value should be measured for 5 ROI (1 cm^2 each), distributed as shown in Fig. 17.2: one at the centre of the image and the other 4 at the centre of each quadrant [22].

Frequency

Following equipment service to tube or detector and more frequently as required by protocol. Within the UK: Every 6 months by technicians/physicists and monthly by Radiographers.

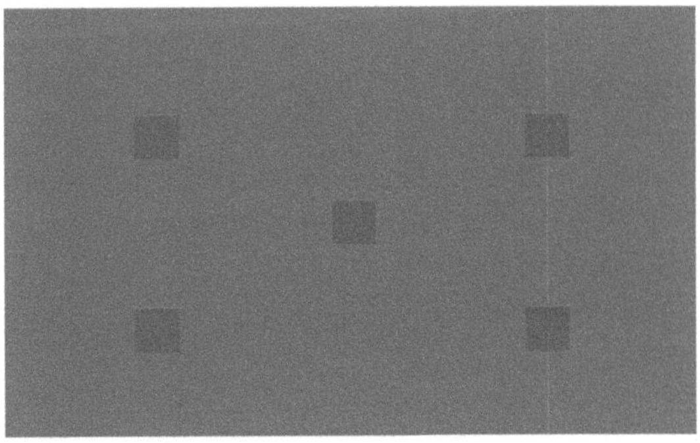

Fig. 17.2 Reference ROIs for uniformity measurements

Expected Results

Mean SNR, calculated for all 5 ROIs should present a maximum deviation of ≤15 % [4].

The images can be assessed for artefacts. Image artefacts can have different origins, including client, practitioner and equipment-related.

The artefacts related to the client can be caused by motion or due to the anatomical characteristics (for instance the thin breast artefact (<20 mm) that is caused because it is possible that during compression, the paddle edges may be included at the corners of the image creating the artefact) [24].

The practitioner can introduce artefacts during the positioning of the breast, improper detector handling (CR systems) and inadequate screen cleaning procedures (CR systems) than can cause white dots due to dust and parts of the coating of the cassette [25].

The most common artefacts related to the equipment are those related to software processing errors and those that are caused by the specific architecture of the detector, namely geometric distortion due to incorrect stitching of sub-images and inhomogeneities towards the lateral sides of the image. Absence of detector calibration can also cause artefacts due to imperfections and differences in gain of each individual segments of the detector. The grid lines can also appear causing artefacts due to the stopping or slowing down of grid and also misplacement and vibration [23–25].

Frequency

Weekly, following an equipment service in which the image acquisition system was modified or following correction software [9, 23]. Within it is every 6 months.

Expected Results

The images should be artefact free. Importantly, dead pixels, missing lines or columns should not be visible in the area that is clinically relevant.

Test to Evaluate Image Retention (Ghosting)

In some digital imaging systems signal retention in the image receptor may be observed following radiation exposure, e.g. a ghost image superimposed on the subsequent image. This effect may cause artefacts and degrade image quality.

Procedures and Materials

Image retention can be tested by irradiating a rectangular PMMA phantom with dimensions $18 \times 24 \times 45$ mm^3, using typical clinical exposure settings with grid in.

The first image should be produced with the phantom positioned with the longest side perpendicular to the chest wall edge, covering half of the perspex it is not positioned on the image receptor but on top of breast support platform. A second image is obtained with the phantom repositioned, centred in the breast platform covering it as much as possible with an 0.1 mm thick Al sheet placed (centred) on top to generate a low contrast signal. A time interval of one minute should occur between both exposures and the 2 images need to be acquired in raw format (no processing).

The mean pixel value is measured in 3 ROI (1 cm^2), within the area attenuated by the Al foil and in the surrounding background as illustrated in Fig. 17.3. The measured pixel values need to be corrected with STP data and then used to calculate an image retention factor:

$$Image\,retention\,factor = \frac{\text{mean pixel value}(\text{ROI}3) - \text{mean pixel value}(\text{ROI}2)}{\text{mean pixel value}(\text{ROI}1) - \text{mean pixel value}(\text{ROI}2)} \quad (17.2)$$

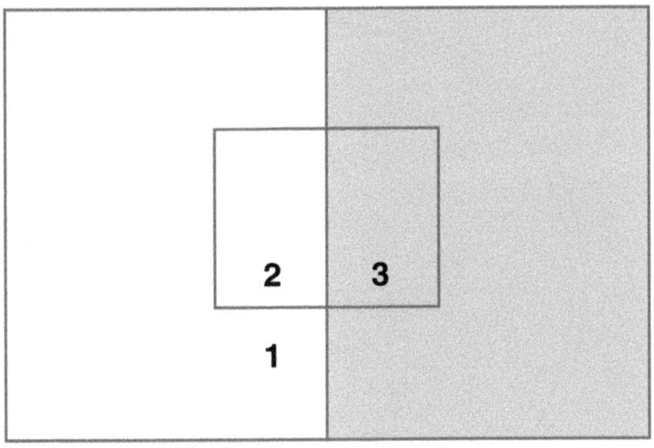

Fig. 17.3 Image retention – positioning of ROI measurements to determine image retention factor. *White area* represents the area with the PMMA attenuation during first exposure

Frequency

Yearly or after detector replacement. Within it is every 6 months

Expected Results

The results can be compared with a reference value of 0.3 as proposed by EP [4].

Image Quality Assessment Using Phantoms

A common method to assess image quality (IQ) uses images produced with test objects and phantoms. This method has limitations due to the models in use. The models do not represent perfectly the breast characteristics and for that reason it is very difficult to establish an acceptable level of diagnostic IQ related to clinical images. However, it is accepted that when a technical image offers adequate quality the clinical image should also be adequate [9]. It is also easier to implement a technical approach with test objects to monitor the quality due to the reproducibility.

There are several phantoms for IQ monitoring. For each, the details that are analysed vary; similarly the methodologies and reference/tolerance values also vary [1].

IQ can be assessed by observers or software. Observer methodologies are outlined in Chap. 16. A limiting factor of observer studies concerns variability; variability is eliminated in software-based approaches. The training of observers is very important to minimise intra- and inter-observer variability; training should also improve validity. Observer studies and software analysis both have a place in IQ analysis.

EFOMP guidelines outline seven different phantoms for mammography image quality (IQ) analysis: American College of Radiology (ACR) mammography accreditation phantom, CIRS Phantom (model 011A), TORMAS, TORMAX, TORMAM, CDMAM and MAM/DIGI. These guidelines are valuable when assisting with the selection phantom for services and also to identify the test methodologies [9]. There are other phantoms, including DMAM2 and QUART, and those dedicated to other breast modalities such as VOXMAX and CIRS (model 020 BR3D for tomosynthesis systems) [26, 27]. Regardless of phantom, it is necessary to define a baseline in order to identify changes over time [9].

Next we will consider a methodology to assess images produced with a phantom that is composed of two parts (1). technical (2). clinical (TORMAM).

Image Quality Assessment with TORMAM (Assessment of Low Contrast Detail)

TORMAM is designed for quick and easy use on a routine basis to provide regular IQ assessment.

One part of the phantom contains a range of filaments, micro-particles and low-contrast detail that aim to mimic pathological features in the breast: 6 groups of multi-directional filaments, 6 groups of micro-calcification in the range 300–100 μm and 6 groups of 3 low-contrast detail subgroups. These details are sensitive to the dynamic range of mammography, noise and unsharpness and can be used to obtain an IQ score.

Another part of the phantom contains a structure that mimics the appearance of breast tissue; it contains micro-calcification clusters, fibrous

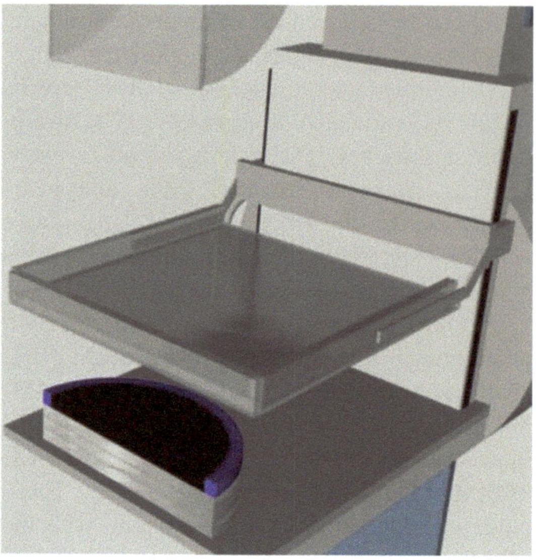

Fig. 17.4 TORMAM phantom on the top of D shaped PMMA for image acquisition (Courtesy of Mário Oliveira)

material and nodules. This part provides a more realistic breast image.

Procedures and Materials

Images should be produced using 3 cm rectangular or D shaped PMMA on breast support and then TORMAM on top of PMMA. A compression force of 60 N should be applied and the images are acquired using the AEC mode in clinical practice (Figs. 17.4 and 17.5).

When TORMAM images are reviewed by observers' ambient light level should be low and the monitor should be free from reflections.

Frequency

Practitioners: Weekly
Physicists/technicians: 6 monthly

Expected Results

There is no established acceptability criteria for this phantom yet the scores are established for the mammography system and compared for any degradation over time.

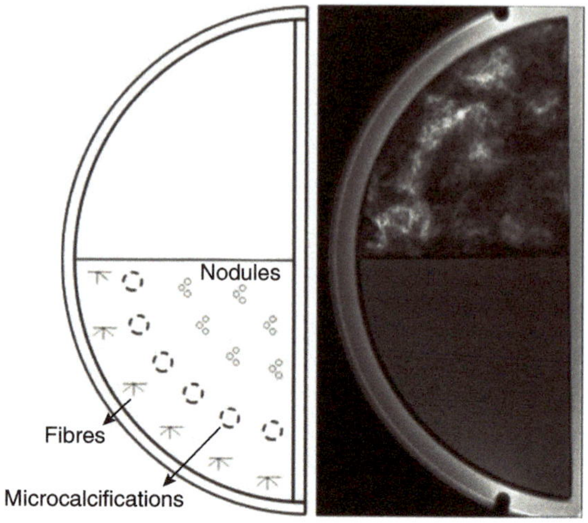

Fig. 17.5 TORMAM phantom: phantom: schematic and radiographic [28]

The maximum possible score is 72 for the fibrous component, 18 for microcalcifications and 54 for nodules. The maximum score is 144.

It is accepted that a higher score corresponds to better IQ. Using CDMAM phantom it is also possible to perform software analysis of IQ, thereby providing an objective and highly reproducible alternative to using observers.

References

1. Reis C, Pascoal A, Sakellaris T, Koutalonis M. Quality assurance and quality control in mammography: a review of available guidance worldwide. Insights Imaging [Internet]. 2013 [cited 2014 Jan 28];4:539–53. http://www.ncbi.nlm.nih.gov/pubmed/23912879.
2. Andolina V, Lyllé S. In: Sabatini P, editor. Mammographic imaging – a practical guide [Internet]. 3rd ed. Baltimore: Wolters Kluwer Health-Lippincott Williams & Wilkins; 2011. p. 1–610. http://wk-trusted-auth.ipublishcentral.com/services/trusted-auth/reader/isbn/9781605470313?partnerKey=w1WcOVItAWsvkr2CoOOemMyBXE6EFM/yNbWMX+Gkk7o=&userID=eswyJCiLE26c9AecOR7noM3XN0JfIOReRnBtBC7nuadNdiW+8BB4hEt48lhJ1KPcjPMg40qOlB3jRFAxfyjAng==.
3. International Atomic Energy Agency. Quality assurance programme for digital mammography. Young. Vienna: International Atomic Energy Agency; 2011.

4. European Communities/EUREF. In: Perry N, Broeders M, de Wolf C, Törnberg S, Holland R, von Karsa L, editors. European guidelines for quality assurance in breast cancer screening and diagnosis [Internet]. 4th ed. http://www.euref.org/european-guidelines. Luxembourg: European Communities; 2006 [cited 19 Jan 2012]. p. 1–432. http://www.euref.org/european-guidelines.
5. National Health Care Breast Screening Programme. Commissioning and routine testing of full field digital mammography systems – NHSBSP equipment report 0604. London; 2009. p. 1–58.
6. National Breast Screening Quality Assurance. In: Moore AC, Dance DR, Evans DS, Lawinski CP, Pitcher EM, Rust A, et al., editors, The commissioning and routine testing of mammographic X-ray systems. York: Institute of Physics and Engineering in Medicine; 2005. p. 1–146.
7. Bosmans H, Engen R van, Heid P, Lazzari B, Schopphoven S, Thijssen M, et al. EUREF type testing protocol. Nijmegen: European Communities/EUREF; 2011. p. 1–20.
8. Lelivelt H, Ongeval C van, Jacobs J, Bun P, Bosmans H, Engen R van, et al. EUREF type testing – clinical evaluation protocol. Nijmegen: European Communities/EUREF; 2010. p. 1–12.
9. European Federation of Organisations for Medical Physics: Working Group on Mammography. Quality Control in Digital Mammography [Internet]. Press. 2014. http://www.efomp.org/index.php/ct-menu-item-3/112-science/246-working-group-on-mammography.
10. Ciraj-Bjelac O, Faj D, Stimac D, Kosutic D, Arandjic D, Brkic H. Good reasons to implement quality assurance in nationwide breast cancer screening programs in Croatia and Serbia: results from a pilot study. Eur J Radiol [Internet]. Elsevier Ireland Ltd; 2009 [cited 19 Jan 2012];78:122–8. http://www.ncbi.nlm.nih.gov/pubmed/19896314.
11. Thierens H, Bosmans H, Buls N, De Hauwere A, Bacher K, Jacobs J, et al. Typetesting of physical characteristics of digital mammography systems for screening within the Flemish breast cancer screening programme. Eur J Radiol [Internet]. 2009 [cited 16 May 2011];70:539–48. http://www.ncbi.nlm.nih.gov/pubmed/18374533.
12. Ng K-H, Jamal N, DeWerd L. Global quality control perspective for the physical and technical aspects of screen-film mammograph--mage quality and radiation dose. Radiat. Prot. Dosimetry [Internet]. 2006 [cited 16 May 2011];121:445–51. http://www.ncbi.nlm.nih.gov/pubmed/16709704.
13. Avramova-Cholakova S, Vassileva J. Pilot study of patient and phantom breast dose measurements in Bulgaria. Polish J Med Phys Eng [Internet]. 2008 [cited 5 Aug 2011];14:21–32. http://versita.metapress.com/openurl.asp?genre=article&id=doi:10.2478/v10013-008-0003-3.
14. Zdesar U. Reference levels for image quality in mammography. Radiat Prot Dosim [Internet]. 2008 [cited 30 Mar 2011];129:170–2. http://www.ncbi.nlm.nih.gov/pubmed/18375465.
15. Nikodemová D, Horváthová M, Salát D. Implementation of QA and QC standards in radiology in Slovakia. Radiat Prot Dosim [Internet]. 2005 [cited 16 May 2011];117:274–6. http://www.ncbi.nlm.nih.gov/pubmed/16461525.
16. Shannoun F, Schanck JM, Scharpantgen A, Wagnon MC, Ben Daoud M, Back C. Organisational aspects of mammography screening in digital settings: first experiences of Luxembourg. Radiat Prot Dosim [Internet]. 2008 [cited 20 Dec 2010];129:195–8. http://www.ncbi.nlm.nih.gov/pubmed/18448438.
17. Hemdal B, Herrnsdorf L, Andersson I, Bengtsson G, Heddson B, Olsson M. Average glandular dose in routine mammography screening using a Sectra MicroDose Mammography unit. Radiat Prot Dosim [Internet]. 2005 [cited 14 Dec 2011];114:436–43. http://www.ncbi.nlm.nih.gov/pubmed/15933152.
18. Committee on New Approaches to Early Detection and Diagnosis of Breast Cancer; National Cancer Policy Board; Board on Science, Technology and EPP and GAD. Saving Women's Lives: Strategies for Improving Breast Cancer Detection and Diagnosis. In: Joy JE, Penhoet EE, Petitti DB, editors. Economic policy. Washington: The National Academies Press; 2005. p. 1–362.
19. National Healthcare System Breast Screening Programme (NHSBSP). Guidance notes for equipment evaluation: protocol for user evaluation of imaging equipment for mammographic screening and assessment NHSBSP equipment report 0703. Sheffield; 2007. p. 1–54.
20. International Atomic Energy Agency. In: International Atomic Energy Agency, editor. Quality assurance programme for screen film mammography. Vienna: International Atomic Energy Agency; 2009. p. 1–158.
21. The National Cancer Screening Service. In: The National Cancer Screening Service Board, editor. Guidelines for quality assurance in mammography screening [Internet]. 3rd ed. Natl Cancer Screen Serv Dublin: Members of the Quality Assurance Committee/The National Cancer Screening Service Board; 2008. p. 1–163. http://www.ncbi.nlm.nih.gov/pubmed/21586679.
22. Mackenzie A, Doylo P, Honey I, Marshall N, O'Neil J, Smail M. Measurements of the performance characteristics of diagnostic X-ray system: digital imaging system – IPEM report 32 Part VII. York; 2010. p. 1–125.
23. Bick U, Diekmann F, editors. Digital Mammography [Internet]. Berlin/Heidelberg: Springer; 2010 [cited 19 Mar 2014]. p. 1–222. http://www.springerlink.com/index/10.1007/978-3-540-78450-0.
24. Ayyala RS, Chorlton M, Behrman RH, Kornguth PJ, Slanetz PJ. Digital mammographic artifacts on full-field systems: what are they and how do I fix them? Radiographics [Internet]. 2008 [cited 20 May 2012];28:1999–2008. http://www.ncbi.nlm.nih.gov/pubmed/19001654.
25. Van Ongeval C, Jacobs J, Bosmans H. Artifacts in digital mammography. JBR-BRT. 2008;91:262–3.

26. Leeds. Leeds test objects. TOR MAs TOR MAX [Internet]. North Yorkshire; 2011;1–3. www.leedstestobjects.com.
27. Brunner CC, RJ, Acciavatti MB, Bakic PR, Maidment ADA, Williams MB, Kaczmarek R, Chakrabarti K. Breast Imaging. In: Maidment ADA, Bakic PR, Gavenonis S, editors. 11th Int. Work. IWDM 2012, Philadelphia, 8–11 July 2012. Proc. Pennsylvania: Springer; 2012. p. 284–91.
28. Leeds Test Objects Ltd. Products Mammography TOR MAM [Internet]. Leeds Test Objects. 2014 [cited 3 Mar 2014]. http://www.leedstestobjects.com/modules/products/product_setup/file_library/TORMAMproductspecifications.pdf.php?module_name=products/product_setup&product_name=TOR MAM&group_name=Mammography.

Radiation Dose in Mammography

18

Ingrid Helen Ryste Hauge

Introduction

A certain proportion of the radiation energy which is generated in the x-ray tube will penetrate the breast and an image (mammogram) based on the density variations inside the breast is formed. The beam of x-rays that does not penetrate the breast and reach the detector is absorbed in the breast in different ways as a radiation dose. The radiation dose within the breast decreases rapidly with increasing depth. The transmitted photons that reach the detector are carriers of diagnostic information.

The radiation dose is measured for several reasons: (a) to assess the performance of mammographic imaging equipment, (b) to compare imaging systems, (c) to comply with regulations and techniques, (d) in order to perform benefit-risk analysis, (e) to answer questions regarding dose level from patients and physicians and (f) as an important part of mammographic quality control [1–3].

In mammographic screening there is a strict demand on quality assurance. The reason for this is that apparently healthy women are being invited to an x-ray examination. A compromise between keeping the doses as low as possible and obtaining adequate image quality needs to be fulfilled [4, 5]. The principle of keeping the doses as low as possible is known as the ALARA principle ("as low as reasonably achievable") within radiation protection.

Radiation effects on female breast cancer rates have been widely studied [6–14]. The reason for this is that breast tissue appears to be relatively radiosensitive and further because breast cancer is the most common cancer among women worldwide [15].

Definition of Kerma and Absorbed Dose

Kerma (kinetic energy released per unit mass) is defined as the initial kinetic energy of all secondary charged particles *liberated* per unit mass at a point of interest by uncharged particles [16]. For x-rays used for medical imaging the kerma is usually expressed in air (K_a).

The absorbed dose, D, is defined as the mean energy *deposited* (or imparted) after interaction with ionising radiation per unit mass of the matter (medium). The SI unit of absorbed dose is J/kg and this unit has been assigned the name *gray* (Gy). In mammography the doses are in the mGy (milligray ($0.01\,Gy$)) area. The absorbed

I.H.R. Hauge
Section for diagnostic physics, The Intervention Centre, Oslo University Hospital, Rikshospitalet, 4950 Nydalen, N-0424 Oslo, Norway
e-mail: inheha@ous-hf.no

P. Hogg et al. (eds.), *Digital Mammography: A Holistic Approach*,
DOI 10.1007/978-3-319-04831-4_18,

dose is a very useful quantity for the prediction of biological effects, and it is the basic physical quantity in radiation biology, radiology, and radiological protection [17]. Further, it is used for all types of ionising radiation.

Under special conditions, which are assumed to occur when measuring the radiation doses in mammography, kerma is numerically equal to the absorbed dose [16]. The most common method for specifying output (radiation dose) of x-ray tubes used for medical imaging is to measure the air kerma free-in-air on the central axis of the x-ray beam at a specific distance from the focal spot.

Tube Output and Radiation Dose

The output (radiation dose) from a generator is related to kilovolts (*kV*), tube current (*mA*) and exposure time (*s*): there is a linear relationship between the current-time-product (*mAs*) and radiation output for each kilovoltage setting [18]. The dose increases with increasing *kV* and increasing *mAs*.

Patient Dose in Mammography: The Definition of Mean Glandular Dose (MGD)

The proliferative tissue or stem cells within the terminal ductolobular units is the most radiation sensitive tissue [19–22]. As a result, there is agreement that the average dose to the glandular tissue, or the mean glandular dose (MGD), is the most appropriate dosimetric quantity to predict the risk of carcinogenesis [22, 23]. The MGD gives an indication of the degree of ionisation of glandular tissue in the breast due to exposure from x-rays.

Some assumptions are made in order to determine the MGD: (a) that compression is applied, (b) that there is an outer layer of adipose tissue surrounding the breast, and (c) that the breast contains a uniform mix of adipose and glandular tissue [1]. The glandularity, glandular fraction or mammographic density of the breast refers to the simplified partition between glandular tissue (the radiation-sensitive component) and adipose tissue. A breast composed of half adipose tissue and half glandular tissue would have a glandularity of 50 %.

The MGD is affected by

- Depth from the entrance surface of the compressed breast
- Compressed breast thickness (compression)
- Breast composition (fibroglandular/glandular content, adipose content, etc.)
- Beam quality (target, filter, *kV*)
- Tube current (*mAs*)
- Detector characteristics

Estimating the Mean Glandular Dose (MGD) for Screen Film Mammography (SFM) and Full-Field Mammography Units (FFDM)

The MGD cannot be measured directly, but needs to be estimated based on the entrance surface air kerma and so-called conversion factors:

$$MGD = entrance\,surface\,air\,kerma \\ \times conversion\,factors$$

In practice, the entrance surface air kerma is measured with a dosimeter at the top surface of the breast, without backscatter, for each exposure. The conversion factors, or the normalised glandular dose, are the amount of effective ionisation in the breast per unit entrance surface air kerma. These factors are based on simulations of photon transport in tissue; so-called Monte Carlo techniques [1, 2, 23, 24].

In order to estimate the conversion factors a compressed breast phantom is used [25]. A computer programme simulated each photon and the conversion factors were established based on the paths and energy deposition of the photons. With the emergence of new target-/filter-combinations the technical parameters and imaging protocols have changed over the years, and there-

Table 18.1 Typical target-/filter-combinations applied in mammography

		Target		
		Mo	**Rh**	**W**
Filter	**Mo**	Mo/Mo	Mo/Rh	
	Rh		Rh/Rh	W/Rh
	Al			W/Al
	Ag			W/Ag

fore new conversion factors have had to be established. Different conversion coefficients have been developed by different research groups [22, 25–29]. EUREF[1] uses the conversion factors published by Dance et al. in 1990, 2000 and 2009 for estimations of the MGD [25, 28–30].

The conversion factors depend on physical qualities of the radiated breast (compressed breast thickness, glandular content) and the radiation quality (represented by the measured half value layer (HVL)). The HVL, which is measured in mm aluminium (Al), has to be measured for each applied radiation quality (target, filter, *kV*) when exposing the women to radiation. Typical target-/filter-combinations are shown in Table 18.1.

In accordance with Dance et al. the MGD can be expressed as:

$$D = Kgcs$$

K is the kerma measured in air at the entrance surface of the compressed breast, without backscatter (entrance surface air kerma), while *g*, *c* and *s* are the conversion factors, which are tabulated in published papers [25, 28].

The radiation output is measured for a specific breast thickness (45 mm) and then the inverse square law is applied in order to find the kerma for any other applied compressed breast thicknesses. The radiation output is measured in *mGy/mAs* (or *μGy/mAs*), and for each exposure the radiation output must be multiplied with the applied *mAs* for that exposure, in order to find the entrance dose.

g is the conversion factor from kerma measured in air to MGD [28]. The *g*-factor depends on the compressed breast thickness and HVL (Fig. 18.1). The HVL needs to be measured, while the compressed breast thickness is

[1]EUREF, the European Reference Organization for Quality Assured Breast Screening and Diagnostic Services, is a pan European organization, widely drawn from different Member States and is operated on a non-profit making basis. At the present time the administrative office is located in Nijmegen where facilities and administrative staff are available. The goal of EUREF is to promote high quality mamma-care in Europe.

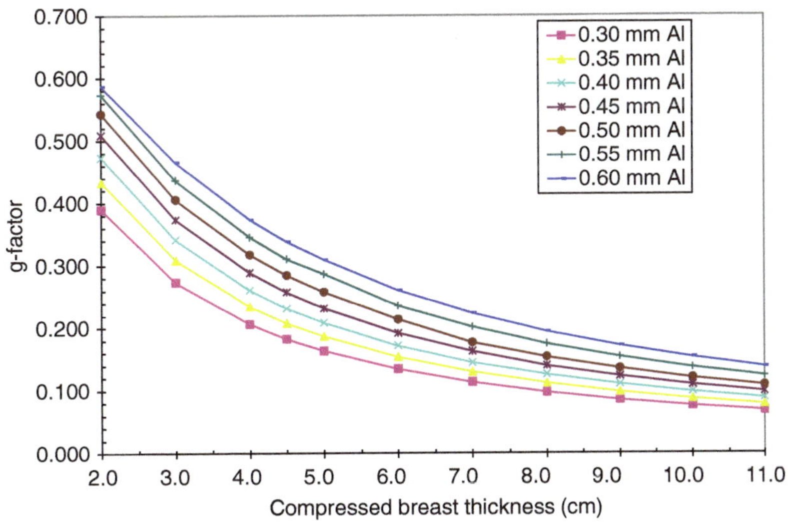

Fig. 18.1 The *g*-factor as a function of half value layer (HVL) and compressed breast thickness (cm). Courtesy of: Kirsti Bredholt, Norwegian Radiation Protection Authority (NRPA), Norway

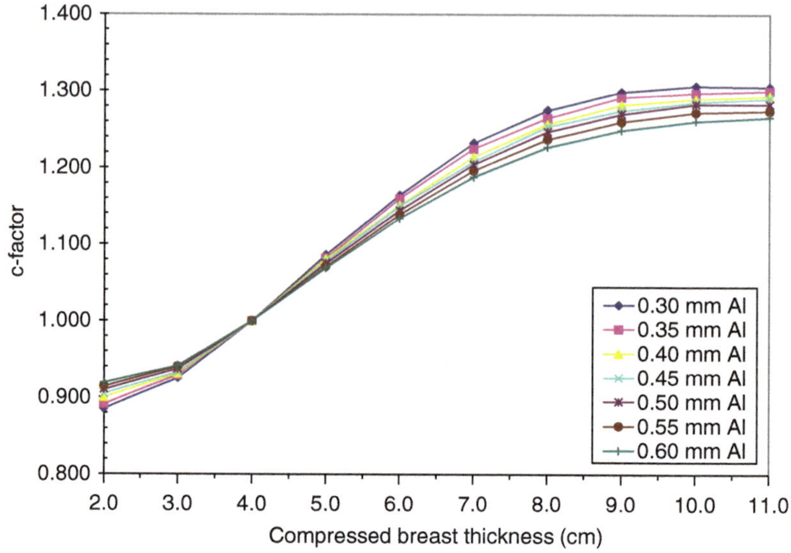

Fig. 18.2 The *c*-factor as a function of half value layer (HVL) and compressed breast thickness (cm) for average breasts for women in the age group 50–64 years

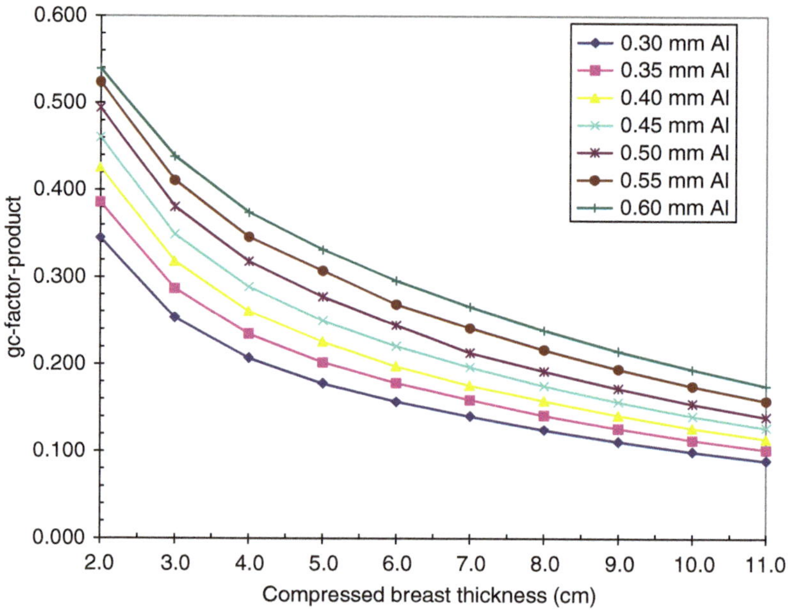

Fig. 18.3 The product of the *g*-factor and *c*-factor as a function of half value layer (HVL) and compressed breast thickness (cm). The *c*-factors used are those for average breasts for women in the age group 50–64 years

displayed on the mammography unit. The displayed and measured compressed breast thickness may not be in accordance with each other, and this will result in uncertainties in the estimation of the MGD [31–36].

c is the conversion factor which corrects for glandular content different from 50 % [25]. The *c*-factor depends on the compressed breast thickness, HVL and glandular content. In order to simplify calculations *c*-factors based on the average glandular content for the two age groups 40–49 years and 50–64 years have been tabulated [25]. The *c*-factors for the age group 50–64 years are shown in Fig. 18.2, and the product of the *g*- and *c*-factors are shown in Fig. 18.3. In the beginning it was assumed that the breast was composed of 50 % fibroglandular tissue and 50 % fat, but this was found not to be the case, and therefore a factor (the

Table 18.2 Tabulated s-factors from Dance et al. [25, 28, 29]

Target	Filter	s-factor
Mo	Mo	1.000
Mo	Rh	1.017
Rh	Rh	1.061
Rh	Al	1.044
W	Rh	1.042
W	Ag	1.042
W	Al	1.069–1.212[a]

[a]Depending on compressed breast thickness [29]

c-factor) was needed that corrects for the variation in glandular content between women. The glandular content has been shown to decrease with increasing age [25, 37, 38]. In order to determine the breast glandularity breasts and tissue equivalent materials of various thicknesses and compositions were exposed using the automatic exposure control (AEC) of the x-ray sets [25]. Then the exposure factors of the breasts and tissue equivalent materials were compared in order to determine the glandularity for the compressed breasts of a given thickness. The glandularity was found to decrease with increasing compressed breast thickness [25].

A study of volumetric breast densities found that the mean compositions, expressed as percent fibroglandular tissue (including the skin), varied from 13.7 to 25.6 % with an overall mean of 19.3 % (BI-RADS[2] category 1) [37]. 95 % of the women had volumetric breast density below 45 % (BI-RADS category 2). Hence, the "50-50" breast is not a representative model of the breast composition.

The s-factor is the conversion factor which corrects for target-/filter-combinations different from molybdenum/molybdenum (Mo/Mo) [25, 29]. Some mammography units choose target/filter/kV based on the compressed breast thickness, while others choose the target/filter/kV based on the breast composition (fibroglandular/glandular content, adipose content, etc.). The s-factor varies with the selected target/filter/kV combination, with the exception of the target-/filter-combination W/Al, for which the s-factor also varies with the compressed breast thickness (Table 18.2).

[2] BI-RADS is an abbreviation of Breast imaging-reporting and data system and is defined by the American College of Radiology. A breast density of less than 25 % glandular tissue is categorised as category 1. Breasts categorised as category 1 are almost entirely made up of fat. Breast densities between 25 % and 50 % glandular tissue are categorised as category 2, and these breasts contain scattered fibroglandular densities.

Estimating the Dose for Digital Breast Tomosynthesis (DBT) Units

DBT uses multiple low-dose radiographic exposures taken at different angles to generate a data set. From this data set 3-dimensional images are reconstructed. The radiation dose for one-view DBT (2.39 ± 0.60 mGy) is approximately equal to a two-view FFDM examination consisting of a CC and MLO view (2.50 ± 0.05 mGy) [39, 40]. In other words a DBT examination roughly doubles the radiation exposure compared with that of a standard examination on a FFDM unit.

The formalism for DBT introduces t-factors for the calculation of breast dose from a single projection and T-factors for a complete exposure series. Dance et al. have proposed the following formalism:

$$D(\theta) = K\,gcs\,t(\theta)$$

The formalism is based on the formalism of the estimation of the 2D breast dose, as explained in the previous section. The dose (D) and t-factor are functions of the projection angle θ. The dose $D(\theta)$ gives the dose for a single projection angle θ. The incident air kerma (K) is measured for the projection angle 0° (no angulation). $t(\theta)$ is fairly independent of breast glandularity and the choice of x-ray spectrum, but varies significantly with projection angle and compressed breast thickness. An increase in projection angle will result in a decrease in $t(\theta)$, due to the changes in geometry. The variation of the factor $t(\theta)$ with compressed breast thickness increases with increasing projection angle. Sechopoulos et al. have used a similar formalism [41].

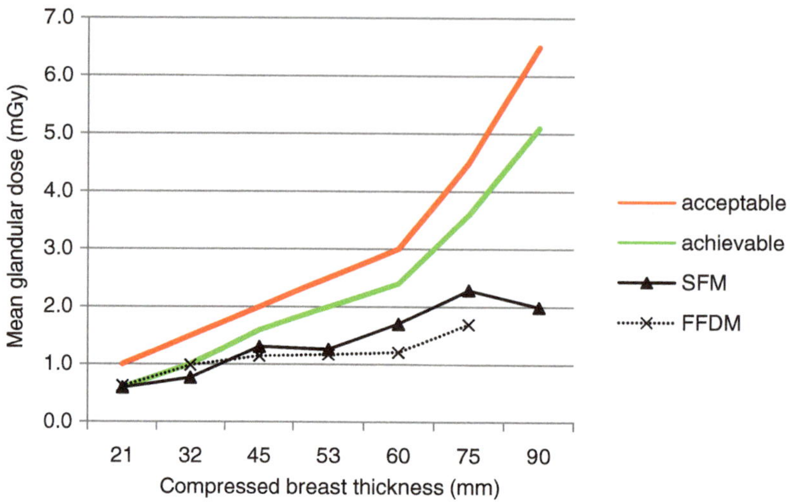

Fig. 18.4 The mean glandular dose as a function of compressed breast thickness for the cranio-caudal (CC) view for screen film mammography (SFM) systems and full-field digital mammography systems (FFDM) used in the Norwegian Breast Cancer Screening Program (NBCSP) [50]. Also, the achievable and acceptable level for the maximum average glandular dose of PMMA breast thickness dose to equivalent breasts as defined by EUREF, the European Reference Organization for Quality Assured Breast Screening and Diagnostic Services, is shown

For a complete examination Dance et al. expresses the 3D dose D_T as [3]:

$$D_T = K_T \, gcs \, T$$

T is a sum over all the projections and the partitions of the tube loading for the examination between the different projections. The *T*-factor is by definition the ratio between the dose for conventional projection mammography and the dose for tomosynthesis if the same tube loading and x-ray spectrum are used.

The previous equations are valid for the Hologic Selenia Dimensions system and Siemens Inspiration, and values for the *T*-factors are tabulated in Dance et al. (2011) [3].[3]

For the Sectra system, which applies a scanning geometry with a narrow beam, the incident air kerma is determined for a complete scan of the system at the same tube loading as the patient exposure. The 3D dose is found from the following equation:

$$D_S = K_S \, gcs \, T_S$$

[3] *T* depend on the number, position and weights of the individual projections, and the tabulated values should only be used when the tube loading for each projection is the same.

The incident air kerma K_S is calculated for a single scan of the Sectra system. The factor T_S is tabulated by Dance et al. [3].

Entrance Dose and Mean Glandular Dose (MGD) Provided by the Mammography Unit

Some SFM and FFDM systems display the MGD value. The different manufacture of mammography units may have used conversion factors from other research groups than Dance et al. [25, 28, 29]. This may result in other values for the MGD compared to using the conversion factors from Dance et al.

National Surveys of Radiation Dose

Dose calculations can be performed based on the exposure parameters (compressed breast thickness, target, filter, kV and mAs) reported for the patient by using software published by the UK Breast Screening Programme [42]. In addition, the tube output and HVL needs to be measured. These measurements are normally performed by a medical physicist.

When estimating the dose in mammography, normally the MGD is estimated for both the CC and MLO view. The MGD per examination is defined as the total dose for all views divided by two, because the breasts are defined as one organ.

National surveys of radiation dose were implemented in the late 1970s [43]. Glandular tissue doses from radiation exposure of the female breast from mammography from 1960 up until the present time has decreased from an average of approximately 12 mGy to approximately 2 mGy [44].

In mammography both SFM and FFDM systems are currently in use. FFDM systems are capable of providing 25–35 % lower radiation doses than SFM systems, depending on breast thickness [5, 45–49]. The systems need to be optimised in order for them to provide lower doses than SFM systems [50].

A survey of patient doses in the UK Breast Screening Programme (NHSBSP) conducted in 2007 to 2009 showed that the average MGD for MLO views for FFDM systems was 1.46 ± 0.02 mGy, approximately 32 % lower than for SFM systems [51].

Dose level for the CC view for different compressed breast thicknesses for SFM and FFDM operating in an organised screening programme are shown in Fig. 18.4. The radiation doses are below the acceptable level proposed by EUREF.

References

1. Rothenberg LN. AAPM tutorial. Patient dose in mammography. Radiographics. 1990;10(4):739–46.
2. Rothenberg LN. Exposures and doses in mammography. In: Haus AG, Yaffe MJ, editors. Syllabus: a categorical course in physics. Technical aspects of breast imaging. 3rd ed. Presented at the 80th scientific assembly and annual meeting of the radiological society of North America, 27 Nov – 2 Dec 1994. Oak Brook: RSNA Publications; 1994. p. 113–9.
3. Dance DR, Young KC, van Engen RE. Estimation of mean glandular dose for breast tomosynthesis: factors for use with the UK, European and IAEA breast dosimetry protocols. Phys Med Biol. 2011;56(2):453–71. doi:10.1088/0031-9155/56/2/011.
4. Beaman SA, Lillicrap SC. Optimum x-ray spectra for mammography. Phys Med Biol. 1982;27(10):1209–20.
5. Fischer U, Hermann KP, Baum F. Digital mammography: current state and future aspects. Eur Radiol. 2006;16(1):38–44. doi:10.1007/s00330-005-2848-0.
6. Shore RE, Hildreth N, Woodard E, Dvoretsky P, Hempelmann L, Pasternack B. Breast cancer among women given X-ray therapy for acute postpartum mastitis. J Natl Cancer Inst. 1986;77(3):689–96.
7. Hildreth NG, Shore RE, Dvoretsky PM. The risk of breast cancer after irradiation of the thymus in infancy. N Engl J Med. 1989;321(19):1281–4. doi:10.1056/NEJM198911093211901.
8. Lundell M, Mattsson A, Hakulinen T, Holm LE. Breast cancer after radiotherapy for skin hemangioma in infancy. Radiat Res. 1996;145(2):225–30.
9. Lindberg S, Karlsson P, Arvidsson B, Holmberg E, Lunberg LM, Wallgren A. Cancer incidence after radiotherapy for skin haemangioma during infancy. Acta Oncol. 1995;34(6):735–40.
10. Mattsson A, Ruden BI, Hall P, Wilking N, Rutqvist LE. Radiation-induced breast cancer: long-term follow-up of radiation therapy for benign breast disease. J Natl Cancer Inst. 1993;85(20):1679–85.
11. Thompson DE, Mabuchi K, Ron E, Soda M, Tokunaga M, Ochikubo S, Sugimoto S, Ikeda T, Terasaki M, Izumi S, et al. Cancer incidence in atomic bomb survivors. Part II: solid tumors, 1958–1987. Radiat Res. 1994;137(2 Suppl):S17–67.
12. Boice Jr JD, Preston D, Davis FG, Monson RR. Frequent chest X-ray fluoroscopy and breast cancer incidence among tuberculosis patients in Massachusetts. Radiat Res. 1991;125(2):214–22.
13. Howe GR, McLaughlin J. Breast cancer mortality between 1950 and 1987 after exposure to fractionated moderate-dose-rate ionising radiation in the Canadian fluoroscopy cohort study and a comparison with breast cancer mortality in the atomic bomb survivors study. Radiat Res. 1996;145(6):694–707.
14. Lundell M, Mattsson A, Karlsson P, Holmberg E, Gustafsson A, Holm LE. Breast cancer risk after radiotherapy in infancy: a pooled analysis of two Swedish cohorts of 17,202 infants. Radiat Res. 1999;151(5):626–32.
15. United Nations Scientific Committee on the Effects of Atomic Radiation (UNSCEAR): volume I: report to the general assembly. Scientific annex A. Epidemiological studies of radiation and cancer. New York: United Nations; 2006. http://www.unscear.org/docs/reports/2006/07-82087_Report_Annex_A_2006_Web_corr.pdf. Accessed 11 Oct 2013.
16. ICRU. Patient dosimetry for X rays used in medical imaging. J ICRU 5(2). Report 74. In: International commission on radiation units and measurements. Oxford: Oxford University Press; 2005.
17. ICRU. Fundamental quantities and units for ionizing radiation. ICRU report 60. In: International commission on radiation units and measurements, Bethesda, 1998.
18. Dowsett DJ, Kenny PA, Johnston RE. The physics of diagnostic imaging. London: Hodder Arnold; 2006.
19. Institute of Physical Sciences in Medicine (IPSM). The commissioning and routine testing of mammographic x-ray systems. 2nd ed. Report No. 59. Institute of Physical Sciences in Medicine, 1994.

20. O'Leary D, Rainford L. A comparison of mean glandular dose diagnostic reference levels within the all-digital Irish national breast screening programme and the Irish symptomatic breast services. Radiat Prot Dosimetry. 2013;153(3):300–8. doi:10.1093/rpd/ncs112.
21. Al-Hajj M, Clarke MF. Self-renewal and solid tumor stem cells. Oncogene. 2004;23(43):7274–82. doi:10.1038/sj.onc.1207947.
22. Klein R, Aichinger H, Dierker J, Jansen JT, Joite-Barfuss S, Sabel M, Schulz-Wendtland R, Zoetelief J. Determination of average glandular dose with modern mammography units for two large groups of patients. Phys Med Biol. 1997;42(4):651–71.
23. Hammerstein GR, Miller DW, White DR, Masterson ME, Woodard HQ, Laughlin JS. Absorbed radiation dose in mammography. Radiology. 1979;130(2):485–91.
24. Dance DR, Skinner CL, Carlsson GA. Breast dosimetry. Appl Radiat Isot. 1999;50(1):185–203.
25. Dance DR, Skinner CL, Young KC, Beckett JR, Kotre CJ. Additional factors for the estimation of mean glandular breast dose using the UK mammography dosimetry protocol. Phys Med Biol. 2000;45(11): 3225–40.
26. Wu X, Gingold EL, Barnes GT, Tucker DM. Normalized average glandular dose in molybdenum target-rhodium filter and rhodium target-rhodium filter mammography. Radiology. 1994;193(1):83–9.
27. Boone JM. Normalized glandular dose (DgN) coefficients for arbitrary X-ray spectra in mammography: computer-fit values of Monte Carlo derived data. Med Phys. 2002;29(5):869–75.
28. Dance DR. Monte Carlo calculation of conversion factors for the estimation of mean glandular breast dose. Phys Med Biol. 1990;35(9):1211–9.
29. Dance DR, Young KC, van Engen RE. Further factors for the estimation of mean glandular dose using the United Kingdom, European and IAEA breast dosimetry protocols. Phys Med Biol. 2009;54(14):4361–72. doi:10.1088/0031-9155/54/14/002.
30. van Engen R. European protocol for the quality control of the physical and technical aspects of mammography screening. 4th ed. European Commission, Luxembourg, 2006. http://www.euref.org. Accessed 03 Apr 2014.
31. Highnam RP, Brady JM, Shepstone BJ. Estimation of compressed breast thickness during mammography. Br J Radiol. 1998;71(846):646–53.
32. Mawdsley GE, Tyson AH, Peressotti CL, Jong RA, Yaffe MJ. Accurate estimation of compressed breast thickness in mammography. Med Phys. 2009;36(2): 577–86.
33. Tyson AH, Mawdsley GE, Yaffe MJ. Measurement of compressed breast thickness by optical stereoscopic photogrammetry. Med Phys. 2009;36(2):569–76.
34. Burch A, Law J. A method for estimating compressed breast thickness during mammography. Br J Radiol. 1995;68(808):394–9.
35. Hauge IH, Hogg P, Szczepura K, Connolly P, McGill G, Mercer C. The readout thickness versus the measured thickness for a range of screen film mammography and full-field digital mammography units. Med Phys. 2012;39(1):263–71. doi:10.1118/1.3663579.
36. Hauge IH, Olerud HM. Uncertainties involved in the estimation of mean glandular dose for women in the Norwegian Breast Cancer Screening Program (NBCSP). Radiat Prot Dosimetry. 2013;155(1):81–7. doi:10.1093/rpd/ncs314.
37. Yaffe MJ, Boone JM, Packard N, Alonzo-Proulx O, Huang SY, Peressotti CL, Al-Mayah A, Brock K. The myth of the 50-50 breast. Med Phys. 2009;36(12):5437–43.
38. Young KC, Ramsdale ML, Bignell F. Review of dosimetric methods for mammography in the UK Breast Screening Programme. Radiat Prot Dosim. 1998; 80(1–3):183–6.
39. Tagliafico A, Astengo D, Cavagnetto F, Rosasco R, Rescinito G, Monetti F, Calabrese M. One-to-one comparison between digital spot compression view and digital breast tomosynthesis. Eur Radiol. 2012;22(3):539–44. doi:10.1007/s00330-011-2305-1.
40. Hauge IH, Bredholt K, Olerud HM. New diagnostic reference level for full-field digital mammography units. Radiat Prot Dosimetry. 2013;157(2):181–92. doi:10.1093/rpd/nct136.
41. Sechopoulos I, Suryanarayanan S, Vedantham S, D'Orsi C, Karellas A. Computation of the glandular radiation dose in digital tomosynthesis of the breast. Med Phys. 2007;34(1):221–32.
42. Young KC. Breast dose surveys in the NHSBSP: software and instruction manual. Version 2.0. In: NHSBSP Report 04 July 2004. 2004.
43. Rothenberg LN, Kirch RL, Snyder RE. Patient exposures from film and xeroradiographic mammographic techniques. Radiology. 1975;117(3 Pt 1):701–3.
44. Thierry-Chef I, Simon SL, Weinstock RM, Kwon D, Linet MS. Reconstruction of absorbed doses to fibroglandular tissue of the breast of women undergoing mammography (1960 to the present). Radiat Res. 2012;177(1):92–108.
45. Gennaro G, di Maggio C. Dose comparison between screen/film and full-field digital mammography. Eur Radiol. 2006;16(11):2559–66. doi:10.1007/s00330-006-0314-2.
46. Hermann KP, Obenauer S, Marten K, Kehbel S, Fischer U, Grabbe E. Average glandular dose with amorphous silicon full-field digital mammography – Clinical results. Rofo. 2002;174(6):696–9. doi:10.1055/s-2002-32221.
47. Moran P, Chevalier M, Ten JI, Fernandez Soto JM, Vano E. A survey of patient dose and clinical factors in a full-field digital mammography system. Radiat Prot Dosimetry. 2005;114(1–3):375–9. doi:10.1093/rpd/nch514.
48. Obenauer S, Hermann KP, Grabbe E. Dose reduction in full-field digital mammography: an anthropomorphic breast phantom study. Br J Radiol. 2003;76(907):478–82.
49. Bick U, Diekmann F. Digital mammography: what do we and what don't we know? Eur Radiol. 2007;17(8):1931–42. doi:10.1007/s00330-007-0586-1.

50. Hauge IH, Pedersen K, Sanderud A, Hofvind S, Olerud HM. Patient doses from screen-film and full-field digital mammography in a population-based screening programme. Radiat Prot Dosimetry. 2012; 148(1):65–73.

51. Oduko JM, Young KC, Burch A. A survey of patient doses from digital mammography systems in the UK in 2007 to 2009. Paper presented at the In: Proceedings of the 2010 International Workshop on Digital Mammography, Girona, 16–18 June.

Mammographic Density

19

Solveig S.H. Hofvind, Gunvor Gipling Waade, and Sue Astley

Background

Mammographic density (MD) refers to the radiographic density of the breast on the mammogram. The risk of developing breast cancer is 4–5 times higher for women with the highest compared to lowest MD. The increased risk is related to biological mechanisms and the decreased sensitivity of mammography in women with dense breast (tumour masking effect). MD has mainly been used for risk estimation in an epidemiological approach. Selecting women for additional imaging and/or screening intervals based on their MD might be the future in screening programmes for breast cancer. MD can be measured subjectively, semi-automatically and automatically based on the mammogram. Subjective measurement is usually performed visually by a reader. Semi quantitative measurements are performed by a reader and a computer, while automated volumetric measurement is performed objectively, solely by a computer, and requires a digital mammogram.

S.S.H. Hofvind (✉)
Cancer Registry of Norway and Oslo and Akershus University College of Applied Sciences, Fr Nansens vei 19, Oslo 0304, Norway
e-mail: solveig.hofvind@kreftregisteret.no

G.G. Waade
Department of Radiography, University of Salford, Student MSc Biomedicine Oslo and Akershus University College, Oslo, Norway

College of Health & Social Care, University of Salford, Salford, UK
e-mail: gunvorgw@gmail.com

S. Astley
Centre for Imaging Sciences, Institute of Population Health, Manchester Academic Health Science Centre, The University of Manchester, Stopford Building, Oxford Road, Manchester M13 9PT, UK
e-mail: sue.astley@manchester.ac.uk

Introduction

Mammographic density (MD) refers to the radiographic density of the breast [1]; the amount of parenchymal and connective tissue which appears white on the mammogram [1–7]. Cancerous tissue also appears white on a mammogram. Tumours can thus be difficult to perceive amongst dense tissue, in which the sensitivity of mammography is less in dense versus fatty breasts. As a woman ages, particularly after the menopause, the breast tissue usually involutes, becoming more fatty, and the sensitivity of mammography typically increases. The risk of developing breast cancer is 4–5 times higher for women with the highest MD (>75 % parenchyma) compared to women with fatty breast (<25 % parenchyma) [8–10]. The increased risk is related to biological mechanisms [11] and the decreased sensitivity of mammography (tumour masking effect) [12].

Until now, MD has mainly been used for risk estimation in an epidemiological approach [13, 14]. Clinical application has been hampered by inability to automatically and objectively measure, lack of MD included in risk models, and limited options for

P. Hogg et al. (eds.), *Digital Mammography: A Holistic Approach*,
DOI 10.1007/978-3-319-04831-4_19, © Springer International Publishing Switzerland 2015

additional or other screening tests for women with dense breasts. However, a wider understanding of the sensitivity of mammography in dense breasts is now emerging, and supplementary imaging techniques such as whole breast ultrasound and MRI are considered important adjuncts [15, 16]. Selecting women for additional imaging and/or screening intervals based on their MD might thus be the future in screening programmes for breast cancer. It is worth noting that American women residing in some states receive information about their breast density together with their screening results [17].

Measuring Mammographic Density

MD can be measured subjectively [5, 18–27], semiautomatically [28, 29] and automatically [30–39] based on the mammographic image. Subjective measurements is usually performed by an image reader's visual assessments. Semi quantitative measurements are performed by a reader and by a computer, while automated volumetric measurement is performed objectively, solely by a computer, and requires a digital mammogram.

Subjective Classification

John Wolfe was the first to develop a classification system for mammographic patterns in 1967 [18]. The pattern was divided into four categories; N1, P1, P2, and DY depending on the predominant tissue composition. N1 indicates mammographic lucent tissue with no visible ducts, and a low risk of breast cancer. P1 and P2 refer to linear densities associated with intermediate degrees of risk, where P1 has mostly fatty tissue with ducts occupying up to a quarter of the breast volume, while P2 has ducts occupying more than a quarter of the breast volume. DY describes a breast with diffuse densities, and is representing a high risk of breast cancer.

Norman Boyd described a six class system for subjectively quantifying breast density; this is based purely on amount of dense tissue and contains no descriptors of distribution or pattern [2]. The method has been used widely and is related to breast cancer risk. The classes represented 0 %, <10 %, 10<25 %, 25<50 %, 50<75 % and >75 % density. Boyd's work demonstrated the potential for measures purely based on quantity of dense tissue, and paved the way for later automated methods. The proportion of the breast area occupied by dense tissue has also been measured using subjective assessment with Visual Analogue Scales (VAS); this method has been used in several research studies and related to risk of developing cancer, especially where both views are assessed [19].

In 1997, Laszlo Tabár introduced a five point classification system [20]. The mammograms were classified according to the proportion of four components; nodular density, linear density, homogeneous fibrous tissue, radiolucent adipose tissue. Density I included mammograms with a balanced proportion of all components of breast tissue with a slight predominance of fibrous tissue; density II comprised predominant fatty breast; density III fatty tissue with retroareolar residual fibrous tissue; and density IV included nodular and fibrous tissue (dense breast). Patterns I, II and III were considered as low-risk, while patterns IV and V were considered as high-risk.

The 5th edition of BI-RADS (Breast Imaging-Reporting and Data System of the American College of Radiology (ACR) is the most commonly used system for classification of MD today [5]. Category A refers to entirely fat tissue; B is scattered fibroglandular densities; category C is heterogeneously dense breast, which could obscure detection of small masses, and D: extreme dense breast tissue, which lowers the sensitivity of mammography.

Despite the quantitative and objective definitions, all these measurements and assessments are highly subjective and show significant observer variability [21–27]. Because of the subjectivity and labour intensive nature of these methods, semi-automated and automated objective volumetric techniques have been developed.

Semi-automated Methods for Assessing MD

Developing semi-automated methods, also called computer-assisted methods, was a natural step to decrease the subjectiveness of the assessment of mammographic density. Computer-assisted methods require mammograms on a digital form. Since most of the work on computer-assisted measurement pre-dated the widespread use of Full Field Digital Mammography (FFDM), such methods involved a digitisation step, where film images were scanned and converted to pixels, each of which has an associated grey level. The most widely used computer assisted methods are the Madena [28] and the Cumulus [29]. The programme requires the user to delineate the breast by applying a threshold to the pixel values, allowing correction and removal of the pectoral muscle area where necessary, and then to select another threshold that subjectively separates the dense fibroglandular areas in the image from the fatty regions. The software operates by counting pixels in the breast area, and in the threshold dense tissue regions. The output is thus the percentage density based on the relative proportion of the breast area occupied by dense tissue, and an absolute area of density. Cumulus has been very widely used and for many years regarded as the gold standard for density assessment due to its unequivocal relationship with breast cancer risk. Despite this, it suffers from the dual limitations of being subjective (since the user defines the threshold for each image) and area-based. Mammograms are projection images, and the area of density depends on the compression of the breast.

Fully Automated Methods of Assessing MD

The introduction of FFDM brought the opportunity to compute breast density directly from the images without human intervention. The appearance of a mammogram depends on the physical properties of the breast tissue, the X-ray spectrum and exposure factors, properties of the detector and any image processing that has been applied. Automated methods aim to eliminate variability in mammographic appearance attributable to the imaging process and thus measure the volumes of fatty and dense tissue (including glandular tissue, the acinar and ductal epithelium and associated stroma, all of which have similar X-ray attenuation properties) in the breast. Such methods are referred to as 'volumetric' and generally output a relative measure (the proportion of the breast volume occupied by dense tissue) as well as absolute volumes of dense and fatty tissues.

Calibration-based and physics-based methods are the two main volumetric approaches. In calibration-based methods (Cumulus V [30, 31], Single X-ray Absorptiometry [32], and the Manchester Method [34]) an object such as a step-wedge calibration using tissue-equivalent material is imaged. The calibration enables accurate density measurement, but the requirement of imaging a calibration object and the inability to retrospectively analyse images acquired without one, represent disadvantages. In the physics-based methods (Quantra™ and Volpara™) [34, 35] knowledge about tissue attenuation coefficients and the physics of the imaging process are used. All methods require knowledge of compressed breast thickness; whilst this is relatively straightforward in the region where the breast is in contact with the compression plate, it is much more difficult to accurately measure the uncompressed breast edge. However, since this region mainly comprises skin and subcutaneous structures with little dense tissue, such inaccuracies do not usually have a great impact on overall density measures.

Currently the physics-based measures most widely used build on the work of Highnam and Brady [36] in which they developed a model for measuring volumetric density in digitised analogue mammograms. For example, in 2008 Hartman et al. published validation data and described ways in which the commercial software Quantra™ was improved in comparison to the original method [37]. Both Quantra™ and Volpara™ are fully automatic and can be used prospectively or retrospectively, provided that raw (unprocessed) mammogram data are available. Both methods have been validated and are currently in use worldwide both clinically and for research purposes [37–38]. One of the main differences between these two techniques is that Volpara™ uses a relative physics model, similar to that described by van Engeland et al. in 2006 [39]. This has the advantage of reducing the need for accurate imaging physics data, but depends on identifying a suitable fatty reference area within the image [38, 39].

Volumetric measures of breast density such as these are intuitively better at describing breast composition than area-based methods (which are susceptible to variation depending on the positioning and compression of the breast) or subjective techniques, which demonstrate significant inter-observer variability. To date most of the validation data linking increased density to risk of developing cancer has used methods which are both subjective and area-based, due to lack of availability of longitudinal data sets of FFDM images. The issue is set to change, and more detailed data about the relationship of increased breast density to risk will soon become available. Other areas under exploration are automated measures of image texture, which aim to capture structure as well as quantity. Early results indicate that these may complement volumetric breast density measures.

References

1. Kopans D, editor. Breast imaging. 3rd ed. London: Lippincott Williams & Wilkins; 2007.
2. Boyd NF, Byng JW, Jong RA, et al. Quantitative classification of mammographic densities and breast cancer risk: results from the Canadian National Breast Screening Study. J Natl Cancer Inst. 1995;87(9):670–5.
3. Ginsburg OM, Martin LJ, Boyd NF. Mammographic density, lobular involution, and risk of breast cancer. Br J Cancer. 2008;99(9):1369–74.
4. Vachon CM, van Gils CH, Sellers TA, et al. Mammographic density, breast cancer risk and risk prediction. Breast Cancer Res. 2007;9:217.
5. Sickles EA, D'Orsi CJ, Bassett LW, et al. American College of Radiology, et al. ACR BI-RADS® mammography. In: ACR BI-RADS® atlas, breast imaging reporting and data system. Reston: American College of Radiology; 2013.
6. White J. Breast density and cancer risk: what is the relationship? J Natl Cancer Inst. 2000;92(6):443.
7. Alonzo-Proulx O, Jong R, Yaffe MJ. Volumetric breast density characteristics as determined from digital mammograms. Phys Med Biol. 2012;57(22):7443–57.
8. McCormack V, dos Santos SI. Breast density and parenchymal patterns as markers of breast cancer risk: a meta-analysis. Cancer Epidemiol Biomark Prev. 2006;15(6):1159–69.
9. Ursin G, Ma H, Wu AH, et al. Mammographic density and breast cancer in three ethnic groups. Cancer Epidemiol Biomark Prev. 2003;12(4):332–8.
10. Shepherd JA, Kerlikowske K, Ma L, et al. Volume of mammographic density and risk of breast cancer. Cancer Epidemiol Biomark Prev. 2011;20(7):1473–82.
11. Lisanti MP, Tsirigos A, Pavlides S, et al. JNK1 stress signaling is hyper-activated in high breast density and the tumor stroma: connecting fibrosis, inflammation, and stemness for cancer prevention. Cell Cycle. 2014;13(4):580–99.
12. Checka CM, Chun JE, Schnabel FR, Lee J, Toth H. The relationship of mammographic density and age: implications for breast cancer screening. AJR Am J Roentgenol. 2012;198(3):W292–5.
13. Boyd NF, Martin LJ, Bronskill M, Yaffe MJ, Duric N, Minkin S. Breast tissue composition and susceptibility to breast cancer. J Natl Cancer Inst. 2010;102(16):1224–37.
14. Highnam R, Sauber N, Destounis S, Harvey J, McDonald D. Breast density into clinical practice in breast imaging. In: Maidment A, Bakic P, Gavenonis S, editors. Berlin/Heidelberg: Springer; 2012. p.466–73.
15. Berg WA, Zhang Z, Lehrer D, et al. for the ACRIN 6666 Investigators. Detection of breast cancer with addition of annual screening ultrasound or a single screening MRI to mammography in women with elevated breast cancer risk. JAMA. 2012;307(13):1394–404.
16. Berg WA, Blume JD, Cormack JB, et al. for the ACRIN 6666. Investigators. Combined screening with ultrasound and mammography vs mammography alone in women at elevated risk of breast cancer. JAMA. 2008;299(18):2151–63.
17. Are You Dense Advocacy, Inc. http://www.areyoudenseadvocacy.org/.
18. Wolfe JN. Breast patterns as an index of risk for developing breast cancer. AJR Am J Roentgenol. 1976;126(6):1130–7.
19. Duffy SW, Nagtegaal ID, Astley SM, et al. Visually assessed breast density: the need for two views. Breast Cancer Res. 2008;10:R64.
20. Gram IT, Funkhouser E, Tabár L. The Tabár classification of mammographic parenchymal patterns. Eur J Radiol. 1997;24(2):131–6.
21. Gram IT, Bremnes Y, Ursin G, Maskarinec G, Bjurstam N, Lund E. Percentage density, Wolfe's and Tabár's mammographic patterns: agreement and association with risk factors for breast cancer. Breast Cancer Res. 2005;7(5):54–61.
22. Berg WA, Campassi C, Langenberg P, Sexton MJ. Breast Imaging Reporting and Data System: inter- and intraobserver variability in feature analysis and final assessment. Am J Roentgenol. 2000;174(6):1769–77.
23. Weigert J, Steenbergen S. The Connecticut experiment: the role of ultrasound in the screening of women with dense breasts. Breast J. 2012;18(6):517–22.

24. Harvey JA, Bovbjerg VE. Quantitative assessment of mammographic breast density: relationship with breast cancer risk. Radiology. 2004;230(1):29–41.
25. Ciatto S, Visioli C, Paci E, Zappa M. Breast density as a determinant of interval cancer at mammographic screening. Br J Cancer. 2004;90(2):393–6.
26. Martin KE, Helvie MA, Zhou C, et al. Mammographic density measured with quantitative computer-aided method: comparison with radiologists' estimates and BI-RADS categories. Radiology. 2006;240(3): 656–65.
27. Ren B, Smith AP, Marshall J. Investigation of practical scoring methods for breast density, in digital mammography. In: Martí J, Oliver A, Freixenet J, Martí R, editors. 10th International Workshop, IWDM 2010, Girona, Catalonia, 2010 June 16–18. Berlin/Heidelberg: Springer; 2010. p. 651–8.
28. Ursin G, Ma H, Wu AH, et al. Mammographic density and breast cancer in three ethnic groups. Cancer Epidemiol Biomarkers Prev. 2003;12:332–8.
29. Byng JW, Boyd NF, Fishell E, Jong RA, Yaffe MJ. The quantitative analysis of mammographic densities. Phys Med Biol. 1994;39:1629–38.
30. Pawluczyk O, Augustine BJ, Yaffe MJ, et al. A volumetric method for estimation of breast density on digitized screen-film mammograms. Med Phys. 2003;30(3):352–64.
31. Yaffe MJ, Boone JM, Packard N, et al. The myth of the 50–50 breast. Med Phys. 2009;36(12):5437–43.
32. Malkov S, Wang J, Kerlikowske K, Cummings SR, Shepherd JA. Single x-ray absorptiometry method for the quantitative mammographic measure of fibroglandular tissue volume. Med Phys. 2009;36(12):5525–36.
33. Diffey J, Hufton A, Astley S. A new step-wedge for the volumetric measurement of mammographic density. IWDM 2006, LNCS 4046. Berlin: Springer; 2006. p. 1–9.
34. Quantra. Available from: http://www.hologic.com/en/breast-screening/volumetric-assessment/.
35. Volpara. Available from: http://www.matakina.com.
36. Highnam RP, Brady M. Mammographic image analysis. Dordrecht: Academic; 1999.
37. Hartman K, Highnam R, Warren R, Jackson V. Volumetric assessment of breast tissue composition from FFDM images. Proceedings of IWDM 2008, LNCS 5116. Berlin: Springer; 2008. p. 33–9.
38. Highnam R, Brady M, Yaffe MJ, Karssemeijer N, Harvey J. Robust breast composition measurement – VolparaTM. Proceedings of IWDM 2010, LNCS 6136. Berlin: Springer; 2010. p. 342–9.
39. Van Engeland S, Snoeren PR, Huisman H, Boetes C, Karssemeijer N. Volumetric breast density estimation from full field digital mammograms. IEEE Trans Med Imaging. 2006;25:273–82.

Part IV

Imaging Techniques

20 Recording Clinical and Client Information Prior to Imaging

Bernadette Bickley

Introduction

The mammography practitioner plays a vital role in ascertaining and documenting a relevant, accurate and complete clinical history prior to imaging, ensuring that the imaging workup is justified [1] and tailored to address the clinical need of each individual [2].

The prevalent screen of a client refers to the first screening episode with the NHSBSP, and neither a history of any breast disease/treatment nor indeed any current breast symptoms will be known. The incident screening episode refers to clients who have been screened previously and a limited history may have been documented. However any developing history within the 3 year screening interval or any current breast symptoms that the client may be experiencing will not be known without appropriate questioning.

It may be necessary to recall a client for a clinical assessment given her current clinical symptoms even if the mammographic assessment is normal [2]. It is therefore imperative that the mammography practitioner ensures a current and relevant clinical history is accurately documented at each screening attendance.

B. Bickley
South Staffs Breast Screening,
County Hospital,
Weston Road, Stafford ST16 3SA, UK
e-mail: bernadette.bickley@nhs.net

In the symptomatic setting a request form (electronic or paper) completed by the requesting clinician should accompany the patient. It is the responsibility of the requesting clinician to ensure that this is both legible and accurate. Furthermore, the practitioner must verify that both the patient demographics and the clinical history are relevant and accurate [1] prior to proceeding with the examination.

Initial Client Contact

It is essential that the practitioner firstly introduces themself and gives a relevant explanation of the mammographic procedure, establishing rapport with the client/ patient thus facilitating full co-operation in both obtaining a relevant clinical history and the mammographic examination itself [3].

During this initial contact the individual needs of the client/patient may be assessed. Clients who are anxious, have physical or learning difficulties, or indeed where English is not the functional language, may require additional support and this can be sought prior to the commencement of the examination.

The practitioner must utilise excellent communication skills [4] and verify that the client demographics (name, date of birth and address) are concordant with the request form/client sheet. Documentation to confirm concordance must be completed either by initialling the request form or by making an electronic record.

P. Hogg et al. (eds.), *Digital Mammography: A Holistic Approach*,
DOI 10.1007/978-3-319-04831-4_20, © Springer International Publishing Switzerland 2015

Previous Imaging

Once details have been verified and/or any changes have been made, it must then be established whether the client has undergone any previous breast imaging. If this is the case it must be determined when the imaging occurred. Within the UK, a minimum interval period of 6 months is required for another screen in the screening service [5]. Within the symptomatic setting a 6–12 months interval period between consecutive mammograms is required, dependent upon individual hospital protocol, with the exception of clinically suspicious findings e.g. P4/5 [6]. This information is imperative in order to ensure that a mammogram is the appropriate imaging modality and conforms to both local imaging guidelines and ionising radiation regulations. It is also important to establish where the imaging was performed, thus enabling historical images to be obtained. Comparison with previous images may improve the appreciation of discrete mammographic changes thus increasing sensitivity of breast cancer detection [7].

History Taking

Any history of previous breast surgery must also be ascertained, including when it was performed and the exact location within the breast (depicted with the aid of a breast diagram). A post-operative scar may mimic an architectural distortion suspicious of malignancy [8]. If the previous surgical site is not clearly indicated this may result in avoidable additional imaging or an unnecessary recall, increasing client anxiety. Comparison with previous images is imperative when interpreting the post-operative breast. The density of scar tissue should either remain stable or reduce with time. Any increase in scar density or size would be considered suspicious of loco-regional recurrence and warrant further investigation [9].

Information regarding any history of breast disease (e.g. fibroadenoma or cysts) or previous breast interventional procedure (biopsy proven benign/malignant pathology or possible marker clip in situ) is also essential as this will assist the reporting radiologist/practitioner correlate pre-existing conditions with the corresponding imaging features, thus increasing specificity of diagnosis whilst also reducing unnecessary recall.

Obtaining a history of breast augmentation will enable adaption of imaging technique and exposure parameters ensuring optimal imaging of the residual breast tissue [10]. It is essential that any previous history of injectable fillers be clearly documented with the client being made fully aware of the consequential diagnostic limitations/reduced sensitivity and informed that additional imaging may be required [11].

Documentation of any known skin lesions overlying the breast/axillary tissue (depicted with the aid of a breast diagram) reduces unnecessary recall, for example a sebaceous cyst may mimic a breast lesion whilst dermal calcifications within a skin lesion may result in a diagnostic dilemma [12].

An accurate record of any family history of breast cancer is of importance; age of onset of disease and relationship to client will enable evaluation of the relevance and associated increased risk of breast cancer, identifying those that may be suitable for genetic counselling/ testing and/or increased surveillance or additional use of MRI screening [13].

Where appropriate, documentation of a pacemaker or heart-monitoring device will enable adaptation of mammographic technique, paying special attention not to compress the device during the mammographic examination.

Any current breast symptoms that the client may be experiencing must be carefully documented, specifying the exact location and duration of symptoms [14], paying particular attention to the following:

- Breast lumps
- Skin tethering
- Skin changes, for example *Peau d' orange*
- Nipple discharge
- Changes to the nipple such as recent nipple inversion
- Asymmetrical thickening

Duration of Hormone Replacement Therapy (HRT) or discontinuation of previous use must also be documented, as this information will aid the reporting team when giving consideration to any associated change in breast density between imaging episodes.

Any client limitations or mobility issues that may have a consequence on image quality also requires documentation. Whilst every effort should be made to obtain diagnostic quality images, consideration may be given to any pre-existing limitations. In exceptional circumstances it may be appropriate to record a partial examination, documenting the specific limitations of the examination and fully explaining the diagnostic consequences to the client.

Summary

Key steps for practitioners to remember:

- Establish effective communication
- Check for prior mammography
- Accurate documentation

References

1. IRMER. The ionising radiation (medical exposure) regulations 2000 (online). London: Department of Health; 2000. Available at: https://www.gov.uk/government/publications/the-ionising-radiation-medical-exposure-regulations-2000. Accessed 10 Apr 2014.
2. NHSBSP. Quality assurance guidelines for mammography: including radiographic quality control, Publication 63 (online). Sheffield: Department of Health; 2006. Available at: http://www.cancerscreening.nhs.uk/breastscreen/publications/nhsbsp63.pdf. Accessed 10 Apr 2014.
3. SCoR. Code of professional conduct (online). London: The Society and College of Radiographers; 2013. Available at: http://www.sor.org/learning/document-library/code-professional-conduct. Accessed 10 Apr 2014.
4. Donnelly E, Neville L. Communication and interpersonal skills. Exeter: Reflect Press Ltd; 2008.
5. NHSBSP. Occasional report 02/03: guidance on the justification for repeat screening in the NHSBSP. Sheffield: Department of Health; 2002.
6. Willet AM, Michell MJ, Lee MJR. Best practice diagnostic guidelines for patients presenting with breast symptoms [online]. London: Department of Health; 2010. Available at: http://www.associationofbreastsurgery.org.uk/media/4585/best_practice_diagnostic_guidelines_for_patients_presenting_with_breast_symptoms.pdf. Accessed 10 Apr 2014.
7. Hewang-Kobrunner SH, Dershaw DD, Schreer I. Diagnostic breast imaging. 2nd ed. New York: Thieme; 2001.
8. Shaw de Paredes E. Atlas of mammography. 3rd ed. Philadelphia: Lippincott Williams & Wilkins; 2007.
9. Cardenosa G. Breast imaging companion. 2nd ed. Philadelphia: Lippincott Williams & Wilkins; 2001.
10. Andolina VF, Lillé SL. Mammographic imaging. A practical guide. 3rd ed. Philadelphia: Lippincott Williams & Wilkins; 2011.
11. MHRA. Medical device alert. (online). London: Crown copyright; 2012. Available at: http://www.mhra.gov.uk/Publications/Safetywarnings/MedicalDeviceAlerts/CON149825. Accessed 10 Apr 2014.
12. Barth V. Diagnosis of breast diseases: integrating the findings of clinical presentation, mammography, and ultrasound. New York: Thieme; 2010.
13. NHSBSP. Protocols for the surveillance of women at higher risk of developing breast cancer. Version 4, Publication 74 (online). London: Public Health England; 2013. Available at: http://www.cancerscreening.nhs.uk/breastscreen/publications/nhsbsp74.pdf. Accessed 10 Apr 2014.
14. Ikeda DM. Breast imaging; The requisites. 2nd ed. St. Louis, Missouri: Elsevier/Mosby; 2011.

Practical Mammography

21

Claire E. Mercer, Catherine A. Hill, Allison Kelly, and Helen L. Smith

Introduction

Positioning a client for a mammogram takes a great deal of skill and expertise. Practitioners are required to master a high standard of reproducible positioning skills; incorporating effective compression together with excellent client communication skills. It is deemed essential that practitioners master the art of continual high quality imaging. For any screening and symptomatic service, mammogram images are compared for subtle changes and practitioners need to ensure their images are of high quality and consistent with their peers.

This section illustrates a step by step guide to the basic positioning techniques required to produce high quality mammogram images. A 'handy hints' section will provide key points throughout.

Prior to Imaging

Aside the information gathered, indicated in Chap. 20, the practitioner should:

- Explain the procedure to the client
- Ask the client to remove evidence of deodorants or talcum powder
- Ask the client to remove jewellery (large earrings, large necklaces) and spectacles

Remember, your client will feel vulnerable and putting them at ease is a priority; this will assist in achieving high quality images.

Your client should then be asked to undress from the waist up. Whilst doing so the appropriate paddle size should be selected. The following views, cranio caudal (CC) view and medio lateral oblique (MLO) view, are then performed. The practitioner should observe the breast to check for sores or rashes (see Chap. 15) and record these in the appropriate format following your service procedures (see Chap. 20).

C.E. Mercer (✉)
Breast Imaging, The Nightingale Centre & Genesis Prevention Centre, Wythenshawe Hospital, University Hospital South Manchester, Southmoor Road, Wythenshawe, Manchester M27 9LT, UK
e-mail: claire.mercer@uhsm.nhs.uk

C.A. Hill
Training and Education Lead, Breast Imaging, The Nightingale Centre & Genesis Prevention Centre, Wythenshawe Hospital, University Hospital South Manchester, Southmoor Road, Wythenshawe, Manchester M27 9LT, UK
e-mail: cathy.hill@uhsm.nhs.uk

A. Kelly
Senior Mammographer, Breast Imaging, The Nightingale Centre & Genesis Prevention Centre, Wythenshawe Hospital, University Hospital South Manchester, Southmoor Road, Wythenshawe, Manchester M27 9LT, UK
e-mail: allison.kelly@uhsm.nhs.uk

H.L. Smith
Breast Care Unit, Royal Lancaster Infirmary, University Hospitals of Morecambe Bay NHS Foundation Trust, Ashton Road, Lancaster, Lancashire LA1 4RP, UK
e-mail: helen.l.smith@mbht.nhs.uk

P. Hogg et al. (eds.), *Digital Mammography: A Holistic Approach*,
DOI 10.1007/978-3-319-04831-4_21, © Springer International Publishing Switzerland 2015

Compression Force Application

Breast compression during mammography is one of a number of necessary requirements to produce an image of optimal diagnostic value [1]. Effective compression is said to spread out overlapping tissues to enable better visualisation of breast structures. The application of compression force reduces breast thickness, which would therefore minimise the amount of radiation required for imaging. However compression force has the potential to cause the client pain and discomfort which may ultimately deter them from attending for routine screening mammography (see Chap. 14) [2, 3].

It is acknowledged that one of the most important factors in determining the success of a screening programme is screening uptake [4, 5]. The causes of any non-uptake are multifactorial (see Chaps. 9 and 10). Following a systematic review it is evidenced that between 47,000 and 77,000 women in England do not re-attend for breast screening in a year due to pain directly related to a previous mammogram [3].

In order to maximise the number of clients attending screening mammography, pain and discomfort should be minimised. Therefore as practitioners your goal is to achieve optimum image quality with minimal radiation dose and minimal client discomfort. This can be achieved by adopting evidence based mammographic technique, which incorporates effective but not excessive compression force with an equalised balance of force between the image receptor (IR) and the compression paddle [6].

Compression Force and Pressure

At present there can be large variations between practitioners in the compression force they use [7, 8]. This can lead to a wide variation in applied pressure to the breast – *applied pressure is inversely proportional to breast size if the applied compression force is constant* [9]. Further information on the use of pressure to optimise breast compression can be found in Chap. 22.

Achieving Compression Force Balance

The position of the IR when performing the CC projection has a considerable effect on compression force balance between IR and paddle, and size of breast footprint on the IR [6]. It is important to balance compression forces from compression paddle and IR, such that not too much force is exerted from either direction; balancing is likely to minimise pain.

Using pressure mapping technology, left CC 'pressure' images have been created. Firstly, with the IR at the infra mammary fold (IMF) and compression force of 80 N (Fig. 21.1). Secondly (Fig. 21.2), raising the IMF by 2 cm has a demonstrable effect of equalising *compression force balance* together with an increase in *breast footprint* on the IR. The pressure image is represented in a

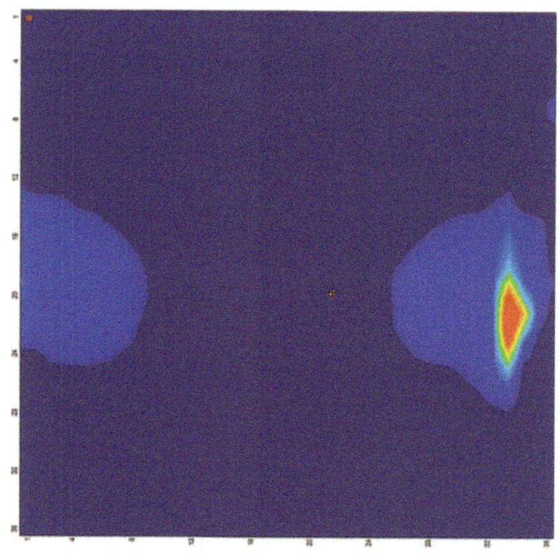

Fig. 21.1 Left CC IR at IMF

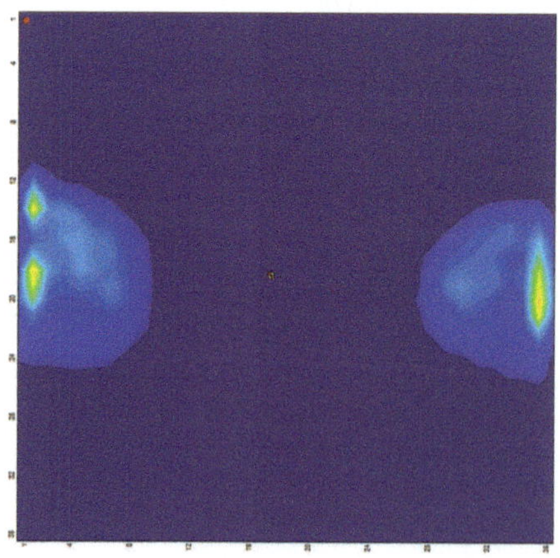

Fig. 21.2 Left CC IMF plus 2 cm

linear colour scale where dark blue represents no pressure and red represents high pressure.

Handy Hints
In order to achieve maximum breast footprint and optimum compression force balance between IR and paddle for the CC projection, you should aim to position the IR approximately 1–2 cm above the level of the IMF.

Cranio-Caudal (CC) View: A Step by Step Guide

Handy Hints
The 5 Ps
Proper **P**lanning and **P**reparation leads to **P**erfect **P**ositioning

- Practitioners should be aware of their postural techniques at all times during positioning to reduce any risk of repetitive strain injury (see Chap. 23).
- Stand the client facing the mammography unit about a hands width back from the IR. Ask the client to stand with their feet hips width apart for stability, with their hand of the side being imaged on their abdomen.
- Stand next to the client, at the contralateral side, and ask the client to turn their head to face you and rest their cheek against the face guard.
- Ask the client to keep their feet in the same position and bend forwards slightly, pushing their bottom back. Lift the breast being imaged, using its natural mobility (Fig. 21.3).
- With a positive hold, using the breasts natural mobility, lift and pull the breast forwards onto the image receptor at the medial and lateral breast sides (Fig. 21.4), adjust so that the nipple is centrally placed. The nipple is a standard and reliable landmark to ensure accurate breast positioning.
- It has been demonstrated that following correct positioning the nipple will fall into profile in at least one view with almost all located along or close to the breast boundary [10, 11].

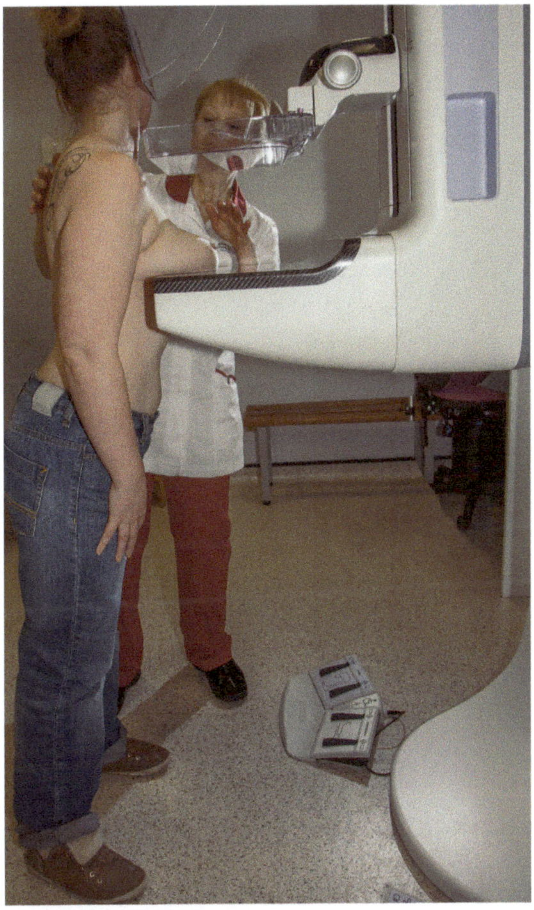

Fig. 21.3 CC view: Initial client position

Raising the Breast

Figure 21.5 highlights the extent to which the breast should be raised prior to positioning for the CC view in the first instance.

Adjust the height of the IR to allow the breast to sit at a 90° angle at the chest wall in the first instance. It is of great importance now to raise the level of the infra mammary fold (IMF) to achieve maximum breast footprint and balance the compression force to the top and bottom of the breast. The amount of uplift will be client dependent; it has been evidenced that an increase in 1–2 cm above the IMF significantly increases breast footprint [6] (Figs. 21.1 and 21.2). It is important to ensure that the IR is not raised too high as this could result in a loss of breast tissue on the image with the nipple inverted down, towards the underneath the breast.

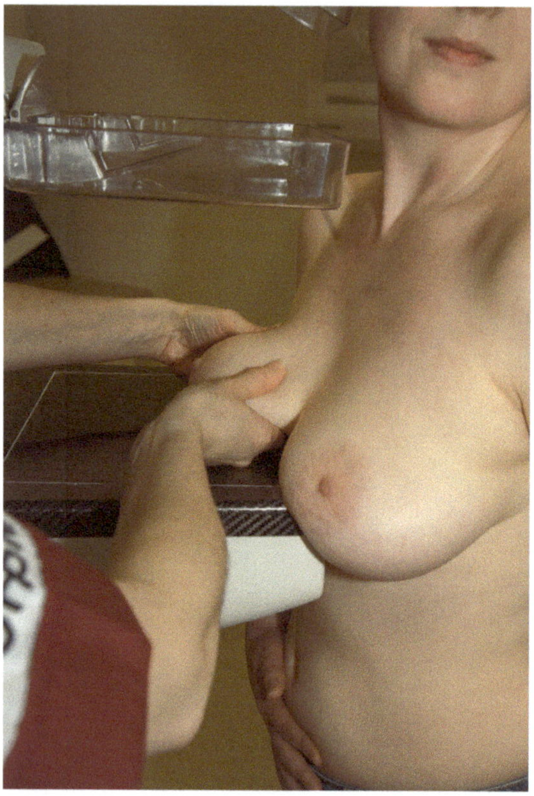

Fig. 21.4 CC view: Placement of breast on Image Receptor

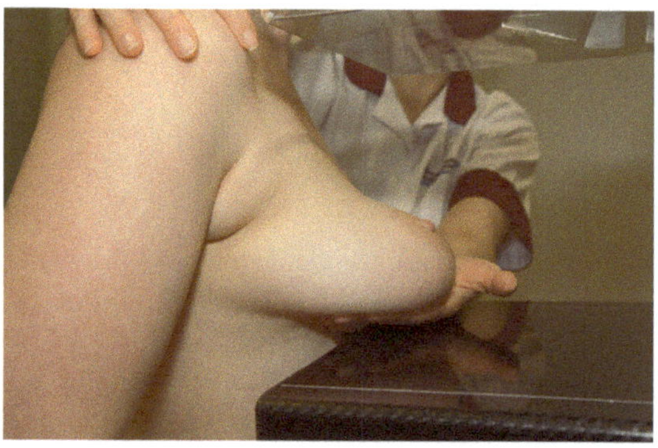

Fig. 21.5 CC view: Raising breast prior to positioning

> **Handy Hints**
> It may occasionally help to place the opposite breast onto the image receptor to encourage the medial breast border to be in the field of view – ensure that the opposite breast is not imaged though

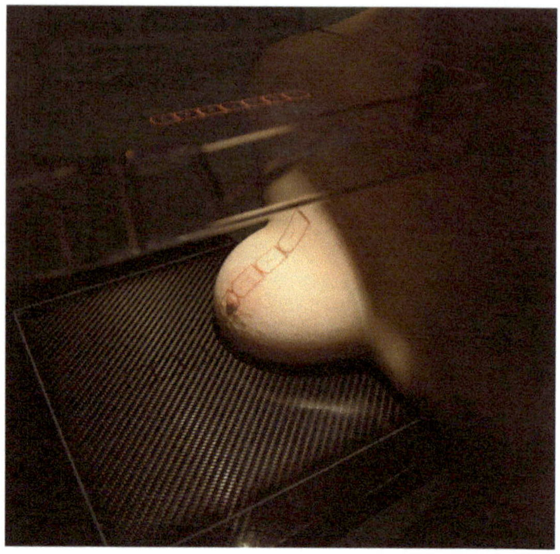

Fig. 21.6 CC view: Nipple position

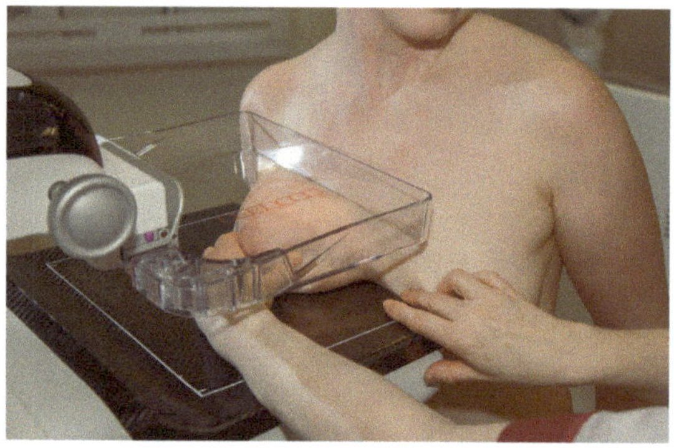

Fig. 21.7 CC view: Compression force application

- Check for creases and air gaps and smooth the breast tissue. Ensure the nipple is in profile (but not at the expense of breast tissue) and central (Fig. 21.6).
- Whilst holding the breast securely with one hand, place one arm around the back of the client and gently guide their shoulder down allowing relaxation of the lateral breast tissue.
- Place your hand positively around the back of the client to encourage a 'leaning forwards motion' followed by compression force application.
- Alert the client that compression is about to commence. Apply compression force slowly and evenly moving your hand towards the nipple as the compression takes over the hand (Fig. 21.7).

> **Handy Hints**
> If your client is unsteady, place their hand, opposite to the breast being imaged, onto the bar of the mammography unit

- If possible, and available on the equipment, the hand compression dial should be used to allow a slow, measured compression force application.
- The breast should be compressed to ensure compression force balance between paddle and IR is achieved; the breast may feel taut and immobile. Client consistency between sequential attendances is imperative [12] and the compression force could be standardised between 90 and 130 Newtons of force [13]. Apply smaller forces if the client experiences discomfort; larger forces if the breast is not immobile.
- Check the medial and lateral borders for skin folds, if present smooth out with fingers ensuring not to disturb any breast tissue (Fig. 21.7). Perform a last check to ensure no artefacts are present on the image detector (i.e.: clients hair, chin)
- Perform the exposure. Following automatic compression release, lower the height of the column slightly prior to imaging the opposing side; this allows for correct breast uplift.

Medio Lateral (MLO) View: A Step by Step Guide

> **Handy Hints**
> Remember the 5 Ps:
> **P**roper **P**lanning and **P**reparation leads to **P**erfect **P**ositioning

- Initial set up: Reduce the height of the IR slightly from the CC view and angle the tube head to 50°.
- Adjust the IR in accordance with the height of the client. It is now of vital importance that the correct angle of the IR is selected. Suboptimal positioning and incorrect angle selection could result in excessive compression force being applied to the chest wall/axilla. This may cause unnecessary discomfort to the client and result in inadequate compression of the breast.

Correct IR Angle Selection

Angle selection for the MLO view is a skill and refinement of the angle selected will be required through positioning. In the first instance a quick observation of the body habitus of the client (Fig. 21.8) will provide a rough indication and enable you to select an appropriate angle to commence.

- The aim on the MLO position is to get the sternal angle and the IR parallel to each other to enable effective compression force balance between IR and paddle with maximum breast footprint on the IR. Figures 21.9, 21.10 and 21.11 illustrate angle positioning for varying body habitus; the parallel lines illustrating correct IR angle selection.
- Incorrect angle selection for the MLO will lead to uneven compression force balance which could increase the levels of pain for the client due to higher pressure points. Figure 21.12 illustrates a right sided MLO with the client positioned at an incorrect 45° angle selection and a correctly selected 55° angle (Fig. 21.13) which highlights correct compression force balance
- Following on from correct angle selection, for stability ask the client to face the machine with feet hips width apart. Standing behind the client place your hand at the bottom of the rib cage of the side being imaged. Move the client forwards until your fingertips are just touching the front and bottom aspect of the IR; the client will be about a hands width back from the IR (Fig. 21.14).
- Height adjustment of the mammography unit can now commence; adjust to the level of the axilla in the first instance. Rest the arm of the client along the top of the IR (Fig. 21.14).
- Standing at 90° to the client place your hand to the lateral aspect of the breast and place your other arm, in a supportive position, around her back (Fig. 21.15).

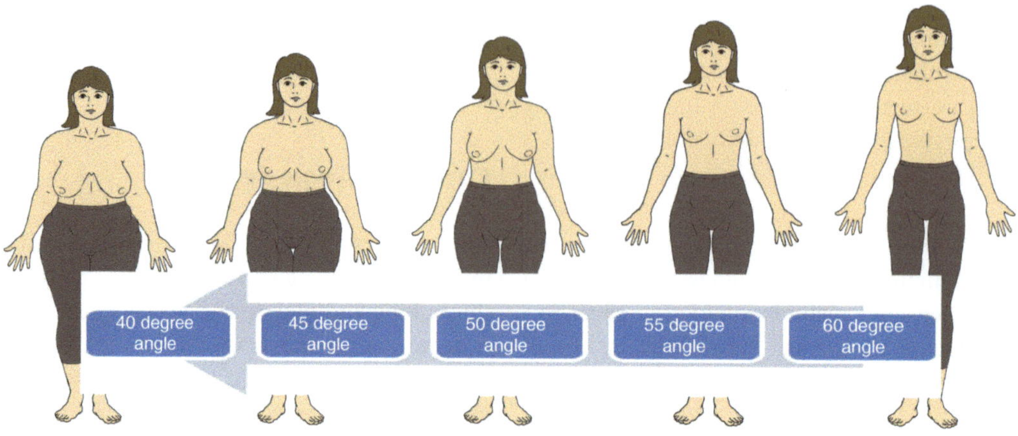

Fig. 21.8 Guide to appropriate angle selection

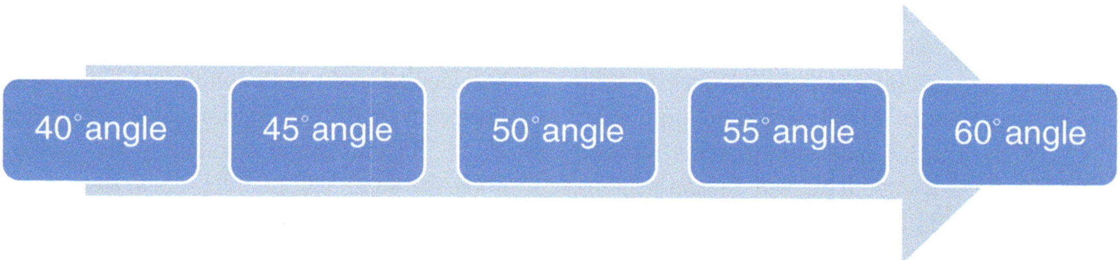

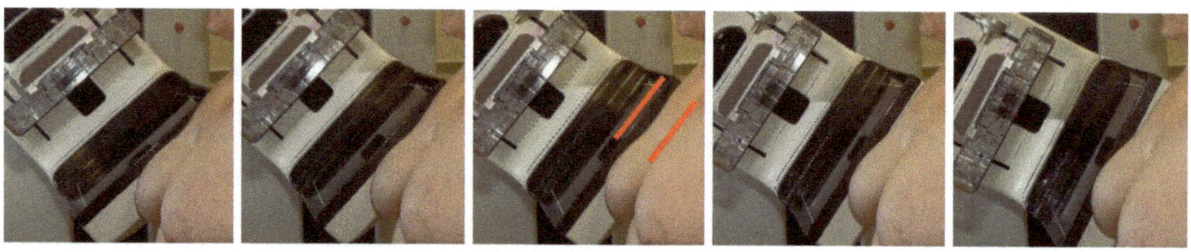

Fig. 21.9 Client would require a 45 or 50 degree angle of the IR

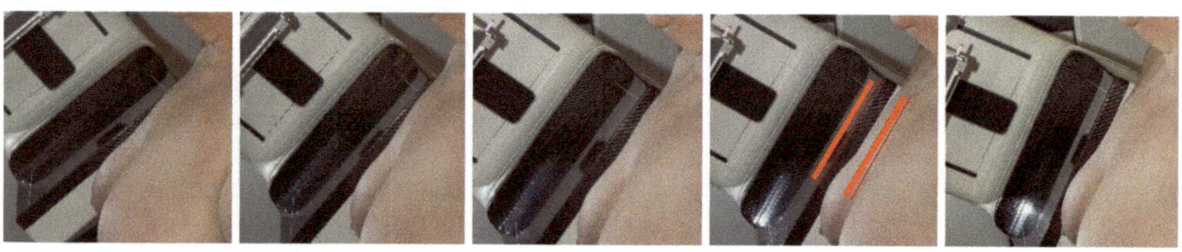

Fig. 21.10 Client would require a 50 or 55 degree angle of the IR

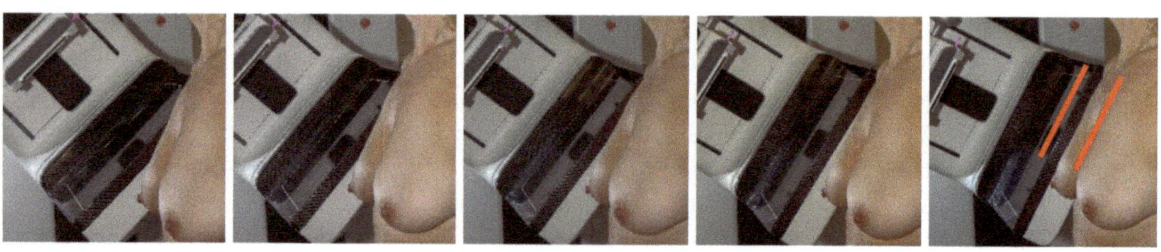

Fig. 21.11 Client would require a 55 or 60 degree angle of the IR

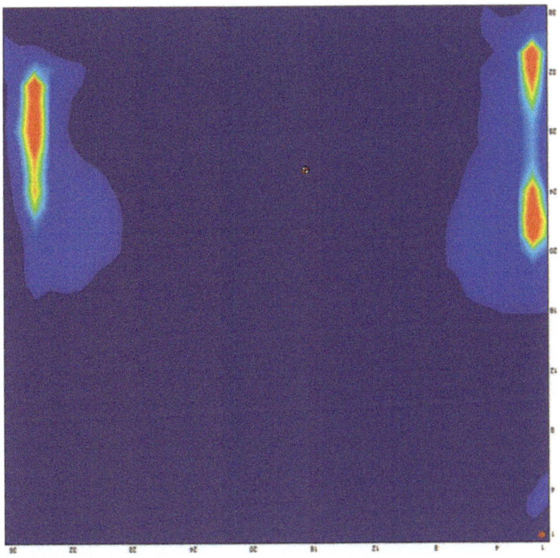

Fig. 21.12 MLO at 45°

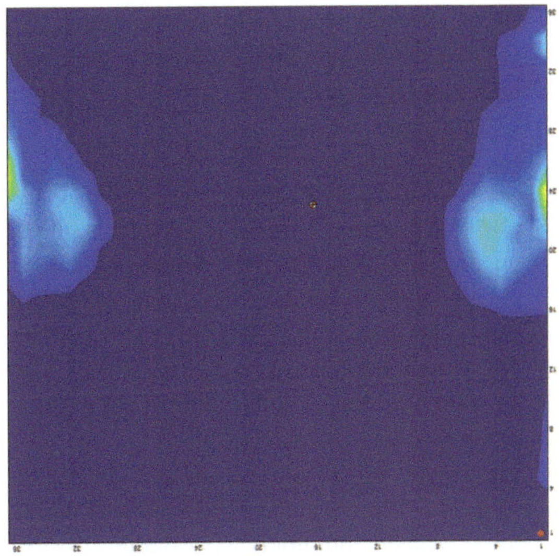

Fig. 21.13 MLO at 55°

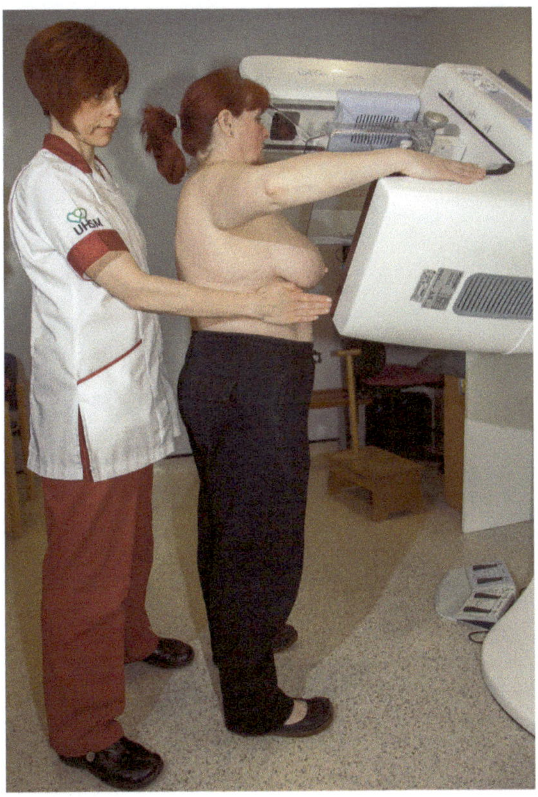

Fig. 21.14 Client position for MLO

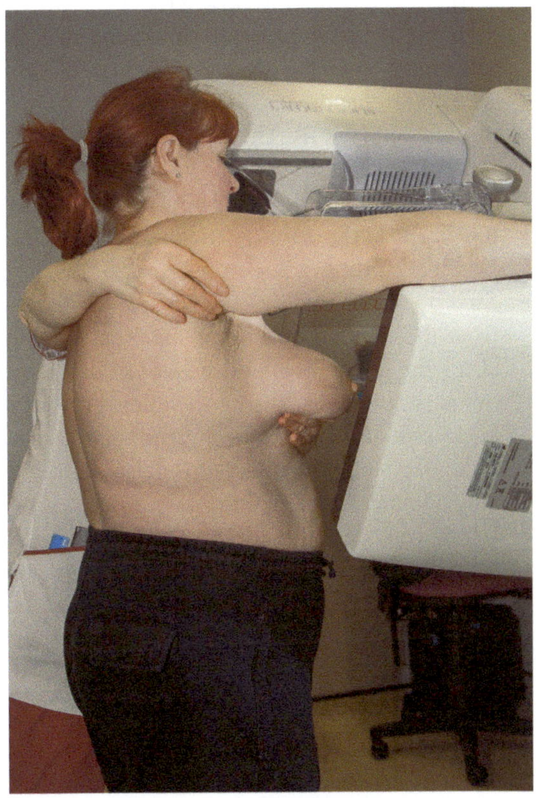

Fig. 21.15 MLO view: Supporting the breast and arm

- Using the natural mobility of the breast, lift the breast with one hand and guide the client into the machine with your other hand. Concurrently, ask the client to bend from their waist and lean towards the side of the IR.
- Move around to the back of the client and position her arm; lifting it upwards, gently reaching the shoulder over the IR. Adjust the height of the machine; the corner of the IR should be seated into the axilla (mid axillary line between the latissumus dorsi muscle and pectoral muscle), or in the space if the axilla is hollow.
- The client can drape her arm over the IR (Fig. 21.16) and rest her hand on the handle of the equipment; but not grasp too tightly as this will cause the pectoral muscle to tense. Ensure the arm of the client is not higher than their shoulder and check that the pectoral muscle is flat and not over stretched.
- Following on, return to the front of the client and sit on an appropriate stool for correct ergonomic positioning (Fig. 21.17).
- Now ask the client to relax down onto the IR and gently ease the shoulder backwards and with both hands carefully pull the breast through onto the IR. The breast should be centrally placed in the IR with the corner of the compression paddle to be seated just below the head of humerus – adjust the column height accordingly if required.
- Sweep your hand down the back of the breast from the axilla to the infra mammary angle checking for creases and ensuring all breast tissue is pulled on. Ensure the clients hips are back and smooth the infra mammary angle. Ask the client to push her hips back slightly if the abdomen is protruding.
- Using your hand lift the breast up and away from the chest wall; the breast is to be imaged at 90° to the chest wall. The nipple should be in profile with no air gaps between the breast and the IR.

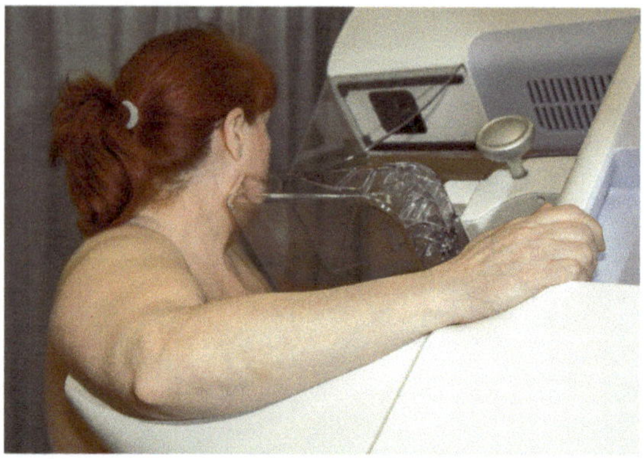

Fig. 21.16 MLO view: Client arm position

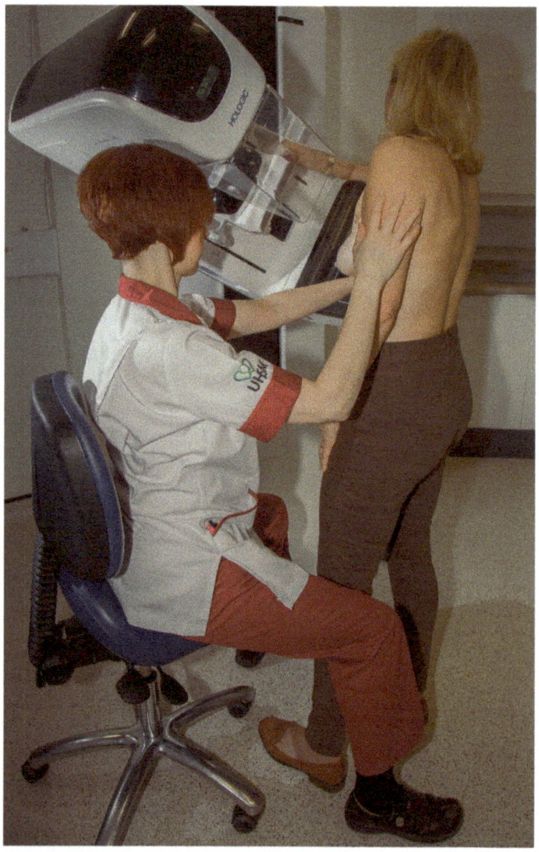

Fig. 21.17 MLO view: Practitioner ergonomic position

- Slowly apply compression force (slowly and evenly) moving your hand towards the nipple as the compression paddle takes over the hand.
- If possible, and available on the equipment, the hand compression dial should be used to allow a slow, measured compression force application.

Handy Hints
When supporting the breast tissue under compression to ensure effective positioning, different hand positions can be used which may reduce your risk of possible repetitive strain injuries (see Chap. 23). Two examples are illustrated in Figs. 21.18 and 21.19.

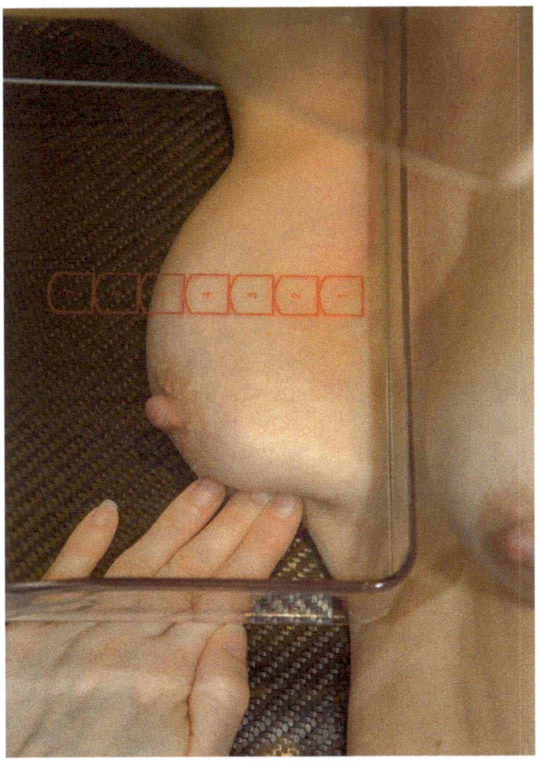

Fig. 21.18 Example One: Hand supportive position

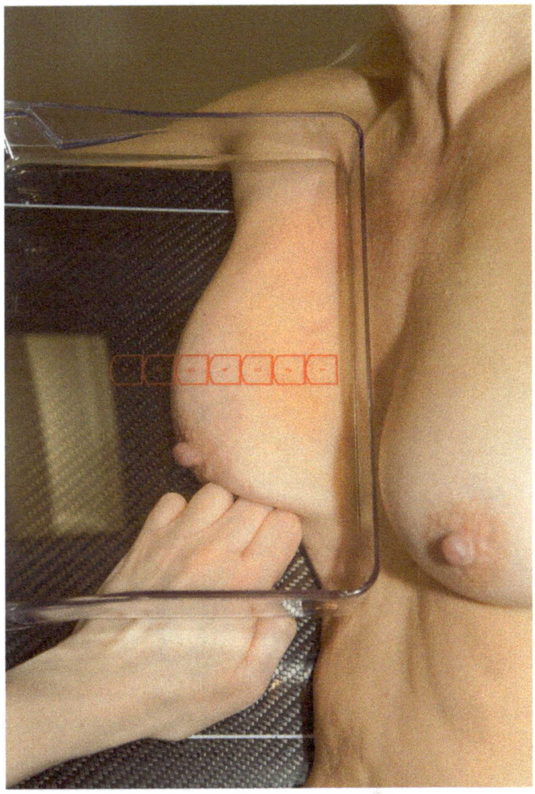

Fig. 21.19 Example Two: Hand supportive position

- The top of the compression paddle should sit just below the clavicle, head of humerus and the inner edge alongside the sternum (Fig. 21.20).
- The breast should be compressed until equal compression force balance between paddle and IR is achieved; the breast may feel taut and immobile. Client consistency between sequential attendances is imperative [12] and the compression force could be standardised between 90 and 130 Newtons of force [13]. Apply smaller forces if the client experiences discomfort; larger forces if the breast is not immobile.
- Ensure the infra mammary angle is open and free from skin folds (Fig. 21.20) and perform a last check to ensure no artefacts are present on the image (i.e.: clients hair, chin, knuckles).

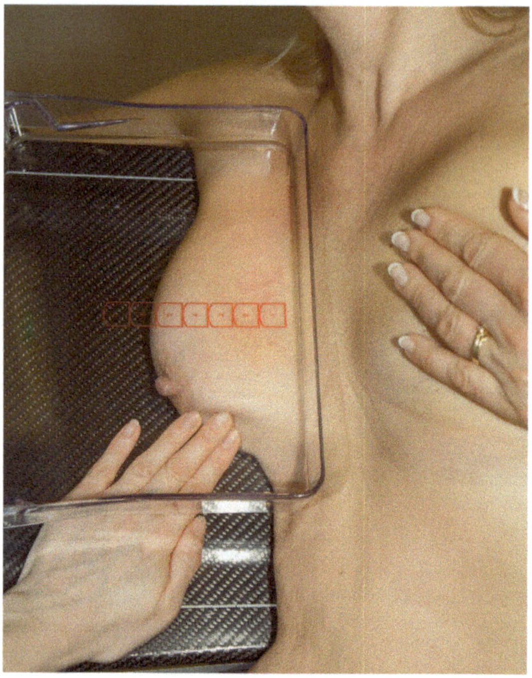

Fig. 21.20 MLO view: Ideal positioning

> **Handy Hints**
> Ask the client to hold her other breast away from the field of view if required and raise her chin slightly

- Perform the exposure. Following automatic compression release, lower the height of the column slightly prior to imaging the opposing side; this allows for effective breast and shoulder placement.

> **Handy Hints**
> Mammogram images are compared for subtle changes and practitioners need to ensure their images are of high quality and consistent with their peers.

Check List and Problem Solving

Rapid Check List

Chapter 36 discusses human observer studies in mammography, including image quality and criteria. Table 21.1 provides an aid to an overview image quality check only.

Table 21.1 Overview check list

View	Checklist
Both	Nipple in profile
	All breast tissue imaged
	Skin fold artefact free
	Symmetrical
	Free from blurring
	Correct exposure parameters used
CC	Back of breast imaged, within 1 cm of the MLO
MLO	Pectoral muscle to nipple level and appropriate width (correct height and angle of IR)
	Infra mammary angle demonstrated

> **P**roper **P**lanning and **P**reparation leads to **P**erfect **P**ositioning

Problem Solving: The CC View

The following information will assist the practitioner to define a solution to a 'problem' before the image has been acquired. If the image has been acquired and the resultant diagnostic image requires a technical repeat or recall, the information below may also assist to define the initial fault and assist the practitioner to identify a solution.

It is important that a decision to repeat an image is only performed following careful consideration and that it will have perceived diagnostic improvements. You should <u>never repeat an image for non-diagnostic reasons</u>.

Problem	Solution
Artefacts on the image	Ensure: Hair is behind ears Earrings are removed Shoulders are relaxed Chin is slightly raised Other breast is being held back
Posterior aspect of breast tissue missing	Check height of image receptor (IR); too high (Fig. 21.21) or too low (Fig. 21.22) the back of the breast will not be imaged. Figure 21.23 illustrates the correct position Ensure the head of the client is facing you and rest it on the face guard; this will ensure that more breast tissue from the back of the breast is imaged The shoulders of the client should be level and relaxed with chin in a neutral position Position client slightly away from the IR to enable client to bend in from the waist; this action moves the ribs and abdomen away and will ensure the back of the breast is imaged Use both hands, one on the medial and one on the lateral side, lift the breast off the IR as you move the breast forward. As compression force is applied keep a firm hand on the breast to prevent any breast tissue slipping out
Creases and air gaps	Check for breast creases medially and laterally before applying compression force If there is an air gap on the medial side gently smooth it out from underneath the IR Check the height of the IR – it may be too low or too high Ensure the client is not reaching up on tiptoes/bent at the knees
Nipples not in profile	It has been demonstrated that following correct positioning the nipple will fall into profile in at least one view with almost all located along or close to the breast boundary [10, 11]. If not: Check height of the IR – it may be too low or too high (Figs. 21.21, 21.22 and 21.23) Ensure the client is not reaching up on tiptoes/bent at the knees Is all the breast tissue pulled through from underneath? Are there any creases on the inferior aspect of the breast?
Symmetry	Is the breast centrally placed on the IR? You can check this by ensuring there is an equal amount of light from the light beam visible on either side of breast (Fig. 21.6)

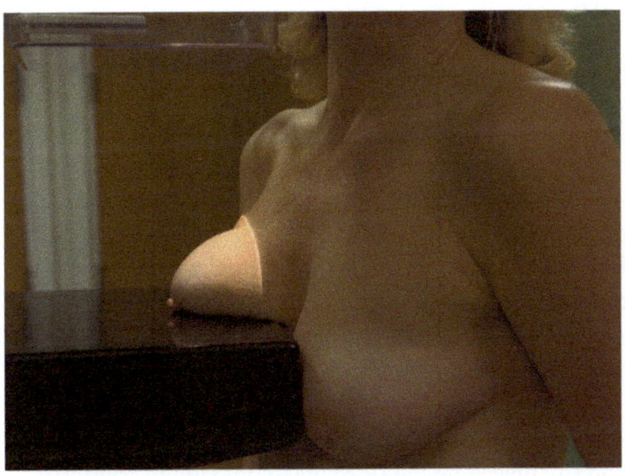

Fig. 21.21 CC view: IR too high

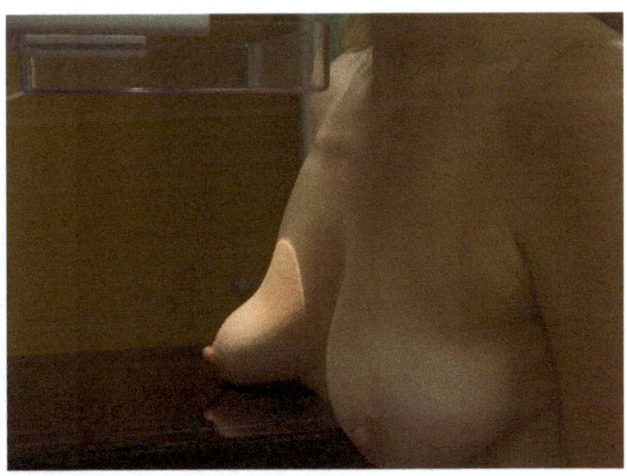

Fig. 21.22 CC view: IR too low

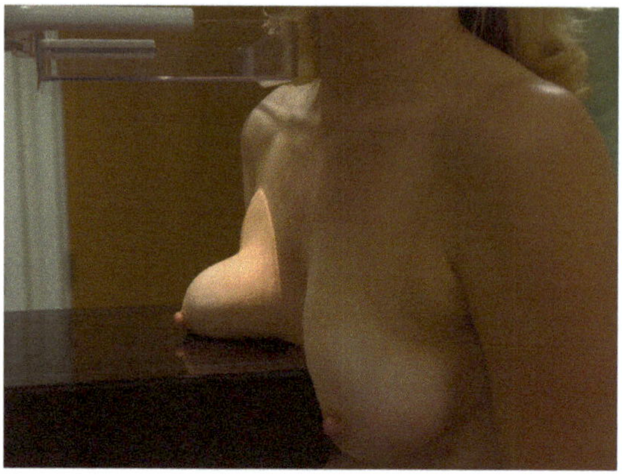

Fig. 21.23 CC view: IR at optimal height, 1 cm above IMF

The following information will assist the practitioner to define a solution to a 'problem' before the image has been acquired. If the image has been acquired and the resultant diagnostic image requires a technical repeat or recall, the information below may also assist to define the initial fault and assist the practitioner to identify a solution.

It is important that a decision to repeat an image is only performed following careful consideration and that it will have perceived diagnostic improvements. You should <u>never repeat an image for non-diagnostic reasons</u>.

Problem Solving: The MLO View

Proper **P**lanning and **P**reparation leads to **P**erfect **P**ositioning

Problem	Solution
Artefacts	Ensure: Hair is behind ears Earrings are removed Shoulders are relaxed back Chin is slightly raised Other breast is being held back
Creases	Ensure client is not standing too close to the IR, bending in from the waist will alter the position of the ribs, smooth out the infra mammary angle and this will eliminate creases behind the breast Perform a 'sweep' of breast tissue, in a downwards motion, behind the breast, starting in the axilla and coming out at the bottom of the breast, keep your hand flat against the IR and your little finger against the rib cage For a slimmer client, ensure the corner of the IR is placed into the axilla at a steeper angle e.g. 55–60°, this will allow the pectoral muscle to lie flat on the IR
Folds across the axilla (Rings of Saturn)	Smooth breast in upwards motion as compression force is applied Before compression force is applied ask client to lift their elbow only on side being imaged, bring down the compression and allow the client's to relax their arm
Height of IR	Ensure that the breast is not too high or too low on the IR The breast tissue should be centrally placed on the IR to obtain maximum comfort for the client and allow optimum pressure distribution over the breast tissue. Correct height placement of the IR will allow the client to relax and flatten the pectoral muscle

Problem	Solution
Infra mammary creases	Ensure that skin folds are removed from behind the ribs prior to compression force application (ask the client to push her hips back whilst you smooth out any creases and then return back in again before the breast is lifted and compressed) Ensure the entire breast is in contact with the IR to avoid any air gaps. It may help to ask the client to bend their knee on the side being imaged Whilst applying compression force, keep the breast uplifted with one hand and smooth the infra mammary with the other When positioning the client ask her to bend forward from the waist and clear the infra mammary area prior to placing the breast on the IR and positioning the arm. This alters the position of the ribs
Missing infra mammary and back of breast	Ensure the client is standing in front of the IR (check position of feet) and that the correct angle is being used for that particular body habitus Has all the breast tissue been pulled on? Use your hand to run down behind the breast, once in position, and pull through all breast tissue
Missing top of breast	If you cannot image the top of the breast and raising the tube does not help, lower the angle of the tube to at least 45
Nipples not in profile	The direction of the nipple will alert you to what portion of the breast would not be demonstrated: If the nipple is facing you it is likely that the client is positioned at the incorrect angle and is facing too far forwards, medially rotate the client towards the IR slightly If the nipple facing inwards towards the IR then probably not enough breast tissue has been pulled through
Position of feet	Ensure the client is standing in the correct place with the feet and ribs in front of the IR With your hand check that the bottom of the ribs are in front and about a palms width away from the IR Slimmer clients can be stood closer to the IR It is useful to ask the client to slightly bend their knee on the side being imaged; the hip will drop which will bring more of the body into contact with the IR
Too wide or too narrow pectoral muscles	*Too narrow*: Check the height of the IR; too high and the muscle will be stretched, tense and not wide enough Always ensure that the corner of the IR is placed to the back of the axilla and the arm stretched across, otherwise the pectoral muscle will be too narrow Ensure the breast is pulled through and the pectoral muscle is flat on the IR with no gaps. Creases will occur if the IR is too far back in the axilla *Too wide*: Check the height of the IR, too low and too much breast tissue will be included around the axilla The IR will be too far back in the axilla, this results in too much breast tissue at the top and insufficient pressure on the main part of the breast
Pectoral muscle not seen to level of nipple:	Alter the angle of the tube to suit the body shape going steeper when necessary (55–60°) for prominent sternums, hollow axillas, slimmer clients
Tube Angle	Use a lower angle 45° or even 40° for clients with short pectoral muscles or 'barrel shapes', 'larger breasts'. HOWEVER: If too much pectoral angle is demonstrated on a client with wide, short pectoral muscles consider increasing your tube angle 50° to reduce the width of the muscle

Acknowledgments The authors would like to pay wholehearted thanks to the professional photographer Gill Brett for her enthusiasm, dedication and commitment without which the photographs within this chapter would not have been possible. We would like to thank our 'staff volunteers' from the University Hospital of South Manchester who gave up their valuable time to pose for the images. Last but certainly not least, the mammography team within the Nightingale Centre, in particular Tina Dunn and Frances Showman for their invaluable knowledge and assistance.

References

1. NHSBSP 63. Quality Assurance Guidelines for Mammography. Apr 2006; 42. ISBN 1 84463 028 5.
2. Poulos A, McLean D. The application of breast compression in mammography: a new perspective. Radiography. 2004;10:131–7.
3. Whelehan P, Evans A, Wells M, Macgillivray S. The effect of mammography pain on repeat participation in breast cancer screening: a systematic review. Breast. 2013;22(4):389–94.
4. Marmot M, Altman DG, Cameron DA, Dewer JA, Thompson SG, Wilcox M. The benefits and harms of breast cancer screening: an independent review. The Lancet. 2012;380(9855):1778–86.
5. Weller DP, Campbell C. Uptake in cancer screening programmes: a priority in cancer control. Br J Cancer. 2009;101 Suppl 2:S55–9. doi:10.1038/sj.bjc.6605391.
6. Smith H, Hogg P, Maxwell A, Mercer CE, Szczepura K. An analysis of the compressed breast area and image receptor/compression paddle pressure balance in different mammographic projections. UKRC 2013 abstract book, Manchester, UK; 2013.
7. Mercer CE, Hogg P, Lawson R, Diffey J, Denton ERE. Practitioner compression force variability in mammography: a preliminary study. Br J Radiol. 2013;86:20110596.
8. Mercer CE, Hogg P, Szczepura K, Denton ERE. Practitioner compression force variation in mammography: a 6-year study. Radiography. 2013; 19(2013):200–6.
9. De Groot JE, Broeders MJM, Branderhorst W, den Heeten GJ, Grimbergen CA. A novel approach to mammographic breast compression: improved standardization and reduced discomfort by controlling pressure instead of force. Med Phys. 2013;40(8): 081901.
10. Pearl O. Breast imaging mammography. Mammography and breast imaging prep, program review and exam preparation. New York: McgrawHill Medical; 2012. p. 213–60.
11. Chuan Z, Chan HP, Paramagul C, Roubidoux MA, Sahiner B, Hadiiiski LM, Petrick N. Computerized nipple identification for multiple image analysis in computer aided diagnosis. Med Phys. 2004;31(10): 2871–82.
12. Mercer CE, Szczepura K, Kelly J, Millington SR, Denton ERE, Borgen R, Hilton B, Hogg P. A call for client consistency in compression. Symposium Mammographicum, Bournemouth, UK; 2014.
13. Hogg P, Taylor M, Szczupera K, Mercer C, Denton E. Pressure and breast thickness in mammography—an exploratory calibration study. Br J Radiol. 2013; 86(1021):20120222.

Bibliography

Dronkers D, Hendricks J, Holland R, Rosenbusch G. The practice of mammography. 5th ed. New York: Thieme Verlag; 2002.

Kopans DB. Breast imaging. 3rd ed. Philadelphia: Lippincott, Williams & Wilkins; 2007.

Lee L, Strickland V, Wilson R, Roebuck E. Fundamentals of mammography. London: WB Saunders Comp. Ltd; 1995.

Prue LK. Atlas of mammographic positioning. Philadelphia: W.B. Saunders Company; 1994.

Tabar L, Dean PB. Teaching atlas of mammography. New York: Thieme Verlag; 1985.

Tucker A, Ng YY. Textbook of mammography. 2nd ed. London: Churchill Livingstone; 2001.

22 Mammographic Compression: A Need for Mechanical Standardisation

Jerry E. de Groot, Woutjan Branderhorst, Ralph Highnam, Ariane Chan, Marcela Böhm-Vélez, M.J.M. Broeders, C.A. Grimbergen, and G.J. den Heeten

Introduction

In mammography image quality is of utmost importance. Good mechanical compression of the breast is one of the essentials of effective mammography. Potential benefits derived from good compression include [1–5]: (1) A more uniform breast thickness resulting in a better fit of the exposure into the dynamic range; (2) Reduced blurring from breast motion; (3) Reduced scattered radiation and improved contrast sensitivity; (4) Reduced radiation dose; (5) Better visualisation of tissues near the chest wall; and (6) Reduced superimposition of overlapping tissues.

However, there is an issue in clinical practice in the sense that "good compression" is not easily defined to be followed routinely. The natural shape of the breast results in varying thickness from the nipple to the chest wall and is a general deterrent to achieving good contrast and visibility without compression. "Good compression" transforms the breast into a more uniform thickness and makes the breast tissue somewhat thinner for better imaging.

All aspects of the mammographic image acquisition process are subject to quality standards [European Guidelines [1], Mammography Quality and Standards Act (MQSA) [2]], but the instructions for compression are too vague to provide any sort of standardisation. To cite the European guidelines literally: "The compression should be firm but tolerable. There is no optimal value known for the force, but attention should be given to the applied compression and the accuracy of the indication." The MQSA only mentions requirements for testing compression devices, but gives no indication on how much force to use in clinical practice. Both guidelines do state an upper limit of 20 decanewton (daN) and all mammographic machines restrict the motor drive to this level. In practice, the amount of compression is guided by approximating the individual pain threshold of the patient and the individual performance of mammographers.

J.E. de Groot, PhD candidate (✉) • W. Branderhorst
C.A. Grimbergen
Post-doctoral researcher, Biomedical Engineering and Physics, Academic Medical Center, Meibergdreef 9, Amsterdam 1105 AZ, The Netherlands
e-mail: jerry.degroot@sigmascreening.com; w.branderhorst@amc.nl; c.a.grimbergen@amc.uva.nl

R. Highnam • A. Chan
Volpara Solutions, Wellington, New Zealand
e-mail: Ralph.Highnam@VolparaSolutions.com; ariane.chan@volparasolutions.com

M. Böhm-Vélez
Weinstein Imaging Associates, Pittsburgh, PA, USA
e-mail: marcelabvelez@gmail.com

M.J.M. Broeders
LRCB Dutch Reference Center for Screening, Nijmegen, The Netherlands

G.J. den Heeten
Department of Radiology, Academic Medical Center, Amsterdam
The Netherlands

LRCB Dutch Reference Center for Screening, Nijmegen, The Netherlands

P. Hogg et al. (eds.), *Digital Mammography: A Holistic Approach*,
DOI 10.1007/978-3-319-04831-4_22, © Springer International Publishing Switzerland 2015

For that reason breast compression is patient- and operator-dependent [6].

Since little is known about compression standardisation, we tried to find information in the literature about compression parameters in the DICOM headers like force and breast thickness. We found that considerable variations exist, especially in the force at exposure [7, 8]. It came to our attention that in different countries different policies are maintained. For example, in the Dutch screening nowadays, a minimum force of 12 daN is maintained, while in the U.S. there seems to be no target force at all.

The Mechanics of Compression

Mechanical compression makes the breast flatter by applying force. One decanewton (daN) of force is equivalent to the weight of approximately 1 kg. Applying a certain force on a small breast has a different effect than applying the same force on a large breast. This is because the force is distributed over different areas of contact. A better comparison is obtained by dividing the applied force by the total breast contact area. This value gives force per unit contact area, also known as contact pressure, which is measured in kilopascal (kPa; 1 kPa = 1 daN/dm^2 ≈ 7.5 mmHg). Applying the same pressure on small or large breasts has the same effect on the tissue because the force is proportional to the breast contact area. This might be relevant because the middle 95 % of breast volumes in the sample of this chapter vary by a factor ten (ca. 0.22–2.2 dm^3). Furthermore, individual breast mechanical properties can differ significantly depending on tissue composition, age and properties of the skin [9].

Recent research in this field showed that it is feasible to use a pressure-standardised compression approach. In addition, that study found that contact area is a significant predictor for pain while compression force itself is not [10]. This makes contact pressure, being the ratio of force and contact area, a better predictor for pain.

Mammographic Monitoring Software

Recently, software for the evaluation of mammogram DICOM information became available (VolparaAnalytics and VolparaDensity, Volpara Solutions, Wellington, New Zealand) enabling cross-comparison of populations. For the first time, this allows for a comprehensive analysis of some of the mechanical parameters of compression of the breast that occur in daily practice in different countries.

The purpose of this chapter is to compare, analyse and visualise the current mammographic compression practice in the Netherlands and the U.S. from a mechanical point of view, and to hypothesise if mechanical standardisation could lead to a more reproducible procedure. This important insight may open the way towards individualised and more reproducible and optimised mechanical compression in mammography.

Methods

The analysis software (VolparaAnalytics (version 1.0) and VolparaDensity (algorithm version 1.5.0), Volpara Solutions, Wellington, New Zealand) calculates breast volume and density, as well as contact area for contact pressure estimates. It also calculates absorbed glandular dose (AGD) using a comprehensive dose model, which enables AGD-comparison between DICOM data from different mammography device manufacturers.

Two large anonymised data sets were available, one from the Dutch breast cancer screening programme ($n = 13{,}610$, August 2012–September 2013), and one from an imaging centre in Pittsburgh, PA, U.S.A. ($n = 7{,}179$, January 2008–March 2014). Figure 22.1 gives an impression of the comparability of breast densities and volumes of women aged 50–75 in both data sets.

Since contact area is the parameter that links force to pressure ($P = F/A$), we will compare parameters as a function of contact area. It is worth mentioning that contact area is strongly correlated with breast volume (Pearson's rho = 0.82, $p < 0.001$). This enabled us to compare

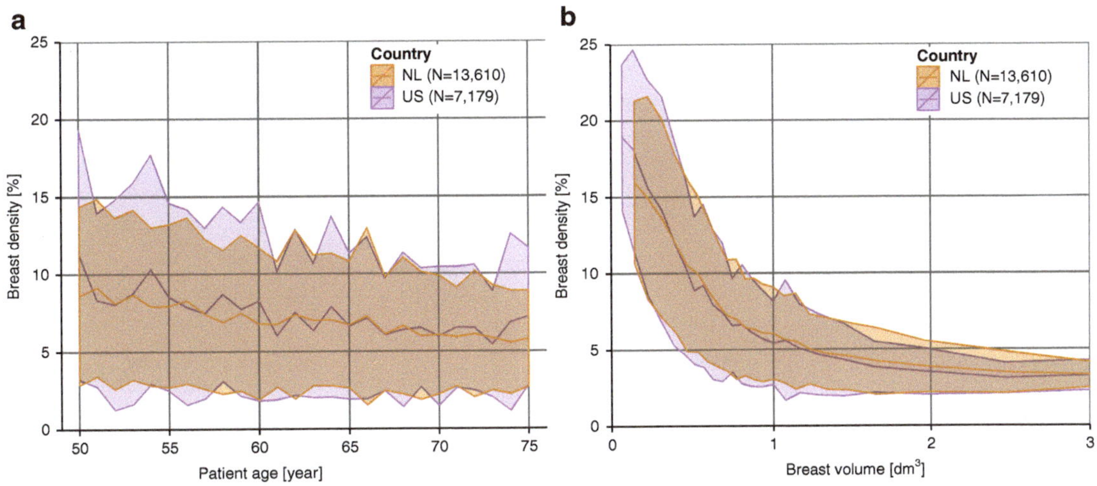

Fig. 22.1 (**a**) Breast density (%) versus patient age (years); plus/minus one standard deviation. (**b**) Breast density (%) versus breast volume (dm^3) mean plus/minus one standard deviation

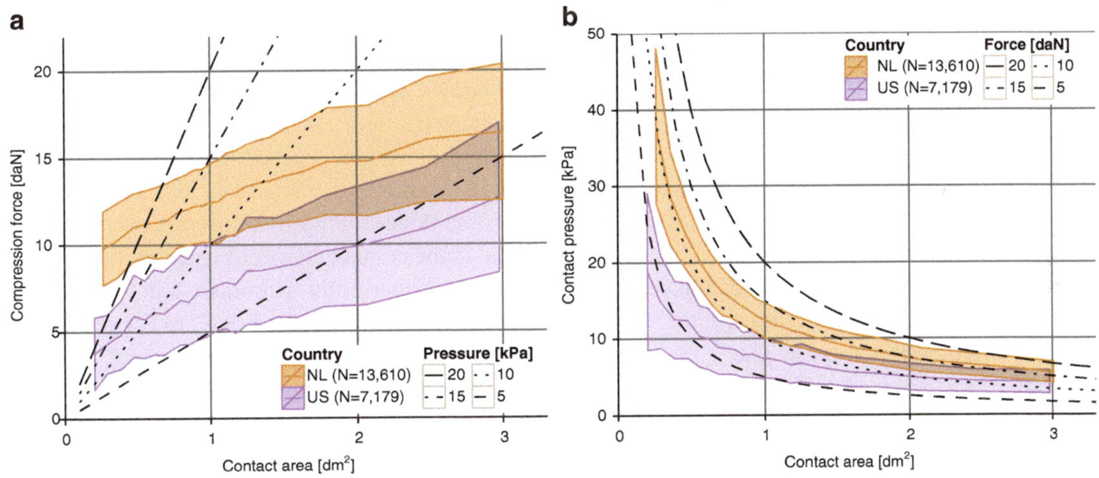

Fig. 22.2 (**a**) Compression force (daN) versus contact area (dm^2); mean plus/minus one standard deviation. (**b**) Contact pressure (kPa) versus contact area (dm^2); mean plus/minus one standard deviation

the variation in compression forces and pressures as function of breast size, as performed by practitioners in two different countries, one with a 12 daN minimum force (The Netherlands) and one without a specific target compression force (U.S.).

Results

Figure 22.2a shows compression force (daN) versus contact area (dm^2) for both data sets. In this figure, four pressure values (5, 10, 15, 20 kPa) are indicated as straight lines: Force (daN) = Pressure (kPa) × Contact area (dm^2). Figure 22.2b shows contact pressure (kPa) versus contact area (dm^2) for the same data. In this figure four force values (5, 10, 15, 20 daN) are indicated as hyperbolas: Pressure (kPa) = Force (daN)/Contact area (dm^2).

It is clearly visible that the applied forces and pressures were considerably higher in the Netherlands, however in both countries similar trends exist as a function of contact area: Smaller breasts received lower forces than larger breasts

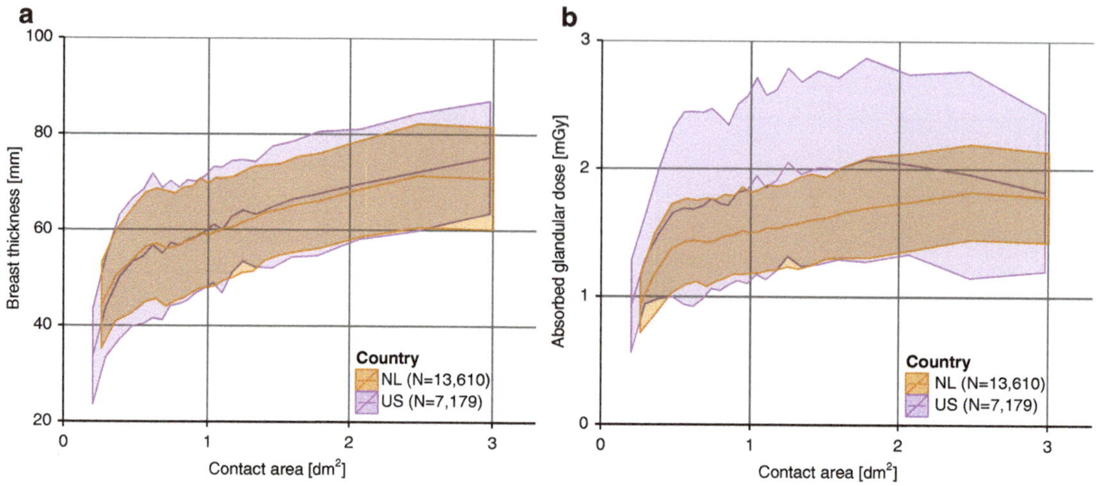

Fig. 22.3 (**a**) Thickness (mm) versus contact area (dm^2). (**b**) Absorbed glandular dose (mGy) versus contact area(dm^2)

in both countries, and pressures were higher for smaller breasts compared to larger breasts.

Comparing the number of high compression forces in both data sets, we see that the Dutch set has 18.6 % ($n=2{,}528$) compressions higher than 15 daN, versus 1.9 % ($n=139$) in the U.S.. In terms of high pressures we find 10.7 % ($n=1{,}458$) compressions higher than 20 kPa in the Netherlands, versus 1.7 % ($n=119$) in the U.S. On the other side of the scale we can compare the number of low compression forces. The U.S. data set contains 23.5 % ($n=1{,}688$) compressions that received less than 5 daN, versus practically none, 0.04 % ($n=6$), in the Netherlands. Lastly, we counted 21.7 % ($n=1{,}555$) compressions below 5 kPa of pressure in the U.S., versus only 0.8 % ($n=114$) in the Netherlands.

Figure 22.3a shows breast thickness (mm) versus contact area (dm^2) for both datasets. The average thickness is nearly identical for both datasets, but the standard deviation in the U.S. data is on average 16 % larger. Figure 22.3b shows absorbed glandular dose (mGy) versus contact area (dm^2). All dose values were recalculated with Volpara's comprehensive dose model, which enables inter-manufacturer comparison. The U.S. data has a higher mean value and a much larger standard deviation compared to the Dutch data. These differences are possibly influenced by the larger variation of the breast thickness in the U.S. set. Another source of variation is that U.S. images were made on mammography machines with various target- and filter materials, whereas the Dutch screening only used machines with Tungsten target and Rhodium or Silver filter.

Figure 22.4 illustrates modelled compressions following a strict force protocol ($F=14$ daN$\pm$5 % standard deviation) and a strict pressure protocol ($P=10$ kPa$\pm$5 % standard deviation). In Fig. 22.4a, the force values for the 10 kPa-protocol are proportional to the contact area until reaching the 20 daN guideline upper limit. The modelled 14 daN-protocol is constant around 14 daN. In Fig. 22.4b the pressure values for the 10 kPa-protocol are constant around the target value of 10 kPa, and again limited to 20 daN of force for contact areas larger than 2.0 dm^2. The strict 14 daN-protocol extends far beyond the scale with a maximum pressure of 120 kPa (900 mmHg) for the smallest breast found in these data sets.

Discussion

The results obtained from this study show that current mammographic compression policies in the Netherlands and in the United States lead not only to a wide range of applied forces but also to a wide range of pressures. We found a large difference between the countries, but also large standard deviations for women with the same breast size within each population. This implicates that from the individual woman's point of view, the procedure is far from reproducible and the amount of applied pressure is unpredictable.

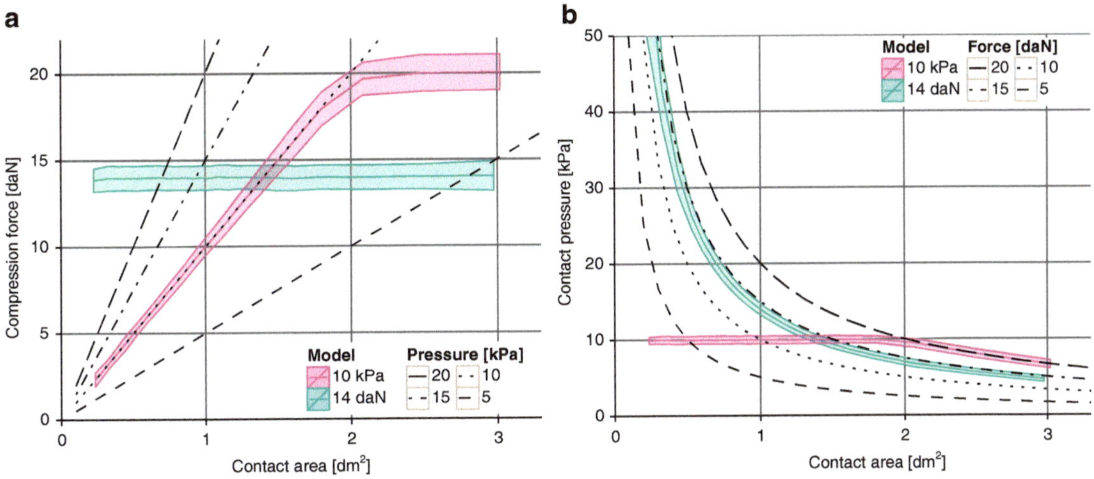

Fig. 22.4 (**a**) Modelled compression force (daN) versus contact area (dm^2) for a strict pressure (10 kPa) and force (14 daN) protocol. (**b**) Modelled pressure (kPa) versus contact area (dm^2) for a strict pressure (10 kPa) and force (14 daN) protocol

This is the first study on breast compression in which not only the applied force but also the contact pressure is compared between two large data sets from different countries. Large variations in applied forces in mammography have been reported before [7, 8] and are a logical result of current compression policies in which practitioners are expected to fixate the breast based on experience, observation of the patient and tautness of the breast tissue [1, 2]. The practitioners thereby subjectively adjust the force to a certain extent compensating for breast size, composition and pain. Since these parameters are highly variable over the population, a large variation in applied forces can be expected. However, if the compression force would be objectively adjusted to breast size and composition (elasticity), this would lead to a similar pressure in all breasts [10]. In the results of this study, we observed that the applied average pressure is highly variable in current mammographic compression practice. The compression force chosen by the practitioner must therefore be predominantly determined by factors other than the breast size and elasticity. In other words, at least from a mechanical point of view, mammographic compression is not standardised. There seems to be only a very weak relation between the biomechanical parameters involved.

On the other hand, mammography has already been employed successfully for decades. Irrespective of the very large variation in compression, there seems to be hardly any noticeable influence on the image quality; it is seldom that mammograms have to be repeated because of insufficient compression. Apparently, there is a large range of pressures in which the resulting images look diagnostically sufficient regardless what pressure is used. However, our data show that current clinical practice leads to strikingly high pressures for women with smaller breasts, particularly in The Netherlands. A recent publication concluded that small breasted women experience more pain [10]. On the other extreme, in the U.S., a large number of women receive alarmingly low pressures, which could be associated with an increased risk of image quality issues and receiving higher dose. In both countries, women will likely endure wide variations in compression over the course of repeated examinations, depending on the performance and training of the practitioners [6].

The absence of compression guidelines, especially in the U.S., may have lead to a gradual decrease of applied compression forces as a measure to avoid pain complaints. This so-called compression creep may unnoticeably affect image quality and dose. We believe that pressure-standardised compression protocols might improve this unwanted situation, but further research is necessary.

Conclusion

Comparing mammographic compression in the Netherlands (maintaining only a 12 daN minimum force) and the U.S. (without a specified target force), forces and pressures are considerably higher in the Netherlands. Variations between women with the same breast size (contact area) are large in both countries.

Standardising with a target force will still lead to large differences between individuals with different breast sizes, and is therefore not an effective standardisation. Standardising with a target pressure, which objectively takes the size of the breast into consideration, effectively leads to a standard tissue pressure and probably less variation in thickness reduction. This could potentially avoid severe pain without putting image quality or breast dose at risk, however, more research is needed.

References

1. Perry N, Broeders M, de Wolf C, Törnberg S, Holland R, Von Karsa L, editors. European guidelines for quality assurance in breast cancer screening and diagnosis. 4th ed. Luxembourg: Office for Official Publications of the European Communities; 2008.
2. Mammography Quality Standards Act of 1992. Mammography facilities requirement for accrediting bodies, and quality standards and certifying requirements. Fed Regist. 1993;58:67565–72.
3. Saunders Jr RS, Samei E. The effect of breast compression on mass conspicuity in digital mammography. Med Phys. 2008;35(10):4464–73.
4. Pisano ED, Yaffe MJ. Digital mammography. Radiology. 2005;234(2):353–62.
5. Heine JJ, Cao K, Thomas JA. Effective radiation attenuation calibration for breast density: compression thickness influences and correction. Biomed Eng Online. 2010;9:73.
6. Mercer CE, Hogg P, Lawson R, Diffey J, Denton ER. Practitioner compression force variability in mammography: a preliminary study. Br J Radiol. 2013;86(1022):20110596.
7. Hendrick RE, Pisano ED, Averbukh A, Moran C, Berns EA, Yaffe MJ, et al. Comparison of acquisition parameters and breast dose in digital mammography and screen-film mammography in the American College of Radiology Imaging Network digital mammographic imaging screening trial. AJR Am J Roentgenol. 2010;194(2):362–9.
8. Sullivan DC, Beam CA, Goodman SM, Watt DL. Measurement of force applied during mammography. Radiology. 1991;181(2):355–7.
9. Gefen A, Dilmoney B. Mechanics of the normal woman's breast. Technol Health Care. 2007;15(4):259–71.
10. de Groot JE, Broeders MJ, Branderhorst W, den Heeten GJ, Grimbergen CA. A novel approach to mammographic breast compression: improved standardization and reduced discomfort by controlling pressure instead of force. Med Phys. 2013;40(8):081901.

Repetitive Strain Injury – RSI

23

Claire D. Borrelli

Introduction

Work-related repetitive strain injury (RSI) and musculoskeletal disorders (MSKD) may encompass a wide range of inflammatory and degenerative diseases and disorders and are a major occupational hazard for mammographers. These conditions are caused by repetitive, forceful, or awkward movements that can result in injury to muscles, nerves, tendons, and ligaments and can include carpal tunnel syndrome, tendonitis, lower back pain and tension neck syndrome [1]. Common areas of the body to be affected by musculoskeletal pain for mammographers include the hands, wrists, elbows, neck, shoulders and lower back, although this list is not exclusive. The repetitive nature of mammographers' work, as well as the awkward postures used while working can cause significant stress on their bodies and the physical strain can cause, or exacerbate these conditions.

It isn't necessarily the nature of a person's movements that cause the musculoskeletal pain (they are often ordinary movements such as bending, straightening, gripping, holding, twisting, clenching and reaching). It is the fact that a person may make the same movements repetitively, often at speed and using force, and with no recovery time between movements that makes them hazardous. This is a particularly important consideration within breast screening with the implementation of the age extension and therefore an increase of women attending the service. To maintain the throughput to meet the demands of the increasing numbers attending, mammographers are likely to adopt unusual postures when pressed for time although positioning should ideally be efficient and timely to reduce the risk of injury [2]. In some cases the person's work environment may be poorly designed which may also mean that their work position or posture is awkward and yet avoidable had consideration been given at the planning stage.

The most common symptom associated with musculoskeletal disorders is pain although some sufferers report joint stiffness, muscle tightness, 'pins and needles' and redness and swelling of the affected area. Musculoskeletal disorders can range from mild to severe and, as they are cumulative in nature, can be measured depending on the severity/longevity of the pain and the extent to which the pain affects a person's ability to work:

Mammography Radiographers and the Risks of Musculoskeletal Disorders

A study conducted in 1997 sought to determine if breast screening radiographers experienced any musculoskeletal discomfort and, if

C.D. Borrelli
St George's National Breast Education Centre,
The Rose Centre, St George's Healthcare NHS Trust,
Perimeter Road, London SW17 0QT, UK
e-mail: claire.borrelli@stgeorges.nhs.uk

P. Hogg et al. (eds.), *Digital Mammography: A Holistic Approach*,
DOI 10.1007/978-3-319-04831-4_23, © Springer International Publishing Switzerland 2015

so, the nature and extent of the problem [3]. The study was extended to investigate and determine the possible occupational, causal, or contributory factors; and proposed a technique for mammography radiographers to adopt to help alleviate discomfort caused by their repetitive actions. In 2007, the National Health Service Breast Screening Program (NHSBSP) in England conducted an ergonomic assessment of different mammography units and reported that repetitive strain injuries affecting thumbs and wrists remains a particular problem [4].

Repetitive strain injuries in mammography radiographers have more recently been described in a professional document published by the Society of Radiographers (SoR) [5]. This document includes a survey of radiographers, in which 62 % indicated that they often or always have to manoeuvre into awkward positions [6]. This, combined with the inevitable time constraints of the job and ever-increasing workload, can lead to a range of symptoms, such as pain, tenderness, swelling, and muscle weakness. These symptoms often result in conditions such as rotator cuff syndrome, carpal tunnel syndrome, tendinitis, and trigger finger or thumb. Ransom [7] states that the aforementioned conditions are progressive and can typically be classified into three categories: mild, moderate or severe stages. At the severe stage, sleep can be disturbed, sometimes leading to an inability to carry out even the most mundane tasks, and can even result in permanent disability. In the SoR's document, SoR CEO Richard Evans states that, "Work-related injury to members of the radiographic workforce is a threat to the health of our members, a threat to their careers and a threat to the services that they have worked so hard to establish" [5].

Equipment design is important in helping to reduce repetitive strain injury to radiographers, as different functions and workflows all play their part in either contributing to or limiting these risks. While the NHSBSP has recommended equipment improvements specifically to address this issue, as yet, no industry standards have been created.

Equipment Considerations

The Column/Gantry

A second major reduction of fatigue and stress results from how rotation is configured. Automatic tube angling is a feature that causes the tube head to move automatically into the oblique position to a pre-set angulation, reducing the amount of stretching required for each examination, and thus decreasing stress on the upper body. However, even with powered rotation, conventional systems require the radiographers to initiate the movement by pressing a button on the tube head and this upper body movement is repetitive during positioning. On older imaging systems, this requires radiographers to raise their arms up to the button height, and to maintain finger pressure on the button as the tube head rotates. To maintain continuous pressure on the button, radiographers have to stretch their arms through the rotations, and if the radiographer did not have correct posture at the initiation of the rotation, this could result in inappropriate twisting. An important ergonomic consideration for the manufacturers is to include automatic tube angulation in all designs and to ensure that movement buttons are strategically placed along the column e.g. tube head, breast platform and bottom of column to suit radiographer's height and positioning stance to ensure ergonomic safety when rotating the gantry (Fig. 23.1).

Easy Height Adjustment of Equipment

Only a light touch should be required to depress buttons and reaching the buttons should be almost effortless. Buttons are replicated both on the tube head and side of the breast platform, so radiographers can use the set of controls that are easiest to access from their position, or alternate between controls to help reduce repetitive movements and the risk of repetitive strain.

The NHSBSP guidelines indicate that it is good practice to offer a choice in how to manipulate the system, and ergonomic development will help vary routine and reduce repetitive strain injuries [3, 4] (Fig. 23.2).

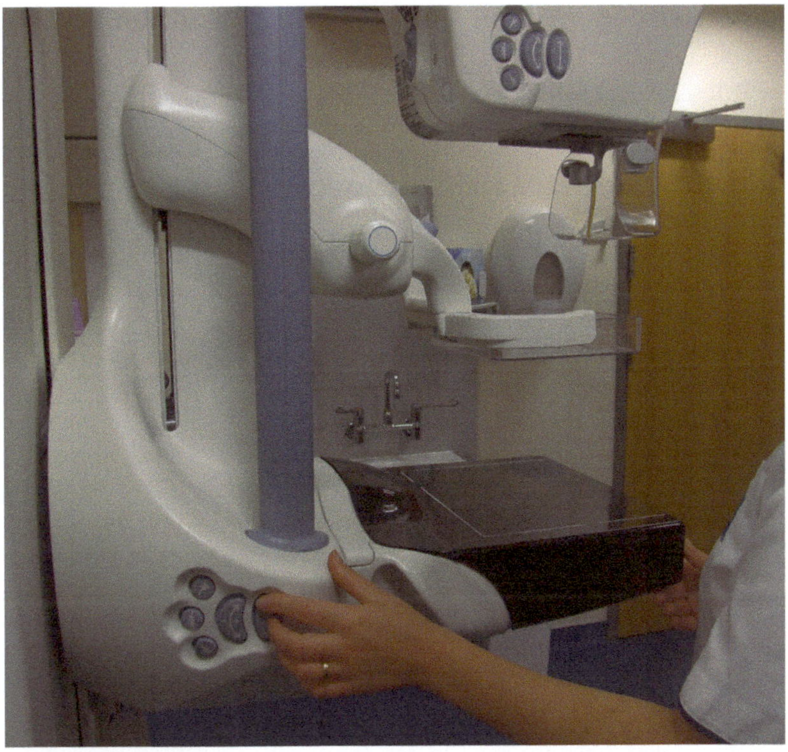

Fig. 23.1 Strategic placement of buttons on the gantry (Source: BreastCheck, Ireland)

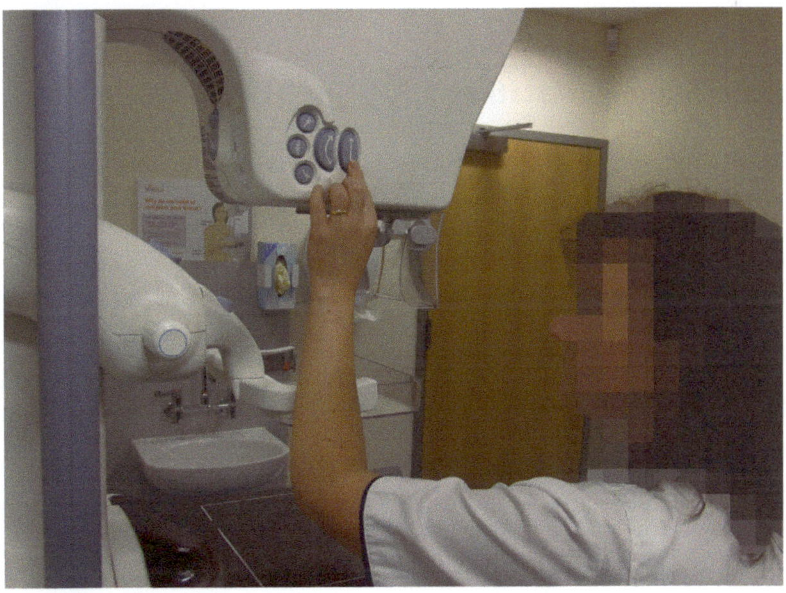

Fig. 23.2 Ease of reaching equipment buttons on tube head (Source: BreastCheck, Ireland)

Motorised Compression

Smooth breast compression technology is achieved by the use of a foot switch, which allows radiographers to use their hands for positioning the breast. A number of features that may help to reduce injury include:

(a) Some units do not require mammographers to make physical changes to the compression paddle between small and large women, thereby reducing the risk of strain.
(b) Where it is not necessary to shift the compression paddle for each oblique view of the smaller breast, demands on the hands and wrists are minimised.
(c) Where hand-controlled compression knobs for fine-tuning the level of compression are avoided, the need for repeated twisting of the wrist is reduced.
(d) Use of a high-edge paddle pushes the contralateral breast back, and supports it away from the field of view. This means that the mammographer does not need to ask (or assist) the client to do this during the oblique projections, thereby reducing the risk of injury.

Acquisition Workstation

Musculo-skeletal injury can be associated with repetitive keyboard use and this can be reduced by limiting the number of steps requiring the use of a mouse or keypad through the mammography process, or by employing touchscreen technology.

Room Design

Careful design of the mammography room can also help to reduce musculo- strains and improve workflow. The working triangle should be as small as possible whilst including considerate choice of equipment. The design of the reporting room should also be considered as many radiographers are now involved in image interpretation as well as mammography. The same principles will apply to radiographers involved in extended roles, such as ultrasound.

Positioning Considerations

1. Adopt good communication skills with the client as this will enable her to move independently rather than being moved.
2. Rather than using the thumb and forefinger to support the whole breast, use the whole hand, or as much of the hand as possible to position the breast (Fig. 23.3).
3. Consider the design of exposure control designs to enable the mammographers to use different fingers and therefore different movements to press the exposure button to avoid injury (Figs. 23.4 and 23.5).
4. The mammographer should be familiar with the full range of the equipment and its controls to adopt a positioning technique that is ergonomically safe and most convenient for repetitive use. Maintaining a good posture throughout the examination is important to minimise strain or injury (Fig. 23.6a–c).

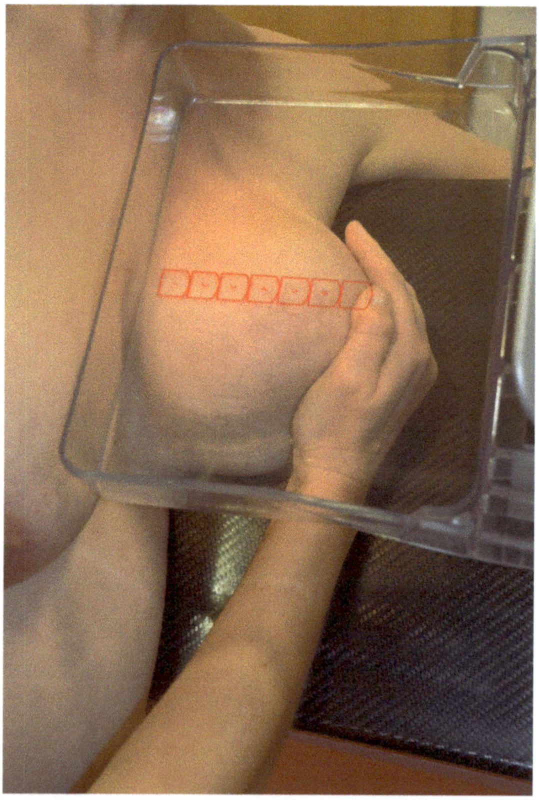

Fig. 23.3 Good hand position for supporting the breast (Source: Kings College Hospital, London)

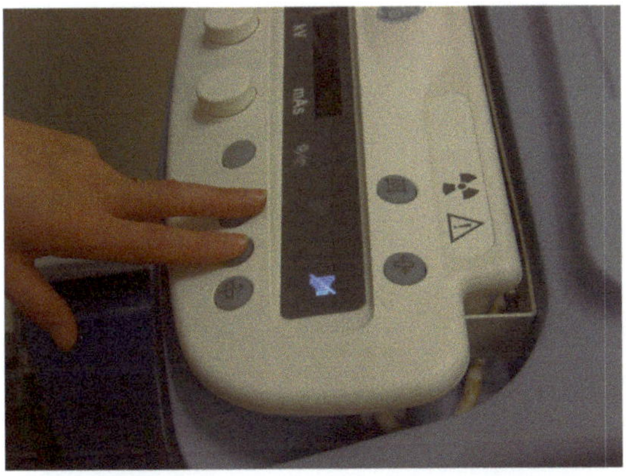

Fig. 23.4 Alternate use of fingers between exposures (Source: BreastCheck, Ireland)

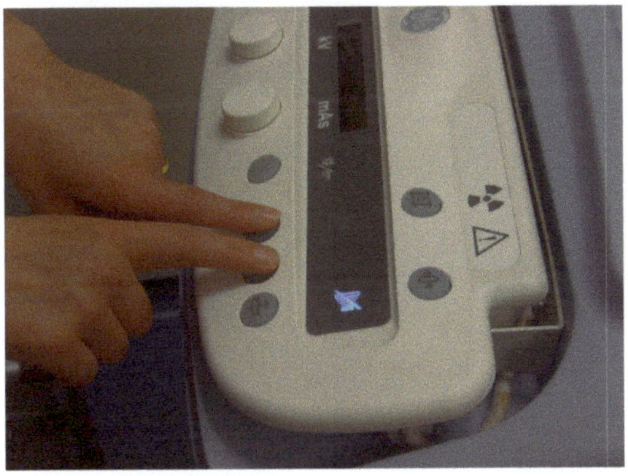

Fig. 23.5 Alternate use of fingers between exposures (Source: BreastCheck, Ireland)

5. Prior to positioning a woman, ensure that the foot pedals are placed correctly so that there is no need to stretch extremities to reduce the risk of injury (Fig. 23.7a, b).
6. Consider the use of a positioning stool for either the client or the mammographer. This will require the provision of suitable chairs and flooring and should be part of the design process for each mammography room. Each mammographer must adjust their seat height and proximity to suit each woman to avoid over-extension of their elbows and shoulders. The wheels on the stool must be selected to give the right level of grip for the type of floor (Fig. 23.8).
7. Additional equipment should be stored at waist height to reduce bending and stretching.
8. Where possible, set the height of the modality acquisition workstation. Some manufacturers have introduced touch screen technology to reduce the use of keyboards.
9. Always have two mammographers available where disabled women or women in wheelchairs are to be screened to ensure health and safety for both client and practitioners.
10. Mammographers' positioning practice should be observed regularly by an experienced colleague. The colleague should identify behaviour and practices that might lead to ergonomic injuries, and advise on alternative approaches. This is a measure of best practice and could serve as CPD activity.
11. Always rotate screening mammography with other tasks to ensure that practitioners have micro-breaks from repetitive tasks [8].

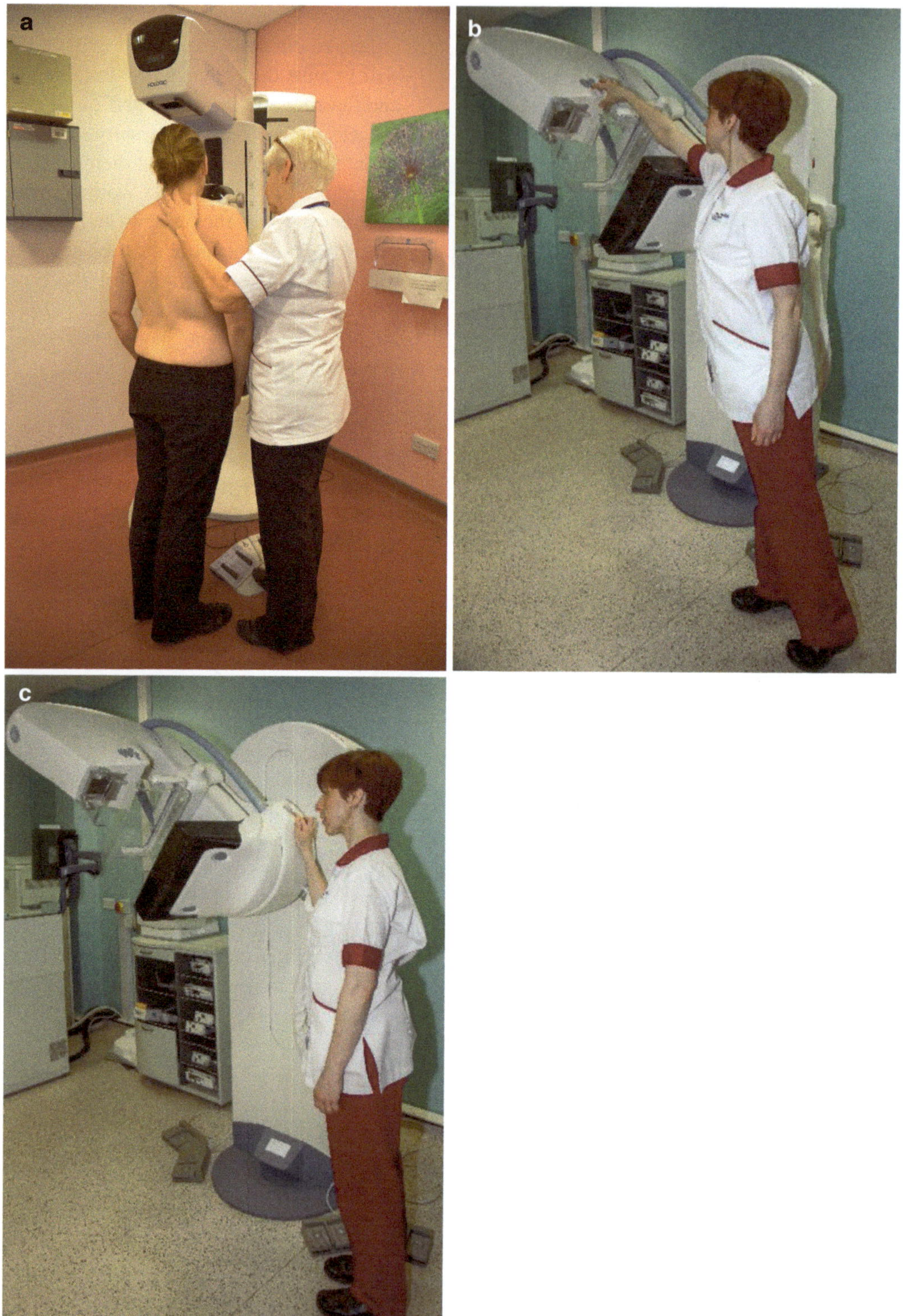

Fig. 23.6 (**a**) Adopt a good posture – straight spine, no over reaching (Source: King's College Hospital, London). (**b**) Over stretching (Source: Nightingale Centre, Manchester). (**c**) Good posture (Source: Nightingale Centre, Manchester)

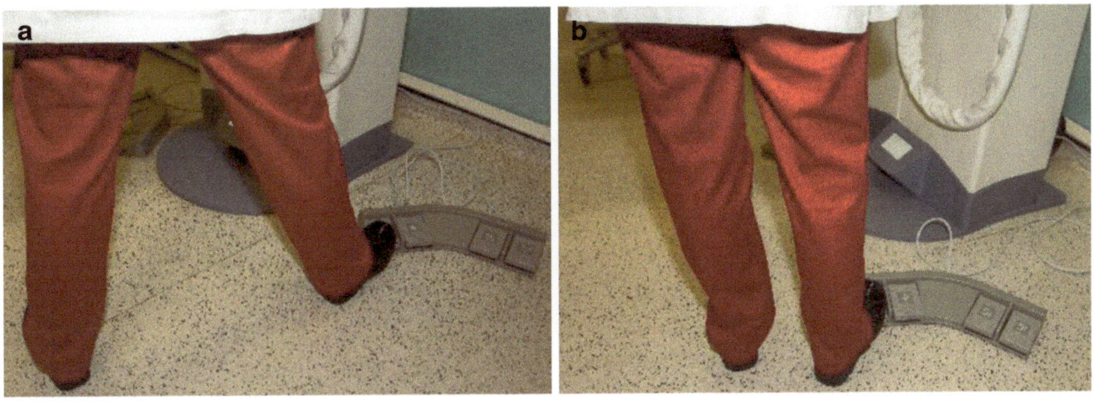

Fig. 23.7 (**a**) Over reaching (Source: Nightingale Centre, Manchester). (**b**) Good foot position (Source: Nightingale Centre, Manchester)

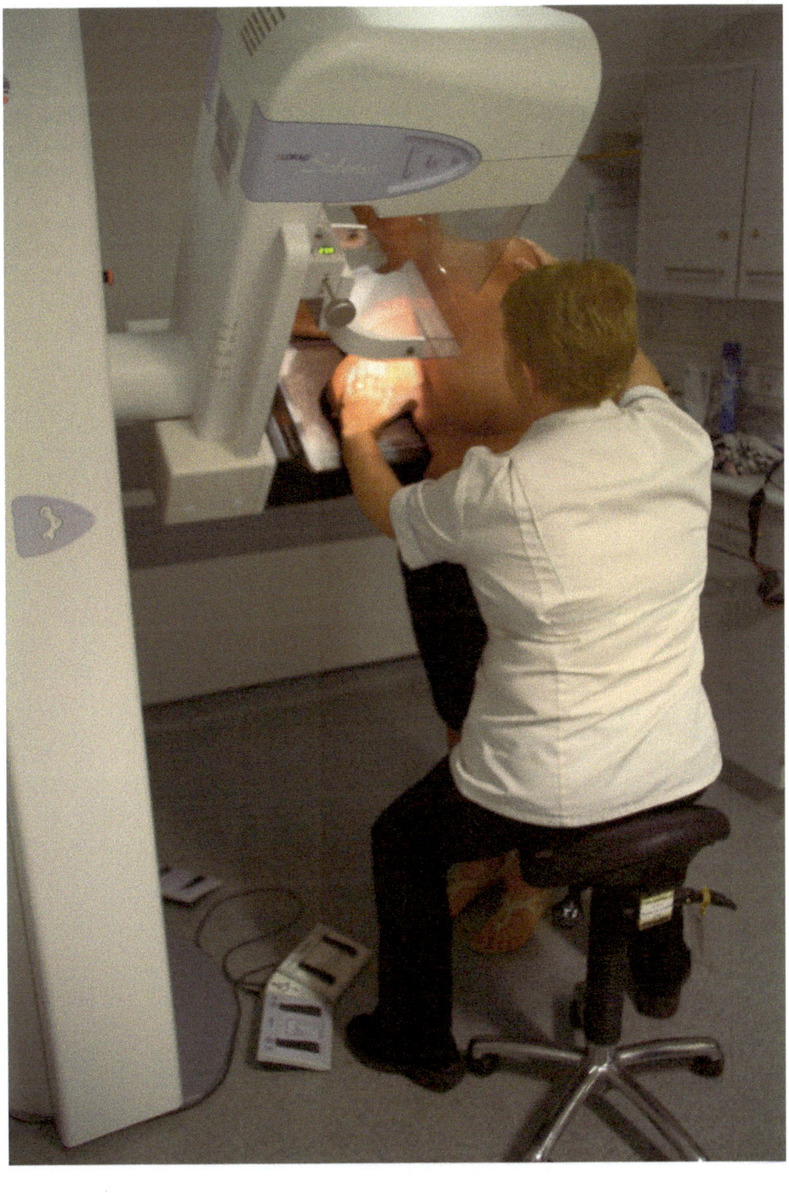

Fig. 23.8 Ergonomic use of a saddle stool for positioning of client (Source: Rose Centre, St George's Hospital, London)

Conclusion

Due to the repetitive nature of breast imaging and the fact that undertaking a mammogram is a notably physical activity, great care should be taken to support the well-being of mammography staff. In deciding which equipment to use, consideration should be given to the ergonomic suitability of the systems. Mammography staff should be familiar in using the equipment effectively and ensure that high image quality is obtained without compromising their own health.

It is the responsibility of individuals for their own health and safety and that of work colleagues to ensure that safe practices are used when performing mammography and undertaking other imaging related duties. The health and safety of all practitioners performing mammograms are critically important, and the Employers' Liability Act makes it the employer's responsibility to care for the health and safety of their employees whilst at work [9].

References

1. Ransom E. The causes of musculoskeletal injury amongst sonographers in the UK. London: Society of Radiographers; 2002. Accessed 5 May 2014.
2. The Cancer Reform Strategy. Policy document. London: Department of Health; 2007.
3. Gale A, May JG. An evaluation of musculoskeletal discomfort experienced by radiographers performing mammography. NHSBSP Publication, 36. 1997.
4. Gale A, Hunter N, Lawton C, Purdy K. Ergonomic assessment of radiographer units. NHSBSP equipment report, 0708. 2007.
5. Wigley L, Dixon A. Musculoskeletal disorders in mammography: a guide to tackling the issues in the workplace. Society of Radiographers Journal: Synergy News. 2009.
6. Interviews with radiographers at Breast Check Ireland and Musgove Park Taunton Breast Screening, 2011, by Miles, J. Breast Check Ireland (BCI): Joanne Hammond, National Radiography Manager, Breast Check Ireland; Catherine Vaughan, Radiographer, Coventry and Warwickshire Breast Screening Centre; Sharon Hoffmeister, Deputy Superintendent Radiographer Musgove Park Taunton Breast Screening: Pat Middleton and her staff. Annemarie Dixon, Senior Lecturer, Leeds University.
7. Ransom E. The causes of musculoskeletal injury amongst sonographers in the UK. London: Society of Radiographers; 2002.
8. Borrelli C, Button M, Dixon AM, Eckersley B, Fretwell AM, Griggs J, Hoffmeiste S, Milnes V, Mumby A, Phillips V, Sellars S, Shaw A, Stanton A, Teape A, Vegnut Z. Reducing the risk of musculoskeletal discomfort in mammography. NHSBSP good practice guide no 138. 2012.
9. HM Government. The Employers Liability Act. 1969.

24 Supplementary Mammographic Projections

Judith Kelly

Introduction

Some breast abnormalities are located in the extreme medial or lateral aspects of the breast. The techniques described in the Practical Mammography chapter for the standard cranio-caudal (CC) and mediolateral-oblique (MLO) projections do not image all the breast tissue in its entirety since these extreme aspects are usually not routinely included. In such cases supplementary projections are necessary to ensure significant abnormalities are not overlooked or misinterpreted in any assessment process. Examples include clinical presentation of a mass within which is not seen on the standard projections or a partially demonstrated perceived abnormality in an asymptomatic woman seen on one standard projection, but not seen on the corresponding projection [1]. Furthermore a factitious appearance may be created by overlapping breast tissue, simulating the appearance of a mass or architectural distortion [2]. Occasionally a perceived mammographic abnormality lies within the superficial skin layers or on the skin surface and projections utilising correlative radiopaque skin markers are required for confirmation of their location.

The availability of various additional supplementary projections within the mammographic armoury is invaluable in assisting to solve some of these diagnostic dilemmas.

This section describes techniques to perform the most commonly employed supplementary projections. The positions for the client are by definition likely to be difficult to maintain and therefore accuracy and efficiency are particularly important practitioner skills.

The ability to decide which supplementary views are appropriate and when to utilise them are important skills that all practitioners should develop under the direction of a healthcare professional trained in mammographic image interpretation [3].

Please note, when performing supplementary projections practitioners are advised to refer to the comprehensive general guidance on positioning, AEC considerations, application of compression force and repetitive strain risk reduction techniques described earlier in this book.

Laterally Extended Cranio Caudal Projection

Region Demonstrated

This maximises visualisation of lateral and axillary tail breast tissue and the medial breast will be excluded. Pectoral muscle should be demonstrated in the lateral aspect of the image and the nipple will point towards the medial.

J. Kelly
Breast Care Unit, The Countess of Chester Hospitals NHS Foundation Trust, Liverpool Road, Chester CH2 1UL, UK
e-mail: judith.kelly2@nhs.net

P. Hogg et al. (eds.), *Digital Mammography: A Holistic Approach*,
DOI 10.1007/978-3-319-04831-4_24, © Springer International Publishing Switzerland 2015

Positioning Technique

The machine angle should be raised from the horizontal approximately 5–10° laterally. Positioning should commence as for a standard CC projection (described in Chap. 21) with the breast lifted onto the image receptor and the nipple in profile. The client is then rotated approximately 60° away from the right or left side (depending on which breast is being imaged). Keeping the client's arm and shoulder as relaxed as possible the lateral breast and axillary region are manipulated into the imaging field and compression applied whilst ensuring the elimination of any skin folds. Care should be taken not to include any aspect of the shoulder or other body part within the region of interest before performing the exposure.

Medially Extended Craniocaudal Projection

Region Demonstrated

This maximises visualisation of medial breast tissue and the lateral breast will be excluded.

Positioning Technique

Positioning commences as for a standard CC projection (Chap. 21) and the breast is lifted onto the image receptor with the nipple in profile. If the left breast is being imaged the breast should be aligned marginally right of centre on the image receptor (the opposite applies for imaging the right breast.) The medial aspect of the right breast should be lifted onto the image receptor to prevent pulling of the left breast and to assist visualisation of the cleavage. Ensure the maximum amount of medial breast tissue is included in the imaging field and eliminate all folds before applying compression and performing the exposure. For the contralateral breast a mirror image of this technique should be performed.

Difficulty may be encountered with this projection in accommodating the client's head around the X-ray tube housing and careful manipulation is therefore required.

Extended Craniocaudal (Cleopatra) Projection

Region Demonstrated

Extreme outer quadrant and axillary tail.

Positioning Technique

Commence as for a standard CC projection and then rotate the client medially to demonstrate the lateral outer quadrant (of whichever breast is under examination). The image receptor may be angled 5–10° laterally to help facilitate the positioning and avoid including the humeral head. The nipple should be placed at the medial aspect of the image receptor as this enables the client to be leaned back onto the lateral aspect, allowing maximum demonstration of the outer breast tissue. Lift the breast onto the image receptor and manipulate into position, eliminate skin creases and apply compression as usual.

Lateral Images: Mediolateral Projection

Region Demonstrated

This also serves to: give an accurate indication of the actual depth of an abnormality; clarify the presence/absence of a possible abnormality seen on one or both standard CC/MLO projections; clearer visualisation of the inframammary angle; post image-guided localisation of a radiopaque marker or wire.

Positioning Technique

The machine should be in a vertical position so the breast will be imaged at a true 90° to the horizontal. Positioning should commence with the client standing (or seated) facing the machine and the lateral edge of the chest (left or right, depending on which breast is to be imaged) parallel to the image receptor. The ipsilateral arm should be raised and rested across the machine (Fig. 24.1).

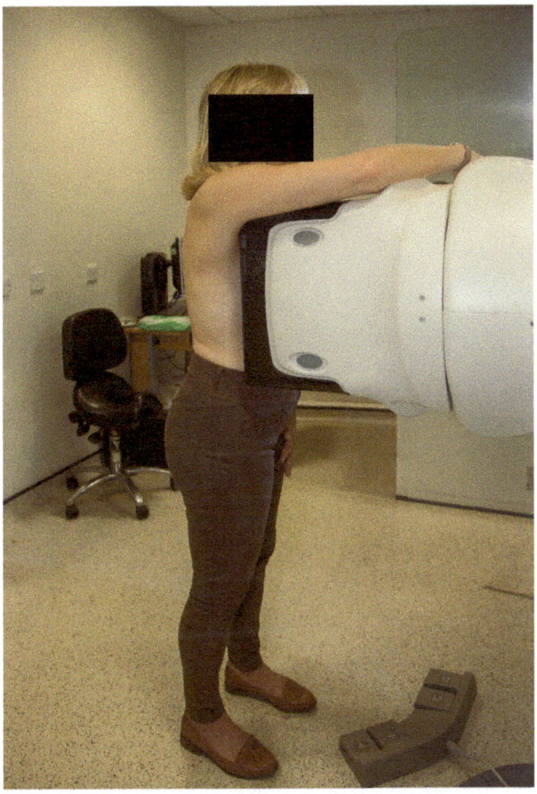

Fig. 24.1 Correct client position for mediolateral projection

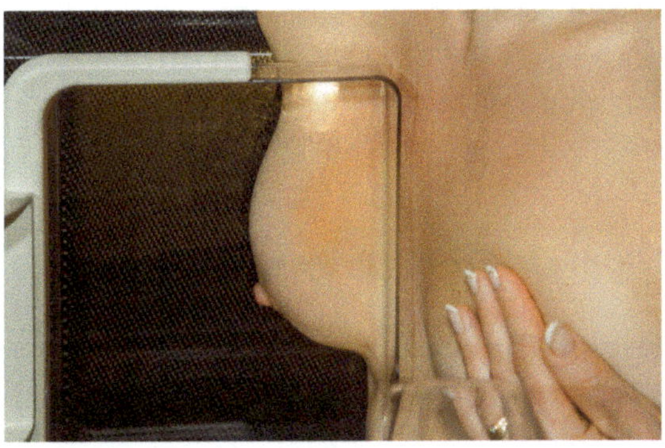

Fig. 24.2 Correct mediolateral positioning

The breast is then lifted upwards and forwards until the lateral aspect is fully resting against the image receptor and the corner is in the axilla. Compression is applied and exposure performed, ensuring the inframammary angle is well demonstrated and nipple in profile.

Fig. 24.2 illustrates positioning technique for this projection

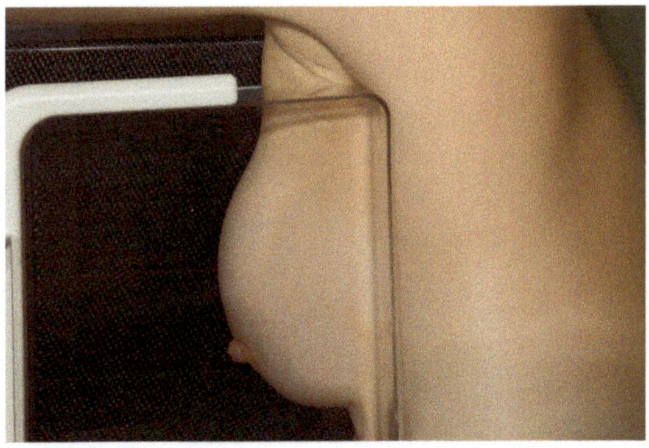

Fig. 24.3 Correct lateromedial positioning

Lateral Images: Lateromedial Projection

Region Demonstrated

The medial breast tissue and inframammary angle.

Positioning Technique

The machine is positioned as for the mediolateral projection. The client is positioned again facing the machine with the image receptor outer edge in line with the sternum. The ipsilateral arm is raised and rested across the machine with the elbow slightly flexed. The breast should be lifted upwards and forwards away from the chest wall until the sternum is resting against the machine and the medial breast in contact with the image receptor. Position the nipple in profile, bearing in mind this can be more difficult to achieve in the lateromedial projection.

Figure 24.3 illustrates positioning technique for this projection.

Cleavage Projection

Region Demonstrated

Maximises the volume of medioposterior breast tissue bilaterally and clearly shows the cleavage.

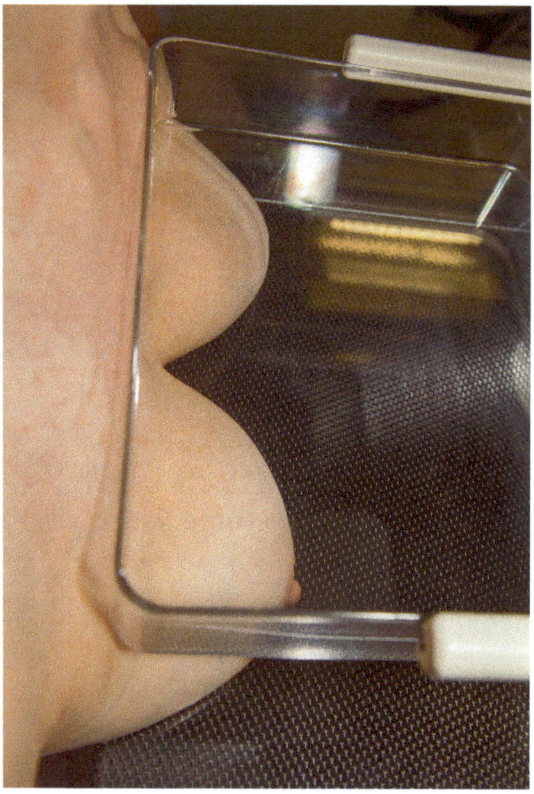

Fig. 24.4 Correct cleavage view positioning

Positioning Technique

Commence positioning as for a CC projection but keep the client centralised rather than off set to one side as is the case when performing separate right or left breast imaging. Lift both breasts forwards separately and rest them onto the image receptor. Lean the client inwards to maximise visualisation of the inner breasts. Place a thumb on each medial aspect and rotate the breasts laterally to demonstrate fully the medial regions while applying compression.

Figures 24.4 and 24.5 illustrate ideal positioning technique for this projection.

NB It is important that a manual exposure is selected (probably guided by a previously recorded CC projection) to avoid the AEC delivering a suboptimal exposure.

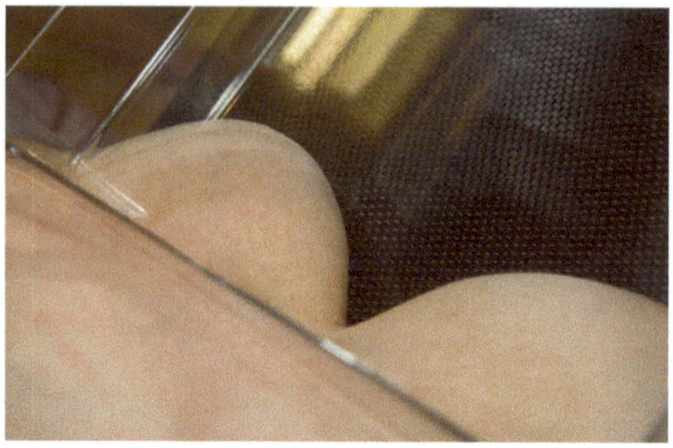

Fig. 24.5 Correct cleavage view positioning

Mediolateral Axillary Tail Projection

Region Demonstrated

The axillary tail, pectoral muscle and low axilla.

Positioning Technique

Set the machine and commence positioning initially for a standard mediolateral oblique projection as described earlier in Chap. 21. The machine height is then raised higher to include more of the breast axillary tail and lower axilla regions. The affected shoulder should be as relaxed as possible and compression applied, making sure the humeral head and clavicle are not caught by the compression paddle.

Nipple in Profile Projection

Region Demonstrated

The nipple should be in perfect profile to demonstrate the subareola structures. Provides clarification that a perceived mass on a standard CC view (where the nipple was not in profile) is in fact the nipple superimposed onto the adjacent breast tissue. Also facilitates accurate orientation, allowing measurement of the location of a perceived abnormality in relation to the nipple.

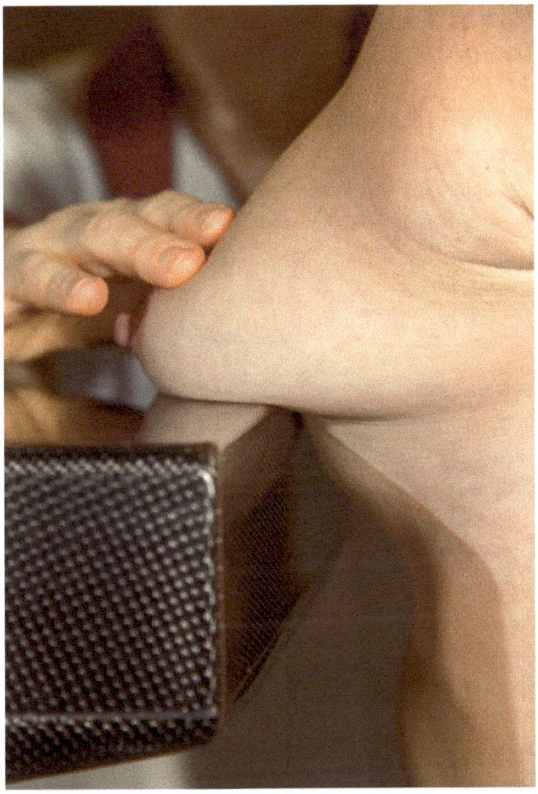

Fig. 24.6 Positioning for nipple in profile

Positioning Technique

Technique should mirror the standard CC (or MLO/ML) positioning initially but concentration should focus on ensuring the nipple is projected in profile. Demonstration of the breast posterior aspect is of lesser importance. Apply compression as described for the standard projections earlier in this chapter.

Figures 24.6 and 24.7 illustrate ideal positioning technique for this projection in the CC view.

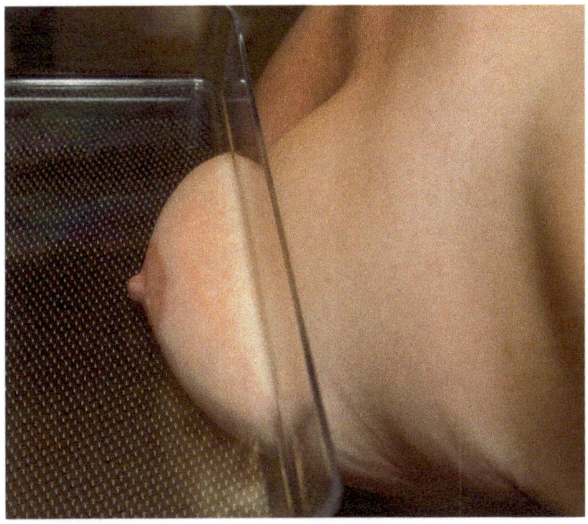

Fig. 24.7 Final nipple in profile position

Inverted Craniocaudal Projection

Region Demonstrated

Demonstrates an inverted CC image of inferior technical quality to a standard CC due to the difficulties involved in physically performing this projection. The posterior aspect of the breast and pectoral muscle are unlikely to be imaged.

NB It is imperative that the image is orientated accurately for image readers to enable the location of perceived abnormalities to be correlated with precision in relation to the other projections performed (i.e. MLO).

Positioning Technique

This technique is seldom used in practice yet indications to perform it are for clients with extreme kyphosis whose head and shoulders would superimpose the breast on a standard CC projection. (The ability of the machine to accommodate this positioning should be ascertained prior to any attempt at client positioning). Commence positioning as for a standard CC view but the breast weight will be supported by the compression paddle therefore careful manipulation is required. This projection requires the involvement of two practitioners due to the technical challenges and the fact that the client may have limited mobility. Aim to maximise the volume of breast tissue included in the imaging field and apply the compression force appropriately whilst supporting the breast. Care should

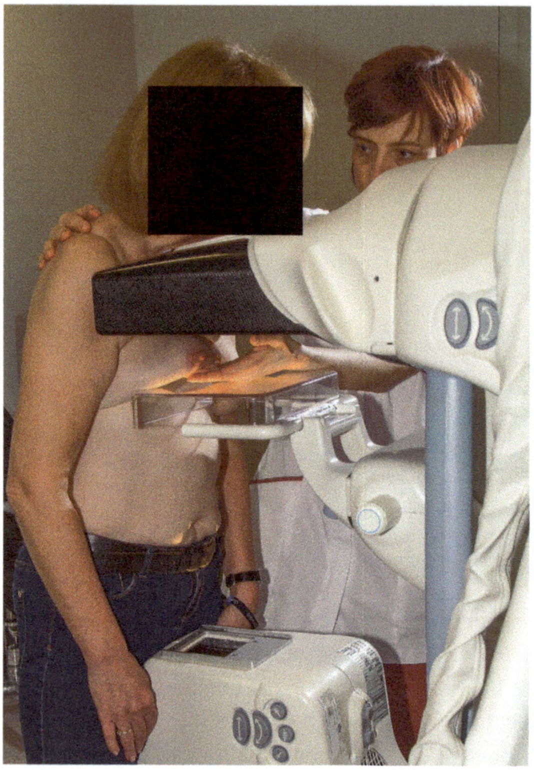

Fig. 24.8 Positioning for inverted craniocaudal projection

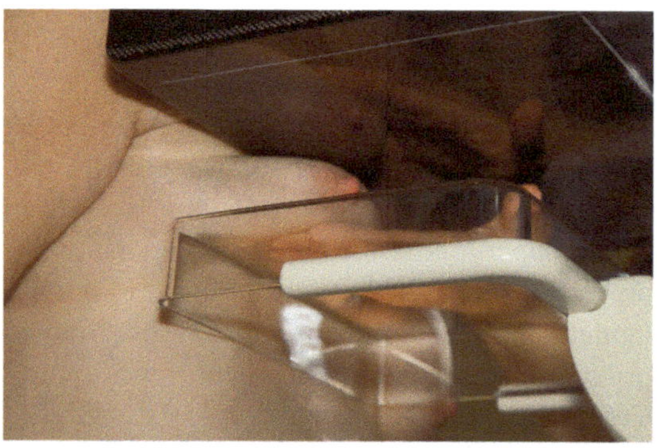

Fig. 24.9 Final inverted craniocaudal position

be taken not to trap practitioner hands within the equipment.

Figures 24.8 and 24.9 illustrate ideal positioning technique for this projection.

NB. Unlikely to be feasible in very large breasted clients.

Projections Using Skin Markers to Localise Skin Lesions

Region Demonstrated

Any area of the breast with surface skin lesions which may be demonstrated on the image.

Positioning Technique

A suitable radiopaque marker (there are multiple varieties available commercially) should be placed on the skin over the lesion in question and an appropriate projection selected to best demonstrate the abnormality which correlates with the original mammogram.

Position and apply compression force as in standard projections.

Rolled Projection

Region Demonstrated

These projections are adapted from the standard CC and MLO positions and are an alternative, effective way to solve equivocal mammography findings by separating overlapping structures from each other and differentiating summation artefacts from genuine lesions [4]. Such projections should be performed under the direction of an individual qualified to interpret mammograms and in conjunction with other additional projections such as coned compression views.

Positioning Technique

The rolled view changes the breast positioning but not the obliquity of the X-ray beams. From the CC position, the breast is rolled in either the medial or lateral direction. For example, while the upper part of the breast is rolled medially (from lateral to medial), the inner part changes its position laterally along the X-axis of the breast. In the MLO position, the breast is rolled in either the inferior or superior direction. The lateral aspect is rolled inferiorly (from superior to inferior) whilst the medial aspect changes its position in the opposite direction.

Compression should then be applied as described for the standard projections.

Acknowledgements The author is most grateful to the professional photographer Gill Brett for her photographic skills and Claire Mercer and her team from the Nightingale Centre, University Hospital of South Manchester for directing and arranging the production of the photographs in this chapter.

References

1. Feig S. The importance of supplementary mammographic views to diagnostic accuracy. Am J Roentgenol. 1988;151(1):40–1. doi:10.2214/ajr.151.1.31.
2. Barbarkoff D, Gatewood MD, Brem RF. Supplemental views for equivocal mammographic findings: a pictorial essay. Breast J. 2000;6(1):34–43.
3. Sickles EA. Practical solutions to common mammographic problems: tailoring the examination. Am J Roentgenol. 1988;151(1):31–9. doi:10.2214/ajr.151.1.31.
4. Alimoglu E, Ceken K, Kabaalioglu A, Cassano E, Sindel T. An effective way to solve equivocal mammography findings: the rolled views. Breast Care (Basel). 2010;5(4):241–5. doi:10.1159/000313904.

Bibliography and Further Reading

Caseldine J, Blamey R, Roebuck E, Elston C. Breast disease for radiographers. London: Wright; 1988.

Hashimoto B. Practical digital mammography. New York: Thieme; 2008.

Lee L, Strickland V, Wilson R, Evans A. Fundamentals of mammography. 2nd ed. London: Churchill Livingstone; 2003.

Pisano ED, Yaffe MJ, Kuzmiak CM. Digital mammography. Philadelphia: Lippincott Williams & Wilkins; 2004.

Shaw De Paredes E. Atlas of mammography. Philadelphia: Lippincott Williams & Wilkins; 2007. ISBN 0781741424, 9780781741422.

Tucker A, Ng YY. Textbook of mammography. 2nd ed. London: Churchill Livingstone; 2001.

Whitman GJ, Haygood TM, editors. Digital mammography. A practical approach. Cambridge: Cambridge University Press; 2012.

Magnification and Compression Views

25

Victoria L. Hipperson

Introduction

Following initial mammography imaging (craniocaudal and mediolateral oblique views) an abnormality may be identified which requires further analysis. Clear mammographic presentation of a lesion or microcalcification is crucial for accurate assessment. Identifiable masses such as cysts, fibroadenomas and larger carcinomas usually proceed to an ultrasound examination without the requirement for further mammographic views [1]. Many masses demonstrated as microcalcification or an asymmetrical density, may not be instantly identifiable on the initial mammograms, and will need further assessment with specialised mammography [2]. The location of the abnormality in the breast can be confirmed by obtaining a lateral view, particularly in the case of microcalcification. This enables the microcalcification to be characterised [3].

Magnification Views

Magnification views are used mainly for the analysis of microcalcification caused by very tiny deposits of calcium phosphate or calcium oxalate resulting from a secretory lesion or malignancy [4]. Microcalcification is minute (50–300 μm) and for an accurate radiological examination the image must be as sharp as possible [2, 4].

Magnification views allow the interpreting practitioner to assess the area of microcalcification for size, shape and distribution of the particles. This informs the next stage of the diagnostic workup process.

Digital mammography allows the images to be manipulated post acquisition. Acquiring geometrically magnified images is preferable to the use of an electronic zoom function because the initial mammograms (contact views) do not always demonstrate all the microcalcification present [5, 6]; the initial mammogram is simply increased in size (zoomed) and may not demonstrate subtle microcalcification which may be better detected on the geometrically magnified views.

Equipment Used

A magnification table is used to create a distance between the breast and the detector, creating a geometrically magnified image. This is attached to the mammography equipment in exchange for the regular platform. The magnification board may be constructed of carbon fibre or polycarbonate and is therefore lightweight; the anti-scatter grid is excluded in this set up.

V.L. Hipperson
Breast Imaging, Whipps Cross Hospital,
Barts Health NHS Trust,
Whipps Cross Road, London E11 1NR, UK
e-mail: Victoria.hipperson@bartshealth.nhs.uk

P. Hogg et al. (eds.), *Digital Mammography: A Holistic Approach*,
DOI 10.1007/978-3-319-04831-4_25, © Springer International Publishing Switzerland 2015

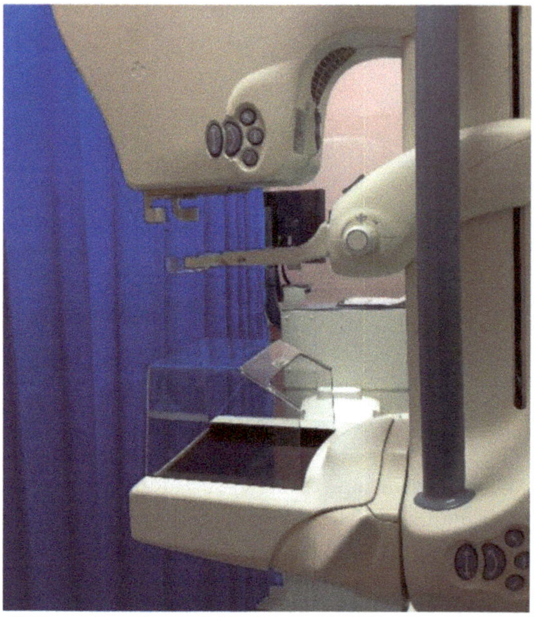

Fig. 25.1 Mammography equipment set up for x1.5 magnification view

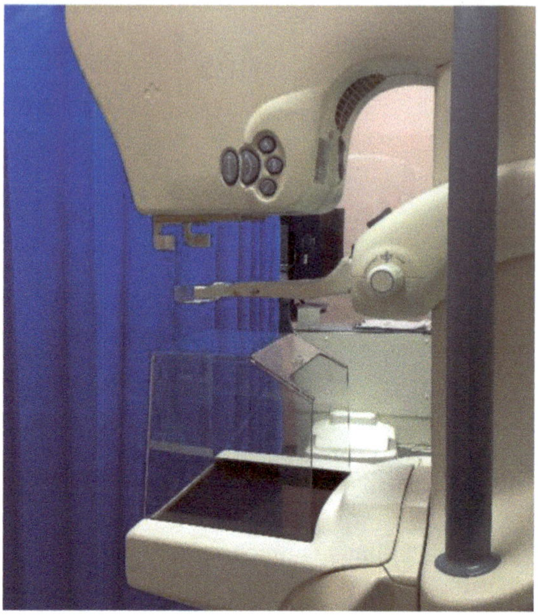

Fig. 25.2 Mammography equipment set up for x1.8 magnification view

Magnification views are subject to some compounding issues. The distance created between the breast and the detector, results in increased geometric unsharpness which may affect the resultant image. In conventional radiography the X-Ray tube focus can be moved further from the object, decreasing the effect of geometric unsharpness; but this is not possible in mammography due to the fixed height of the tube. As a result, there would be increased dose to the breast, therefore a grid is not used. High image resolution is maintained, despite the absence of an anti-scatter grid in the magnification table caused by the air gap between the breast and the detector [7]. The use of a fine focal spot size and the high resolution of the detector also maximises image resolution for this, along with a limited range of magnification factors [6]. These can vary between manufacturers but are usually ×1.5 (Fig. 25.1) to ×2.0 (Fig. 25.2) [8]; a difference in object to detector difference is clearly demonstrated.

When selecting the paddle for magnification views, the practitioner should be aware that they are sometimes different to those used for coned compression views. For some manufacturers the paddle for the magnification view has a ***straight arm***.

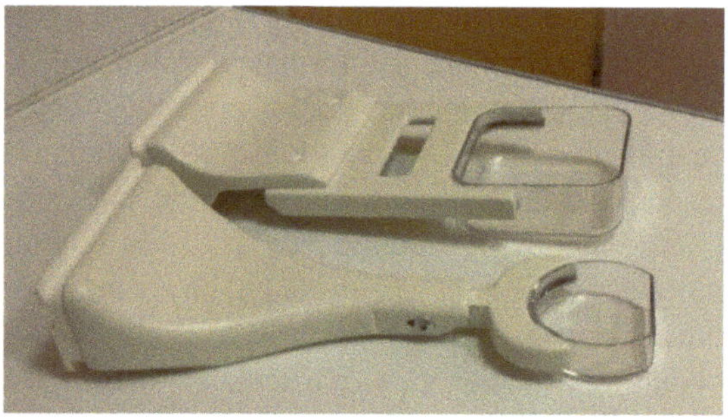

Fig. 25.3 A choice of paddles for magnification views (General Electric)

There are different sized paddles available for use. This allows small and large areas to be focused on appropriately. A small paddle should be chosen for a lesser sized abnormal area, whilst a larger one is reserved for a more extensive abnormality. A larger paddle is used with a lower magnification table, utilising a greater field of view (FOV). An example of the choice of paddles for magnification views are illustrated in Fig. 25.3.

Coned Compression Views

Coned compression views, or paddle views, are another tool in evaluating an abnormality in the breast following initial mammography. This technique is used typically to improve the characterisation of a mass, an asymmetrical density or a parenchymal distortion that was seen on initial imaging.

Equipment Used

The main tool for compression views is the focal compression paddle. It is important to realise that these may differ from those used for magnification views in that the ***arm of the paddle is curved*** (Fig. 25.4).

This allows the paddle to apply focal pressure concentrated on the abnormal area. As with the magnification paddle, there are different sized paddles for coned compression views which allow a smaller or larger area to be focused on. The image is acquired with the breast positioned directly on the usual contact surface (Fig. 25.5).

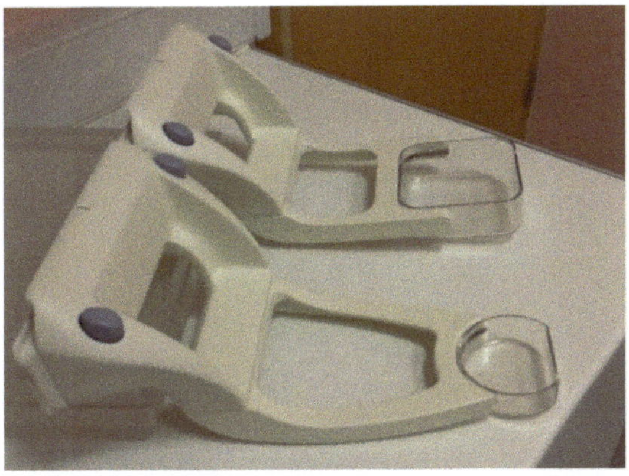

Fig. 25.4 A choice of paddles for coned compression/paddle views (General Electric)

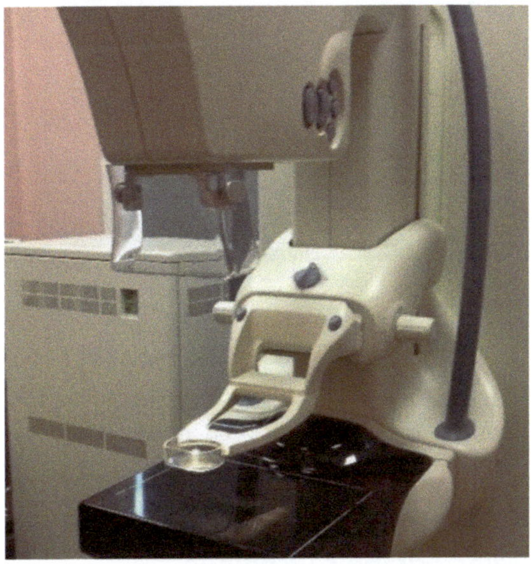

Fig. 25.5 Mammography equipment setup for coned compression/paddle views

Mammographic Technique

The same mammography procedure applies to both techniques; only the equipment set up utilised is different.

Using the initial mammograms, take a measurement using the integrated digital caliper from the nipple to the abnormality. This will need to be done for each orientation. It is useful to write these details down. Measurements obtained, for example, may be as follows: 4 cm deep to the nipple and 2 cm laterally. This is then transferred back to the client to obtain the same location as that seen on the mammograms. If possible, display the images in the imaging room for reference purposes.

Localising the Abnormal Area (See Figs. 25.6 and 25.7)

- Each contact view is uploaded in turn on to the mammographic workstation.
- The abnormal area is confirmed by the reporting practitioner.
- The linear measuring tool is selected.
- A horizontal line is drawn from the nipple posteriorly to the level of the abnormal area. A vertical line (on the image) is then drawn to the abnormality.
- Two measurements will be presented on the screen which should be documented for reference (Figs. 25.6 and 25.7).

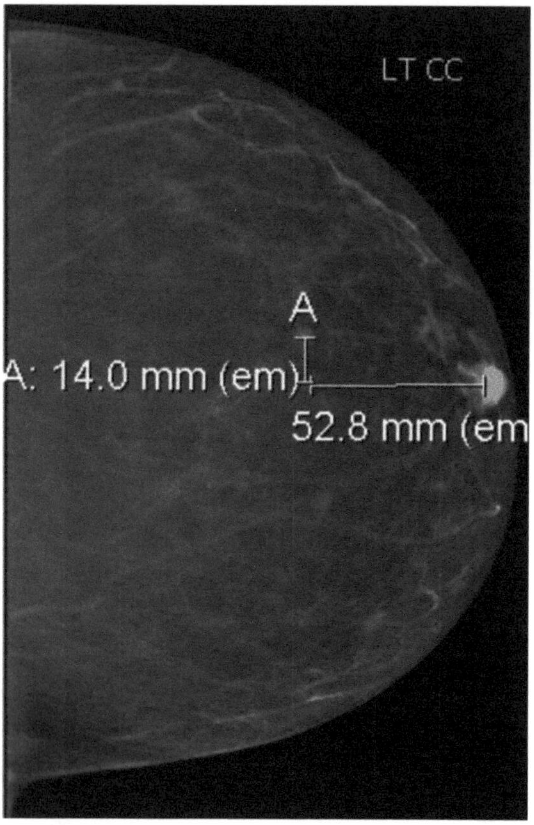

Fig. 25.6 Illustration of lesion localisation measurements in CC projection

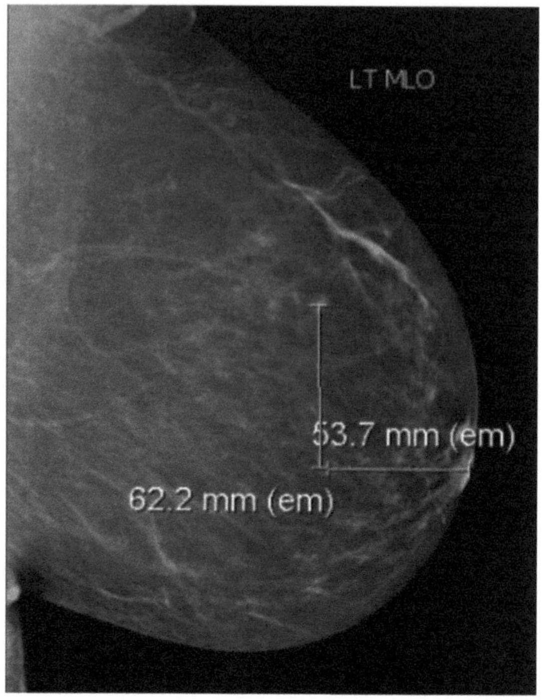

Fig. 25.7 Illustration of lesion localisation measurements in MLO projection

- If two separate further views are required, this procedure should then be repeated for the other projection.

Mammographic Technique

The positioning for coned compression and magnification views is similar to that used for routine mammograms. The technique used for the magnification views will require adaptation due to the height of the magnification table and X-Ray tube head.

The practitioner should prepare the imaging room. The correct identifying details must be selected from the work list at the acquisition station. Digital mammography equipment usually acknowledges the magnification table and the specific compression paddles therefore preselecting an automatic exposure, but this should be confirmed.

The vast majority of clients attending for assessment of a perceived abnormality will be anxious and will require sensitive communication. A member of the breast imaging team will need to explain to the client the reason as to why further imaging is required; this should not provoke anxiety or be over reassuring, as this is not in the best interests of the client [9].

The client should be asked to undress to the waist and the positioning directed as follows:

- Position the client in front of the mammography machine in the same way used for a routine mammogram (Chap. 21) with her feet hips width apart.
- The clients head should be turned away from the affected side, ensuring that there is no superimposition of her ears or hair over the area of interest.
- The light beam diaphragm should be turned on.
- The practitioner should raise the affected breast on to the contact surface or magnification

table (for magnification views) using her opposing hand.

- Locate the abnormal area on the corresponding skin surface of the breast using the previously obtained measurements. It is often useful to identify this with an inked skin mark but consent from the client should be sought first. The practitioner should adjust the position of the breast to align the area of interest within the field of view.
- Apply a small amount of compression to the breast just to hold it in place.
- Re-check the position using the original measurements.
- Once an accurate position has been achieved, the breast can then be compressed for imaging. The breast will feel tense when pressed adjacent to the paddle. This can feel uncomfortable due to the focal pressure, so this should be explained to the client.
- The exposure is done using an automatic selection and not a manual exposure. This is to ensure that the most accurate exposure is given to allow image interpretation, and to avoid repeat X-Ray exposures.

Case Studies

The mammographic positioning is illustrated in the following case studies. These cases demonstrate how the practitioner would identify the location of the abnormality on the mammograms, apply this to the client and position for each image.

Case A: Paddle Views

An asymmetrical density is seen in the upper outer quadrant of the left breast as shown above. The integrated digital caliper is used to measure the distance from it to the nipple. This is so that the practitioner can position the client accurately for imaging. The same procedure is used for each view required; though it often only necessary to image the asymmetrical density in one projection.

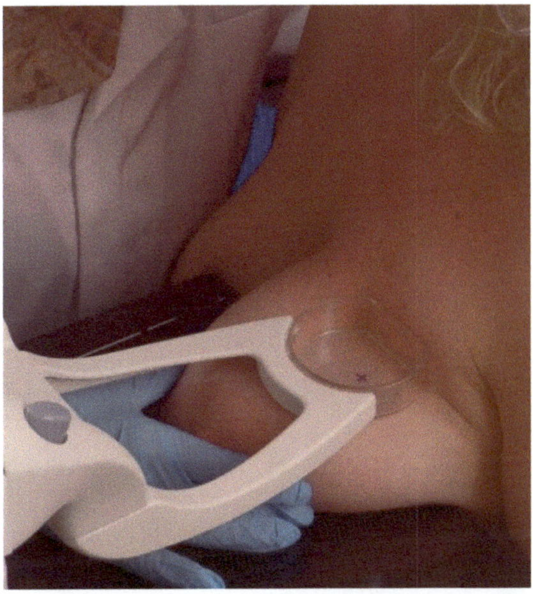

Fig. 25.8 Correct position for coned compression CC view

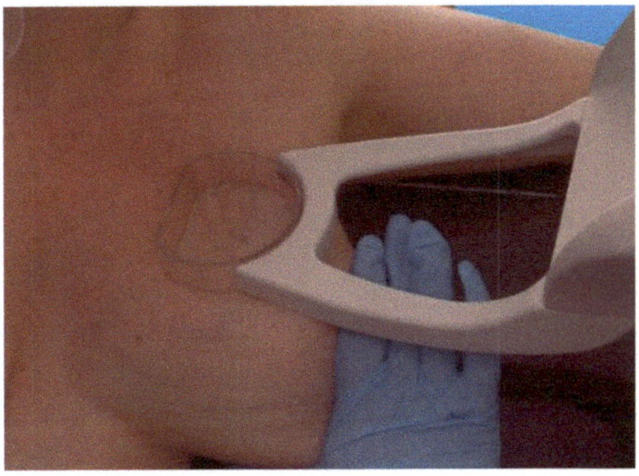

Fig. 25.9 Positioning for MLO view

The breast is manoeuvred so that the correct area of interest (as marked on the skin) is positioned centrally within the field of view (Figs. 25.8 and 25.9). The compression paddle is first applied gently. Once satisfactory positioning is achieved additional compression force can be applied.

The resulting images (Figs. 25.10 and 25.11) should include the area of interest in the centre of the image. It can be demonstrated from this case that the density is a spiculate mass (Figs. 25.10 and 25.11); as this remains during compression with no smooth margins visualised.

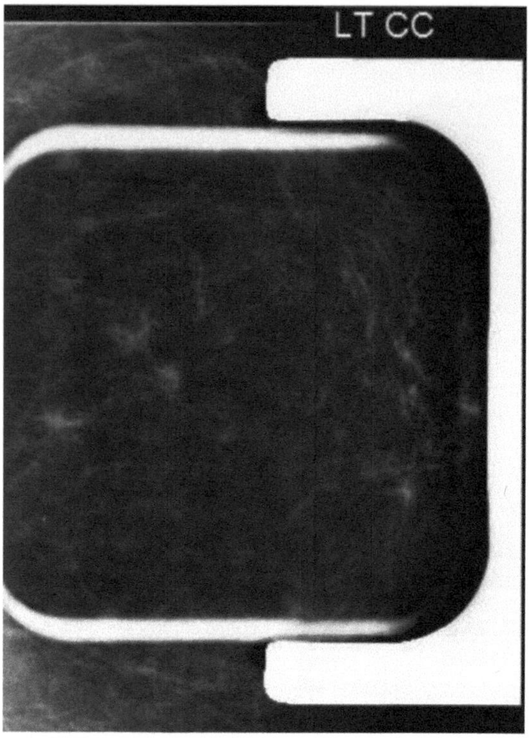

Fig. 25.10 Coned compression craniocaudal image with spiculate mass shown centrally

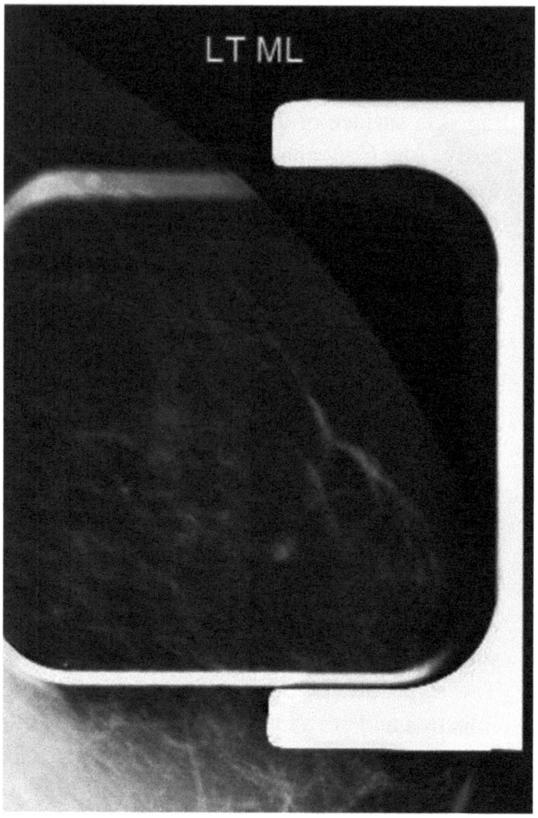

Fig. 25.11 Coned compression image in the MLO position with spiculate mass shown centrally

Case B: Magnification Views

A focus of pleomorphic microcalcification is demonstrated in the lower inner quadrant of the right breast. A lateral view was completed as an additional view. Measurements were then taken from the nipple to the focus of microcalcification, using the CC and lateral views (Figs. 25.12 and 25.13).

The client is then positioned accurately in each position using the measurements. Note: An MLO image should not be used to obtain measurements which are then transferred to a client who is positioned for a lateral view.

The height of the mammography machine will require adaptation once the magnification table is attached. The breast is manoeuvred so that the area of interest, as marked on the skin, can be positioned centrally within the field of view (Figs. 25.14 and 25.15). The compression paddle is firstly applied gently. Once satisfactory positioning is achieved additional compression is then applied.

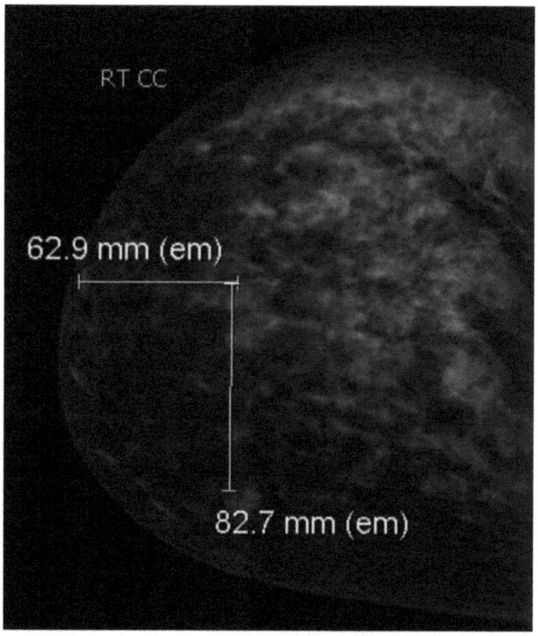

Fig. 25.12 The digital caliper is used on the craniocaudal view to identify the location of the abnormal microcalcification

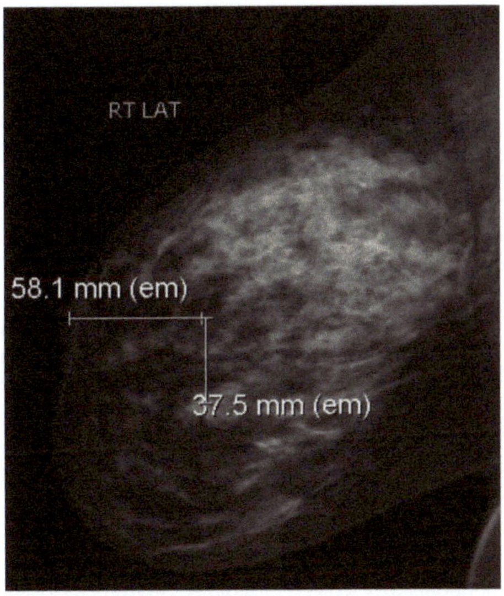

Fig. 25.13 The digital caliper is again used to localise the area of the microcalcification in the lateral position

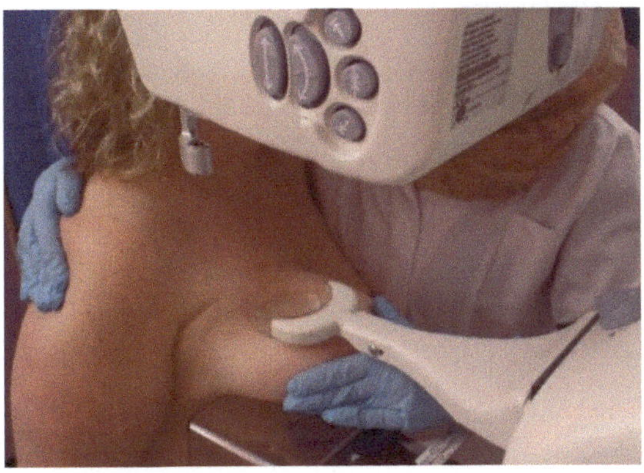

Fig. 25.14 Position for craniocaudal magnification view

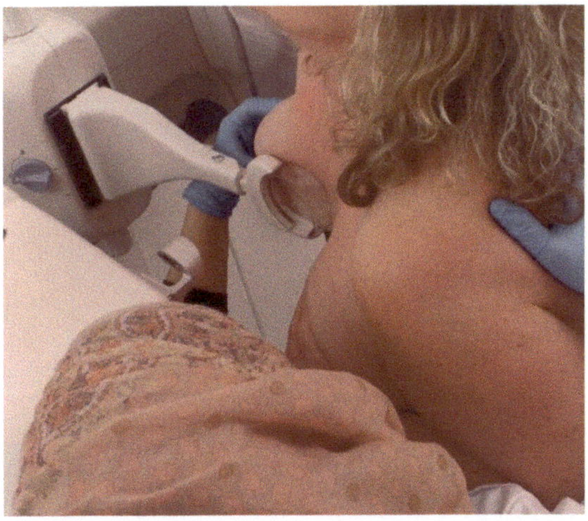

Fig. 25.15 Position for lateral magnification view

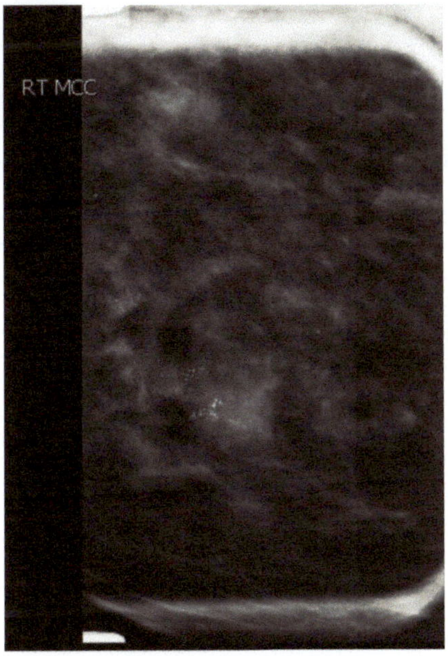

Fig. 25.16 Resultant craniocaudal magnification image showing the abnormal microcalcification positioned centrally within the field of view

The shape and distribution of the focus of microcalcification can now be seen with greater clarity on the resulting images (Figs. 25.16 and 25.17). A larger extent of this calcification can be visualised in these two views, due to magnification of the area and the high resolution of the resultant images. Often only one view is requested for additional imaging.

Sometimes the abnormality will lie deep in the breast and it may be difficult to place the abnormality within the field of view using the typical positioning. In these cases reversing the angle of the mammography machine (as if you were positioning for the other breast) and then positioning the client so that the medial aspect of the breast is closest to the detector, may assist in this.

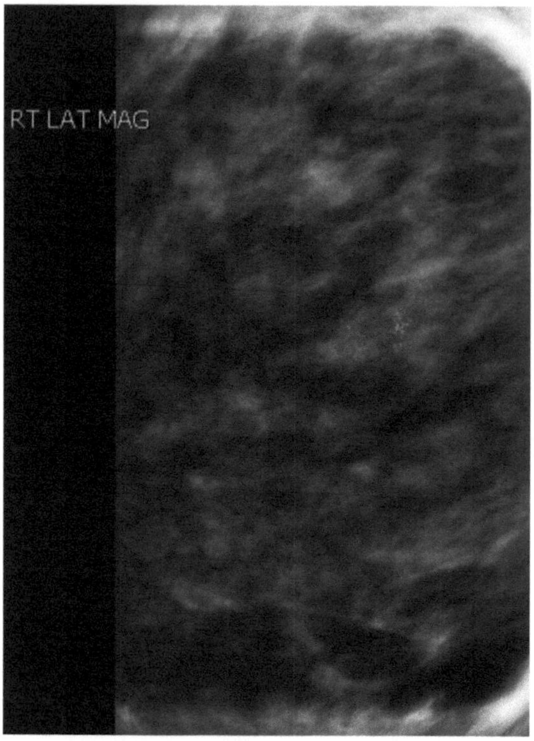

Fig. 25.17 Resultant lateral magnification image showing the abnormal microcalcification positioned centrally within the field of view

References

1. Harris JR, Lippman ME, Morrow M, Osborne CK, editors. Diseases of the breast. 4th ed. Philadelphia: Lippincott Williams and Wilkins; 2010.
2. Michell MJ, editor. Breast cancer. 1st ed. Cambridge: Cambridge University Press; 2010.
3. NHSBSP. Clinical guidelines for breast cancer screening assessment. Publication No. 49 June 2010. 3rd ed. UK: NHS Cancer Screening Programmes; 2010.
4. Tse GM, Tan P, Cheung HS, Chu WC, Lam WM. Intermediate to highly suspicious calcification in breast lesions: a radio-pathologic correlation. Breast Cancer Res Treat. 2008;110(1):1–7.
5. Kim MJ, Youk JH, Kang DR, Choi SH, Kwak JY, Son EJ, Kim E-K. Zooming method (*x*2.0) of digital mammography vs digital magnification view (x1.8) in full-field digital mammography for the diagnosis of microcalcifications. Br J Radiol. 2010;83(990):486–92.
6. Koutalonis M, Delis H, Pascoal A, Spyrou G, Costaridou L, Panayiotakis G. Can electronic zooming replace magnification in mammography? A comparative Monte Carlo study. Br J Radiol. 2010;83(991):569–77.
7. McParland BJ. Image quality and dose in film-screen magnification mammography. Br J Radiol. 2000; 73(874):1068–77.
8. Park H-S, Oh Y, Kim S-T, Kim H-J. Effects of breast thickness and lesion location on resolution in digital magnification mammography. Clin Imaging. 2012; 36(4):255–62.
9. Harvey JA, Cohen MA, Brenin DR, Nicholson BT, Adams RB. Breaking bad news: a primer for radiologists in breast imaging. J Am Coll Radiol. 2007;4(11):800–8.

26 Specimen Imaging

Amanda Coates

Introduction

The X-ray imaging of specimens forms an important part in the diagnostic pathway of breast cancer patients. It provides important information on accurate lesion sampling and radiologic and pathologic correlation [1]. Such imaging is performed using mammographic equipment or dedicated specimen cabinets. By using a magnification table or the compression paddle on a mammography machine, appearances of small lesions can be made clearer [2]. A dedicated specimen cabinet houses an x-ray tube with either an adjustable transparent shelf to place the specimen on or a tray to place the specimen samples in (Fig. 26.1), and an image detector. Specimen cabinets should be subjected to routine (6 monthly) testing by Medical Physics. Image quality is of paramount importance. All specimen images should contain correct client information along with breast laterality.

Types of Specimen Imaging and Reporting

There are three main types of specimen radiography in breast imaging:

1 Core biopsy specimens
2 Surgical excision specimens
3 Fixed pathological specimens

Core Biopsy Specimen Imaging

The imaging of core biopsy specimens, either standard 14 gauge or larger vacuum assisted biopsies, is usually to determine the presence of microcalcifications following stereotactic guided biopsies. This should be carried out prior to removal of the client from the mammography biopsy machine so further sampling can take place if calcification retrieval is inadequate (Fig. 26.2). Adequacy will be determined by the amount of calcification present before biopsy and local protocol. It has been suggested [3] that three or more cores containing calcification, or five flecks or more calcification in total, increases the likelihood of a successful biopsy and a definitive pathological diagnosis. Some pathologists prefer the separation of core biopsy samples containing calcification from those without calcification. This allows the pathologist to concentrate and sample more comprehensively those cores with known calcifications [4].

In core biopsy specimen reports, good practice would include the following:

- the number of core samples obtained
- the number of core samples which contain calcification
- if a marker clip was deployed
- the relationship between the marker clip and the area of calcification.

A. Coates
Breast Imaging, Mid Yorkshire Hospitals Trust, Pinderfields Hospital, Aberford Road, Wakefield WF14DG, UK
e-mail: amanda.coates@midyorks.nhs.uk

P. Hogg et al. (eds.), *Digital Mammography: A Holistic Approach*,
DOI 10.1007/978-3-319-04831-4_26, © Springer International Publishing Switzerland 2015

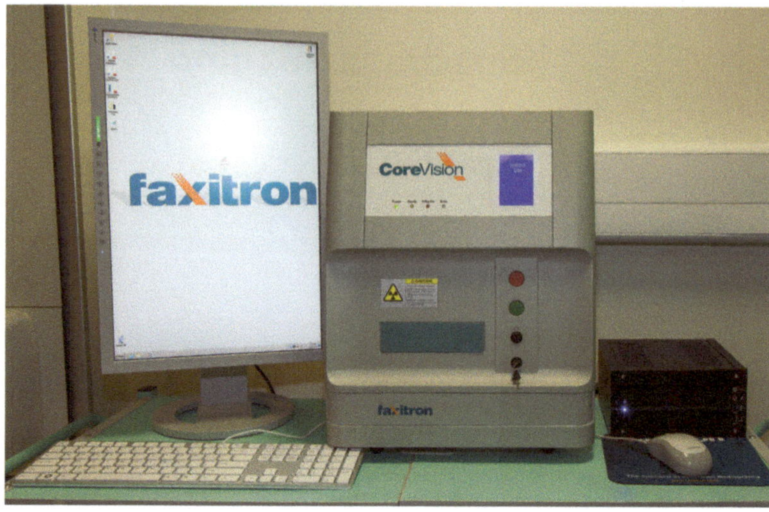

Fig. 26.1 An example of a dedicated specimen cabinet (Photo supplied by Claire Mercer, Lead Radiographer, Nightingale Centre, UHSM)

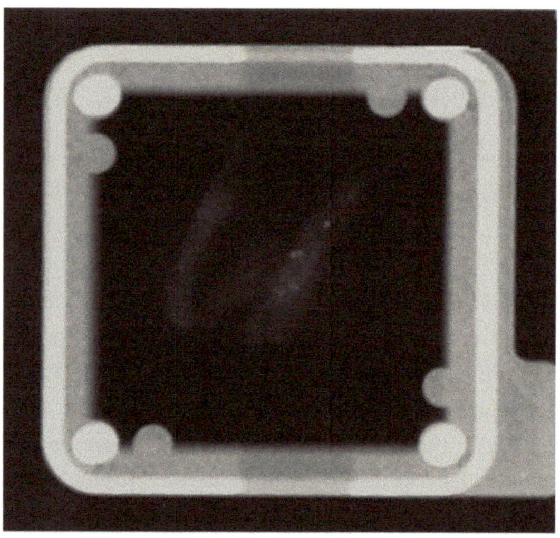

Fig. 26.2 Calcification identified in magnified core biopsy specimens

The report should be available to the pathologist before any multi-disciplinary team meeting (MDT) discussion takes place on future patient management in order to correlate radiologic and pathologic findings.

Surgical Excision Specimen Imaging

Specimen radiography of non-palpable lesions excised during breast conservation surgery should take place before skin closure and be available to the surgeon so that determination of total lesion removal can be achieved. Surgical clips, sutures or colour coded inking are often used to orientate the specimen [5]. If the lesion appears to extend to a margin the surgeon can make an appropriate further excision [6, 7]. An advantageous use of a specimen cabinet located in theatre would allow almost immediate results reducing theatre/anaesthetic time.

As radiography of a specimen is a two dimensional image of a three dimensional object, imaging in more than one plane can be useful but not always easy to do, due to the shape of the specimen. If using a mammography machine, careful and slow use of the compression paddle, can often achieve this (Fig. 26.3a, b).

When reporting excision specimens a description of whether good radiological margins have been observed and, if not, which

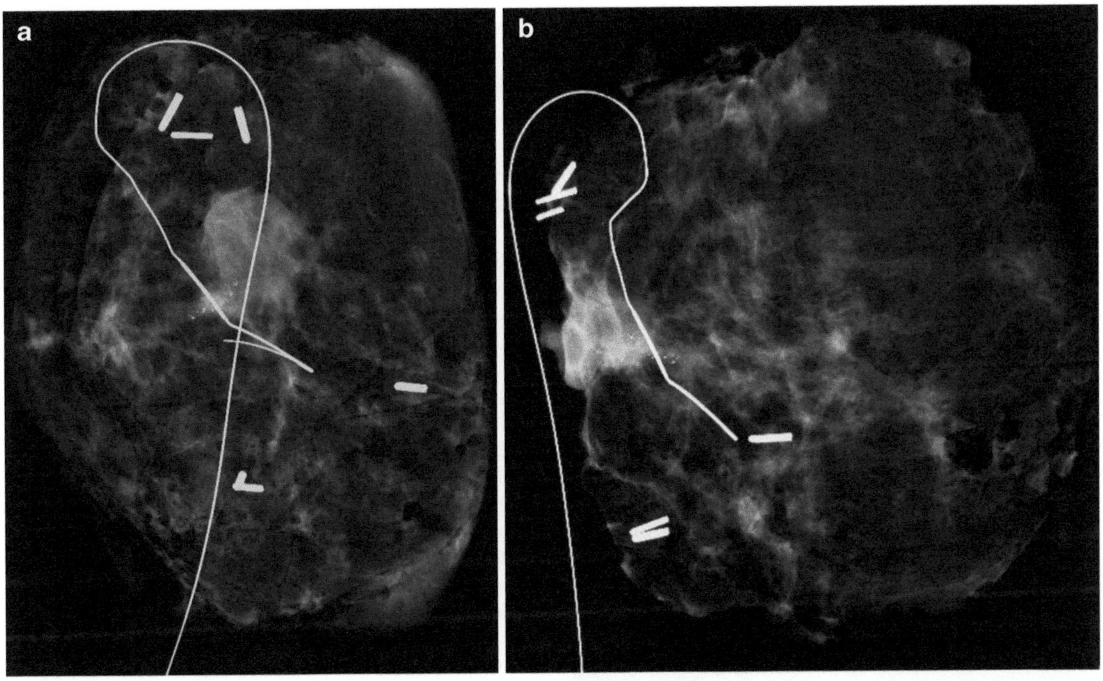

Fig. 26.3 Demonstration of a lesion appearing centrally in the excision (**a**) yet at the margin when an orthogonal view is obtained (**b**)

margin is thought to be involved. It is useful to mention whether a wire and or biopsy marker clip can be seen in the specimen and its relationship to the lesion excised. Lesion/abnormality size can be added if this appears smaller or larger than initially determined on pre-operative imaging. This information will aid the pathologist to further correlate complete lesion excision. A radiological margin of <5 mm is reported as a risk factor for margin involvement by Mazouni et al. [8] however, other work [9], has shown that a radiological margin of <11 mm is 58 % likely to have histologically involved margins.

Often it is necessary to telephone the operating theatre and speak to the surgeon to describe the findings. If this takes place, a notation on the radiology report of '*Theatres informed*' or '*Discussed with…*' can be useful in case there is any uncertainty expressed later.

Fixed Pathology Specimen Imaging

Fixed pathology specimens are usually slices from a mastectomy where perhaps a small lesion in multifocal disease or calcifications cannot be located by pathologist observation [1]. Each slice will be labelled by the pathologist, numerical labelling is common. This may appear on the container the slice arrives in or alternative packaging. In order to match the slice to the image, this identification must be on the image itself, for example, numeric identification, i.e. slice 1, slice 2 is by far the easiest and lead numbers or pieces of lead shot of corresponding amount can be

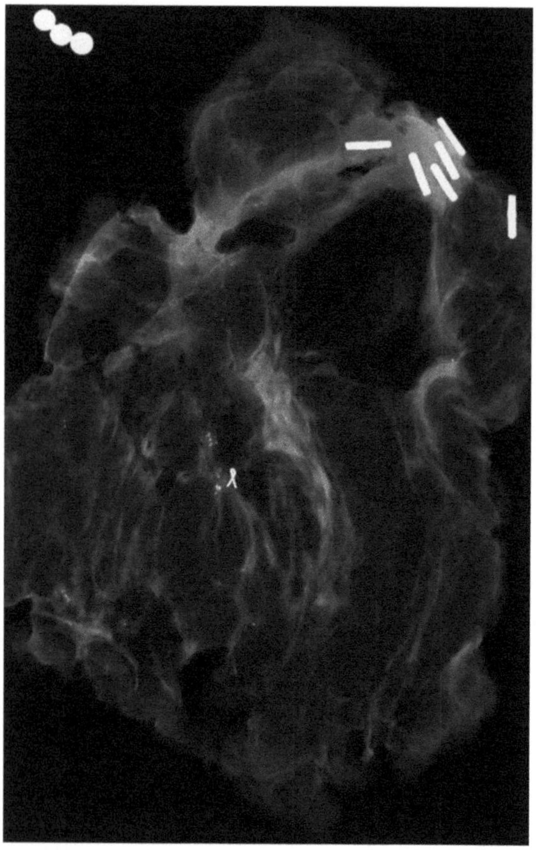

Fig. 26.4 Calcifications and biopsy marker clip demonstrated fixed pathology sliced specimen. Lead shot used to indicate slice number

adhered to the image receptor before X ray exposure. Alternatively free text can be annotated to the image before or after image storage, depending on equipment.

The reporting of fixed specimens usually requires a description of the findings in each slice. This will be determined by the information required, for example '*calcification seen in slices 5 and 6*' or '*5 mm spiculate mass seen in slice 3* (Fig. 26.4).'

References

1. NHS Cancer Screening Programmes. Quality assurance guidelines for breast pathology services, vol. 2. Sheffield: NHS Cancer Screening Programmes; 2011.
2. Morrow M, Strom EA, Bassett LW, Dershaw DD, Fowble B, Harris JR, O'Malley F, Schnitt SJ, Singletary SE, Winchester DP. Standard for the management of ductal carcinoma in situ of the breast (DCIS). CA Cancer J Clin. 2002;52(5):256–75.
3. Bagnall M, Evans A, Wilson A, Burrell H, Pinder S, Ellis I. When have mammographic calcifications been adequately sampled at needle core biopsy? Clin Radiol. 2000;55(7):548–53.
4. Margolin FR, Kaufman L, Jacobs RP, Denny SR, Schrumpf JD. Stereotactic core breast biopsy of malignant calcifications: diagnostic yield of cores with and cores without calcifications on specimen radiographs. Radiology. 2004;233(1):251–4.
5. Volleamere AJ, Kirwan CC. National survey of breast cancer specimen orientation marking systems. Eur J Surg Oncol. 2013;39(3):255–9.
6. Perry N, Broeders M, de Wolf C, Tornberg S, Holland R, von Karsa L. European guidelines for quality assurance in breast cancer screening and diagnosis. 4th Ed. – summary document. Ann Oncol. 2008;19(4):614–22.
7. McCormick JT, Keleher AJ, Tikhomirov VB, Budway RJ, Caushaj PF. Analysis of the use of specimen mammography in breast conservation therapy. Am J Surg. 2004;188(4):433–6.
8. Mazouni C, Rouzier R, Balleyguier C, Sideris L, Rochard F, Delaloge S, Marsiglia H, Mathieu C, Spielman M, Garbay JR. Specimen radiography as predictor of resection margin status in non-palpable breast lesions. Clin Radiol. 2006;61(9):789–96.
9. Britton PD, Li S, Yamamoto AK, Koo B, Goud A. Breast surgical specimen radiographs: how reliable are they? Eur J Radiol. 2011;79(2):245–9.

Imaging the Augmented Breast 27

Claire D. Borrelli

Breast Augmentation: Implants

Breast augmentation is a common surgical procedure and women may undergo breast augmentation with implants for a variety of reasons ranging from aesthetic to reconstructive surgery following mastectomy. Women with breast implants are prone to the same range of diseases as those without implants and the management of those problems is similar.

Whilst mammography remains the gold standard for breast cancer imaging [1], the presence of breast implants in women who have undergone breast augmentation represents an important imaging challenge. Breast implants may interfere with the accurate imaging of breast tissue and could also expose clients to risk factors such as implant rupture during the mammography procedure. Mammography performed by an experienced radiographer reduces the likelihood of rupture and other complications during the mammogram procedure. In addition, techniques are available to achieve successful breast imaging in women with implants.

Considerations for Radiographers

Prior to mammography, women with implants should be advised of the lack of efficacy of breast imaging due to the opaque nature of the implant and the possibility of reduced sensitivity with mammography as the amount of compression force required for an optimal mammography study reduces the likelihood of adequately imaging the breast parenchyma.

A relevant breast history should be taken prior to undertaking the mammogram and information on the type of implant in situ should be obtained from the woman, if possible. The radiographer should observe and record anything considered unusual to include differences in the size of the breasts, position of the nipple, skin colour of the breast and contour of the breast. Any differences should be pointed out and discussed with the client prior to mammography. If a ruptured implant is suspected, it is advisable that mammography is not undertaken and local procedures should be followed.

It is important to gain and record consent when imaging clients with implants. The radiographer must explain the use of minimum compression force and the likelihood that this would not damage the implant. In addition to routine views, the Eklund technique may be used to pull the breast tissue forward from the implant and improve breast tissue visualisation – a full explanation of the imaging technique should be given prior to undertaking the mammogram. Even under ideal circumstances, such as a 'soft' breast and an

C.D. Borrelli
St George's National Breast Education Centre,
The Rose Centre, St George's Healthcare NHS Trust,
Perimeter Road, London SW17 0QT, UK
e-mail: claire.borrelli@stgeorges.nhs.uk

P. Hogg et al. (eds.), *Digital Mammography: A Holistic Approach*,
DOI 10.1007/978-3-319-04831-4_27,

experienced radiographer, approximately 10 % of breast tissue may still be obscured by the implant.

Despite the best efforts to maximise the amount of breast tissue visualised free of the implant, in most clients who have breast implants there will be some compromise in visualisation of all breast tissue. The radiographer should record all details of the examination, for example, views taken, exposure, breast thickness and compression force. A routine post mammography clinical observation should be undertaken. If any changes have occurred the radiologist should be informed and local policy followed.

Women should be informed that they should contact the imaging department for advice if they have any concerns following mammography. As with all women, it is important to emphasise breast awareness and advise them that they should contact their General Practitioner immediately if they have any concerns about new symptoms or are concerned about implant integrity.

Mammographic Imaging

Local protocols on the views should be drawn up. Following a national audit [2], it is recommended that these include:

1. Standard MLO views first to establish the position of the implant (subglandular or subpectoral). This will help with decisions about imaging of that client:
2. Perform standard CC views to get as far back onto the chest wall as possible and demonstrate both medial and lateral borders.
3. Perform Eklund CC views to demonstrate the anterior breast tissue with the implant displaced posteriorly or
4. If the implant is immobile (encapsulated), consider the value of a true lateral view.

Breast Implant Placement

The exact anatomical placement of breast implants can vary but the location of the implant is typically subglandular or subpectoral (Fig. 27.1), should the placement site be known by the client or from previous imaging, this should be documented by the radiographer. Incision sites for implants are usually periareolar, inframammary, or transaxillary. Special considerations may be taken to minimise interference with future breastfeeding or mammography when determining the best incision site and implant placement in individual patients [3]. Implants that are placed below

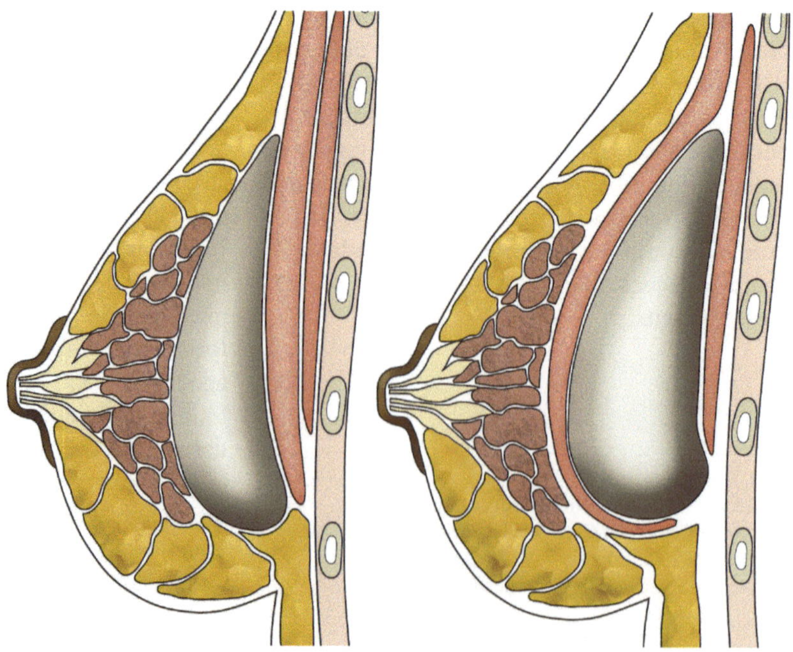

Fig. 27.1 Breast Anatomy demonstrating implant positioning Subglandular implant placement (*left image*) and subpectoral implant placement (*right image*) are options for breast augmentation

the pectoral muscle may be less likely to interfere with mammography imaging [4]. After breast reconstruction surgery, women are encouraged to maintain a normal mammography schedule.

Whilst there is no published guidance on compression force used, typically, a reduced force in this context would be approximately 6–8daN'

Subglandular Placement

In subglandular placement, the implant is positioned posterior to the breast parenchyma and superficial to the pectoral muscle [3]. The subglandular position in patients with thin soft-tissue coverage is more likely to show ripples or wrinkles of the underlying implant.

Subglandular placement can make breast augmentation surgery shorter and reduce recovery time. A possible disadvantage could be having breast implant edges more visibly noticeable under the skin. Imaging during a mammogram can also be more difficult when breast implants are placed by this method (Figs. 27.2 and 27.3).

Subpectoral Placement

In subpectoral placement, the implant is placed under the pectoralis major muscle and over the pectoralis minor muscle [3]. This technique is most commonly used for maximal coverage of implants used in breast reconstruction.

Subpectoral placement may reduce the chances of breast implants being felt through the skin, and it may help reduce the chance of scar tissue hardening around breast implants. It will also make it easier to image breast tissue during a mammogram. Possible disadvantages of this placement choice could be a longer surgery and recovery period (See Figs. 27.1, 27.4 and 27.5).

Implant Displacement: Eklund Views

Implant displacement views, or Eklund views (Fig. 27.6), are used to adequately image breast tissue in women with implants. These views are achieved by pulling breast tissue forward, away

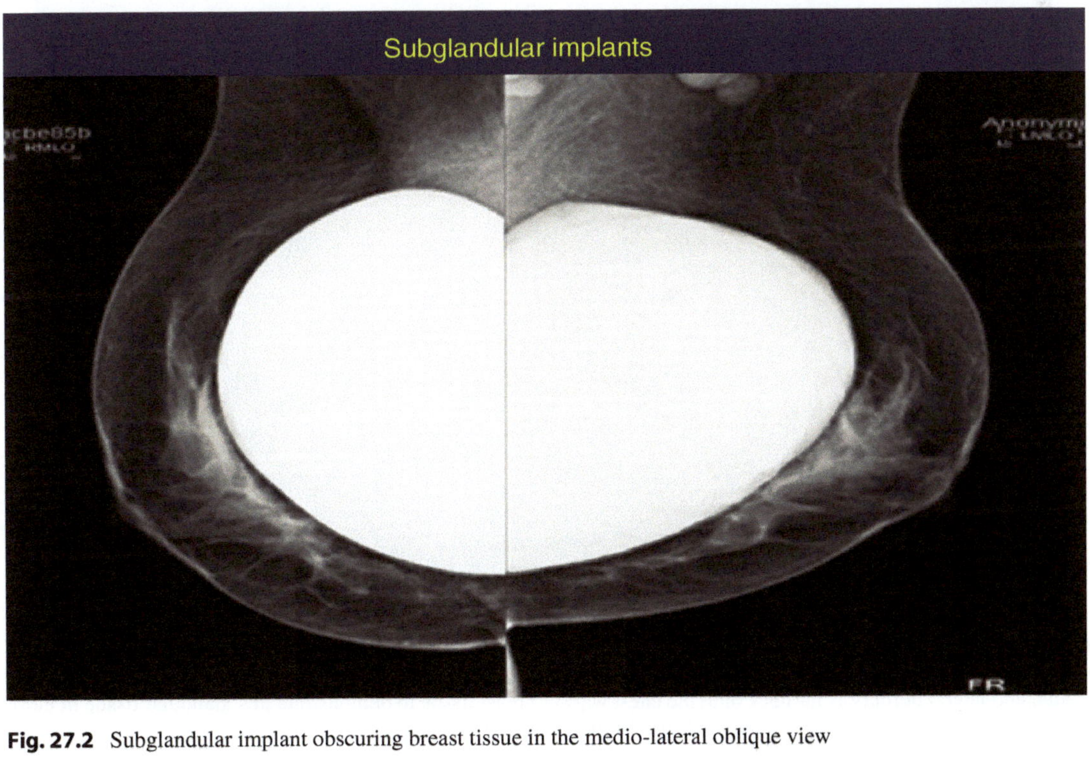

Fig. 27.2 Subglandular implant obscuring breast tissue in the medio-lateral oblique view

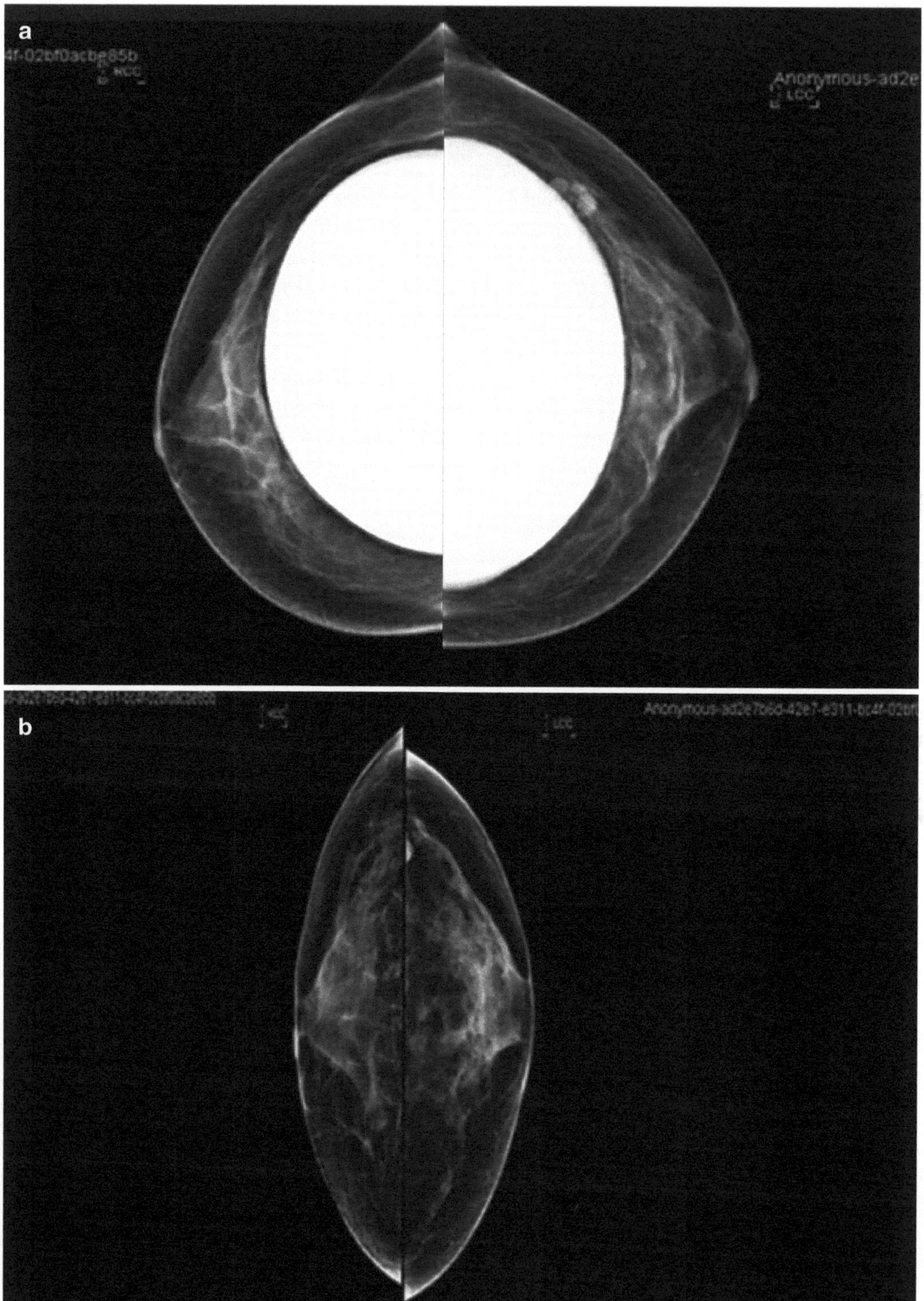

Fig. 27.3 (**a**) Subglandular implant obscuring breast tissue in the cranio-caudal view but demonstrating both medial and lateral borders as far back onto the chest wall as possible. (**b**) Subglandular implant with the Eklund view employed to displace the implant posteriorly onto the chest wall and apply compression to the anterior breast tissue to demonstrate this glandular tissue in more detail

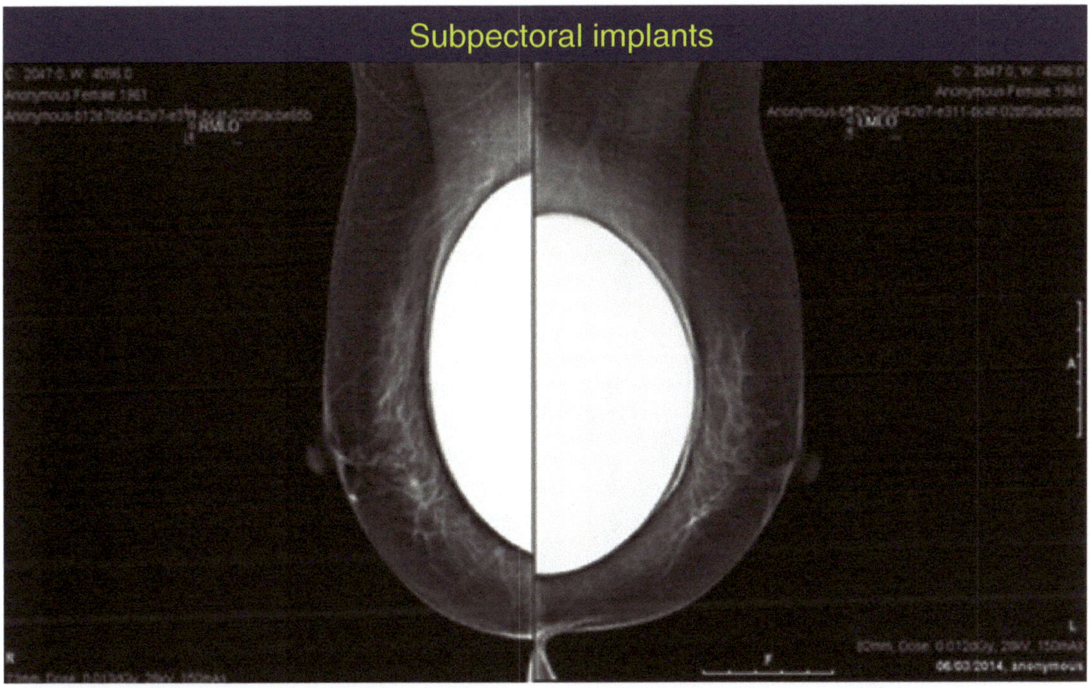

Fig. 27.4 Subpectoral implant seen in the medio-lateral with minimal breast tissue obscured

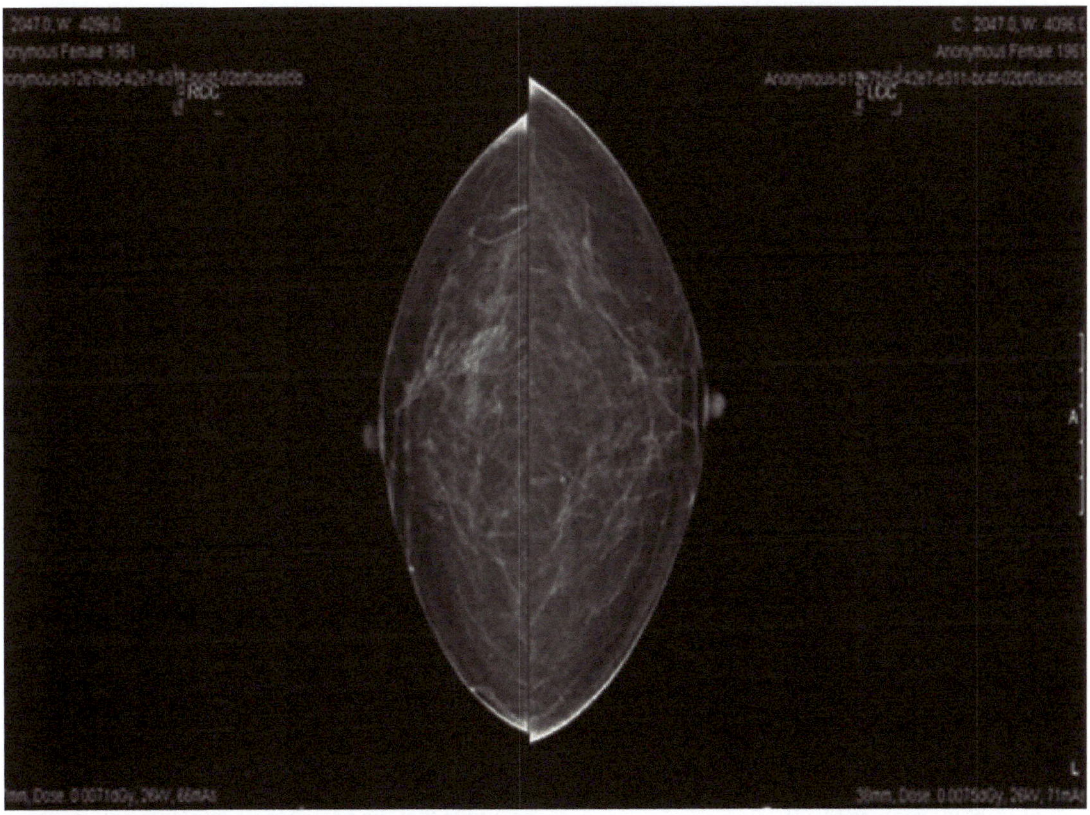

Fig. 27.5 Subpectoral implant seen in the cranio-caudal view at the posterior margin of the breast with minimal breast tissue obscured

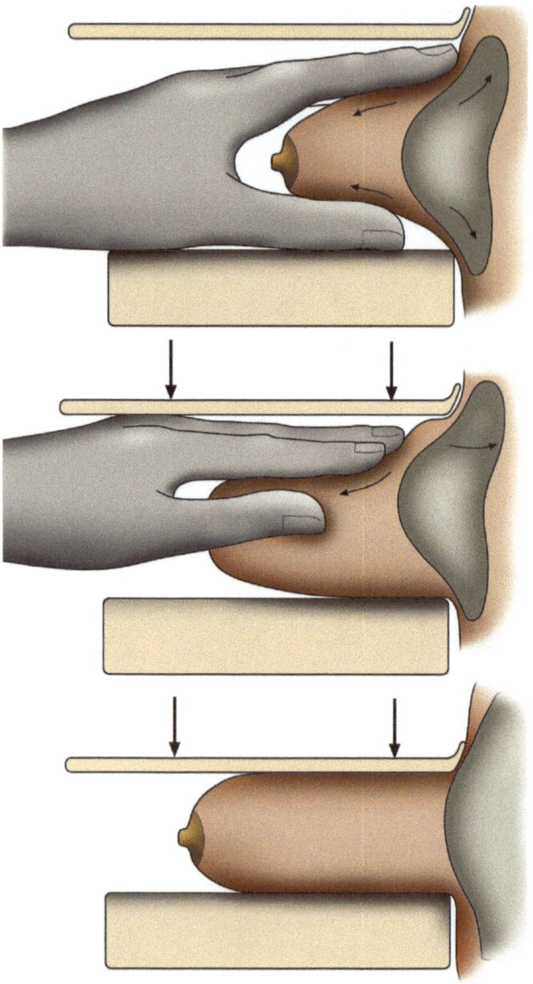

Fig. 27.6 Eklund technique

from the implant. At the same time, the implant is displaced posteriorly against the chest wall so that it is out of the field of view. The radiographer then applies compression force to the tissue in front of the implant [5, 6]. Standard cranio-caudal and mediolateral oblique views are typically taken first. The implant displacement view provides improved imaging of the tissue at the front of the implant, while the standard views provide images of the tissue behind and underneath the implant, as well as the lower axillary area [3]. However, implant displacement views increase the amount of radiation that is delivered during a mammogram procedure and may increase the risk of implant rupture [1, 7].

The quality of imaging studies with implant displacement views and the amount of breast tissue imaged can be impacted by client factors such as breast size, glandularity, and fat content, as well as implant factors such as size, position, and implant-associated complications. Implant position and capsular contracture have the greatest impact on mammography success in clients with implants [3]. Implants placed below the pectoral muscle are less likely to interfere with imaging, resulting in almost twice the amount of breast tissues imaged compared with subglandular breast implants [3, 4].

Standard mammography views are taken first using minimum compression until the skin blanches and to help keep the breast still.

Eklund views are performed with the implant pushed back against the chest wall. The compression paddle is applied to the breast tissue until the skin blanches, which is pulled forward.

Implant Complications

Aside from breast cancer screening, imaging of the breasts in women with implants may be necessary over time to diagnose common complications associated with implants, including implant rupture, silicone extravasation (leakage), gel bleed, polyurethane breakdown, and peri-implant fluid collections. Although imaging with ultrasound and mammography have both been used successfully to evaluate the integrity of implants and detect possible problems over time, MRI is the preferred modality to detect implant rupture [8].

Realistic Client Expectations

While women with implants may be concerned about their implants interfering with adequate breast cancer imaging, the available evidence suggests that implants do not greatly impact clinical outcomes in patients who do develop breast cancer, despite a possible delay in diagnosis [7, 9, 10]. Clients should be aware that the presence of implants will increase the length of their mammography visits and may require breast manipulations to improve the visualisation of the breast parenchyma.

Injectable Enhancements

An alternative to breast augmentation with the use of implants is the option for injectable fillers that may be used for volume restoration and body contouring. A number of products have been offered over the years with varying levels of success. Prior to breast imaging, it is helpful for the radiographer to know in advance if breast fillers or fat transfer have been used as some products may compromise the visualisation of breast tissue and could present as cysts or round masses and may therefore significantly reduce the diagnostic quality of the mammograms which may in turn lead to misdiagnosis.

Summary

Clients who have undergone breast augmentation present an important imaging challenge for the practitioner as the breast implant obscures the breast tissue. Additional mammographic views are required in clients with implants to ensure an effective imaging study to demonstrate maximum breast tissue to enable an accurate diagnosis, but adequate screening is still possible. Despite the challenges for mammography posed by breast implants, clinical outcomes in clients who do develop breast cancer are not noticeably affected in those who have undergone breast augmentation or reconstructive surgery.

References

1. Gutowski KA, Mesna GT, Cunningham BL. Saline-filled breast implants: a Plastic Surgery Educational Foundation multicenter outcomes study. Plast Reconstr Surg. 1997;100:1019–27.
2. Curtis J, Borrelli C. Developing a National Standard. Imaging & Therapy Practice 2013. ISSN: 1360–5518. http://www.sor.org/.
3. Smalley SM. Breast implants and breast cancer screening. J Midwifery Womens Health. 2003;48:329–37.
4. Handel N, Silverstein MJ, Gamagami P, Jensen JA, Collins A. Factors affecting mammographic visualization of the breast after augmentation mammaplasty. JAMA. 1992;268:1913–7.
5. Gorczyca DP, Brenner RJ. The augmented breast: radiologic and clinical perspectives. New York: Thieme; 1997.
6. Eklund GW, Busby RC, Miller SH, Job JS. Improved imaging of the augmented breast. AJR Am J Roentgenol. 1988;151:469–73.
7. Brinton LA, Lubin JH, Burich MC, Colton T, Brown SL, Hoover RN. Breast cancer following augmentation mammoplasty. Cancer Causes Control. 2000;11:819–27.
8. O'Toole M, Caskey CI. Imaging spectrum of breast implant complications: mammography, ultrasound, and magnetic resonance imaging. Semin Ultrasound CT MR. 2000;21:351–61.
9. Brinton LA. The relationship of silicone breast implants and cancer at other sites. Plast Reconstr Surg. 2007;120(7 Suppl 1):94s–102.
10. Smathers RL, Boone JM, Lee LJ, Berns EA, Miller RA, Wright AM. Radiation dose reduction for augmentation mammography. AJR Am J Roentgenol. 2007;188:1414–21.

28 Imaging Bariatric, Post Surgical and Limited Mobility Clients

Lisa Bisset

Introduction

A large proportion of clients have additional requirements that the practitioner must take into account and adapt their technique accordingly. These clients include those with limited mobility, bariatric and those who have had previous surgery. Practitioners should endeavour to produce the best possible images whilst maintaining appropriate care and this requirement is reflected into many professional codes of conduct throughout the world (e.g. The College and Society of Radiographers [1]). This chapter discusses practical ways to achieve good quality images whilst providing appropriate client care in these groups.

Bariatric Imaging

According to the National Cancer Institute (NCI) [2] obesity is associated with an increased risk in breast cancer. There is also a link between increased rates of recall, biopsy and stage of cancer at diagnosis [3]. Consequently this group of clients requires high quality imaging as they are more likely to develop breast cancer [4]. Some studies have shown that such clients are less likely to attend screening [5, 6]. Further studies have demonstrated that there is a higher morbidity rate in obese women [7]. More in depth training into bariatric imaging, which encompasses a sensitive approach to their particular needs, must be considered in order to encourage re-attendance. A relaxed client is more likely to be co-operative and tolerate the examination.

Client Care

Research studies have shown that obese women are less likely to attend for screening; some of the barriers highlighted include insensitive comments about weight and equipment along with gowns that are too small. These factors should be considered by the practitioner so that those who do attend have a positive experience, this should encourage re-attendance for subsequent screens [6].

Technique

The standard imaging views (see Chap. 21) involve cranio caudal (CC) and medio lateral oblique (MLO) positions. Whilst these are the ultimate aim it must be accepted that sometimes standard views are not possible and additional imaging may often be required. It is possible to accidentally exclude the posterior aspect of a large breast off the image receptor (IR) and should a cancer be

L. Bisset
Consultant Radiographer,
Dorset Breast Screening Unit, Poole General Hospital, Longflet Rd, Poole Dorset, BH166FD, UK
e-mail: lisa.bisset@poole.nhs.uk

P. Hogg et al. (eds.), *Digital Mammography: A Holistic Approach*,
DOI 10.1007/978-3-319-04831-4_28, © Springer International Publishing Switzerland 2015

present it risks not being demonstrated. An increased body mass index (BMI) has been associated with greater compressed breast thickness which results in increased geometric unsharpness, decreased image contrast and possibly blur [8, 9]. Where additional exposures are necessary to image the entire breast departmental protocols should be followed along with any statutory regulations (e.g. Ionising Radiation (medical exposure) Regulations 2000 (IRMER)) [10].

Technical points to consider for larger breasts

- For heavier breasts a shallower angle can be useful
- Employ sensible manual handling techniques. Two practitioners may be required.
- Always review previous images, if available.
- Departments should have a protocol for large breasts to aid consistency and comparison with subsequent examinations.
- Mosaic or tiling of images may be necessary.
- When lifting and pulling the breast be careful not to tear skin in IMF (see Chap. 15).

Suggested imaging protocol for larger breasts,

View	Criteria
MLO	Ensure the whole breast is covered. A back of the breast view (posterior) and front of breast (anterior) may be required (nipple in profile in either one or both views)
	Ensure the breast is crease free – particularly in the infra mammary fold (IMF) and the superior breast
	Consider a latero-medial oblique (reverse oblique) for a protruding abdomen
CC	All of the breast needs to be included. This includes the medial and lateral breast as well as the anterior and posterior aspects
	Consider a laterally extended CC for a large breast that appears to 'wrap around'
	It is easy to exclude the posterior aspect of the breast so ensure the breast is pulled on sufficiently
	Nipple should be in profile in accordance with departmental protocol either one or both views

Post-surgical Imaging

All women who have had breast conserving surgery (BCS) should be offered surveillance mammography. This has been shown to improve survival rates by the early detection of local recurrence [11]. The optimal timing and frequency of this is currently a subject of debate and there appears to be no consensus [12]. The current UK NICE Guidance (CG80) [13] states:

> Offer annual mammography to all patients with early breast cancer, including DCIS, until they enter the NHSBSP/BTWSP. Patients diagnosed with early breast cancer that are already eligible for screening should have annual mammography for 5 years
> On reaching the NHSBSP/BTWSP screening age or after 5 years of annual mammography follow-up we recommend the NHSBSP/BTWSP stratify screening frequency in line with patient risk category.

This guidance is open to interpretation and therefore differing breast screening programmes could have different protocols, which can be confusing to patients who move to a new area.

Technique

Postsurgical changes can often overlap with malignant mammographic features. High quality images are essential. Imaging the surgically altered breast poses challenges to the practitioner and the image reader. There are several benign post-surgical features that make both performing and reading the mammogram challenging. These include, scar formation that can mimic cancer, post irradiation changes, oedema, skin thickening, fat necrosis and seromas [14].

Post-surgical calcification develops in about a third of cases which is caused by trauma to breast fat; this can develop 2–5 years after treatment. Skin thickening is the most common finding [14]. Breast oedema gradually diminishes and resolves for many patients by the second year mark but in the interim period this can make mammography uncomfortable as the breast is enlarged and compression may be difficult [15]. It is important the practitioner is aware of these normal post-operative changes that occur so they approach the patient in an empathetic manner allowing for the production of best quality images.

Below are examples of images

The post-surgical changes demonstrated in the Left upper outer quadrant in Fig. 28.1 have

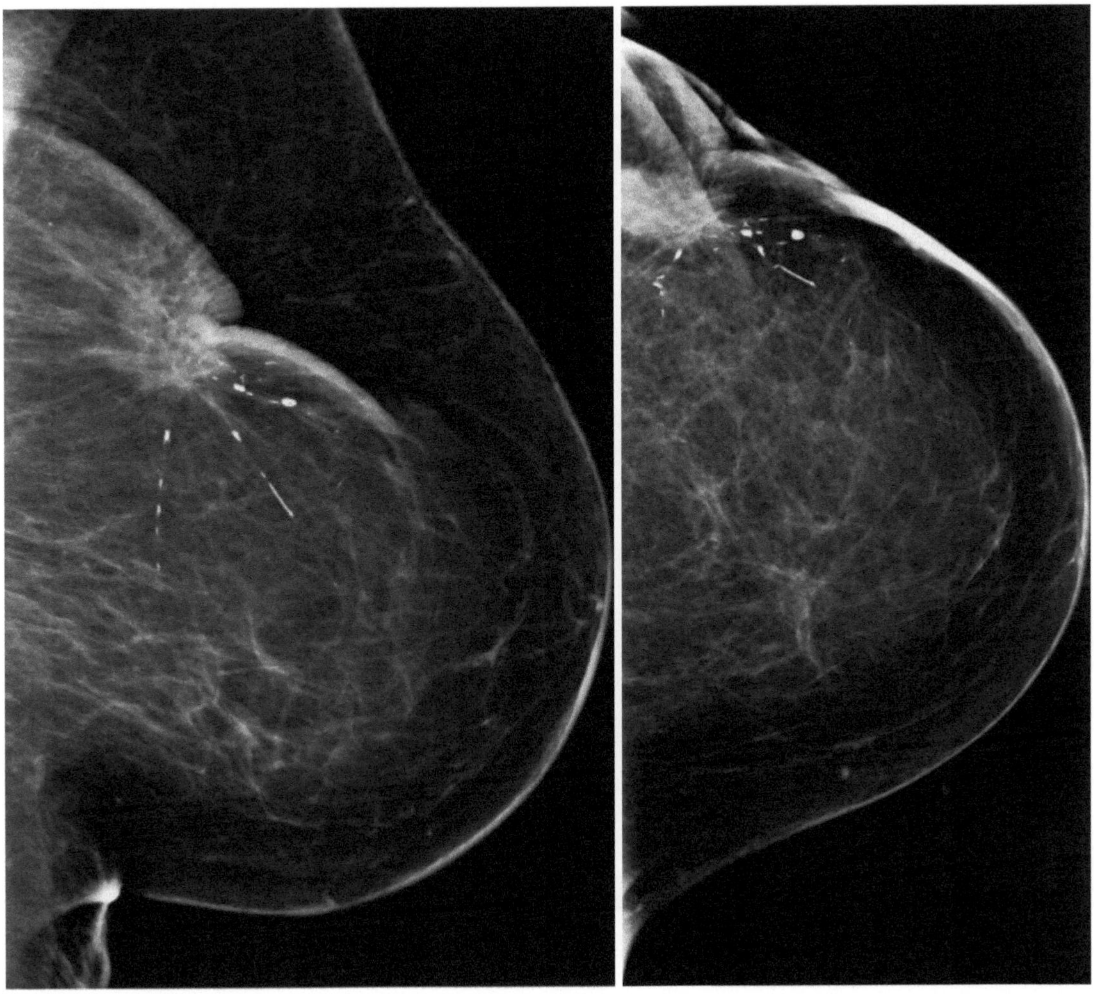

Fig. 28.1 Post surgery mammogram with benign macro calcification and distortion. The *left* image is a *left* medio lateral oblique the *right* is a *left* CC

features which overlap with a carcinoma. There is a clear distortion and skin puckering.

Post surgical changes can create difficulties in positioning the breast with the nipple in profile. There appears to be a well defined mass on the right medio-lateral oblique (MLO) projection in Fig. 28.2 but this represents the nipple. Skin thickening and oedema are also present on these images.

A common feature seen on post surgical mammography is fat necrosis as seen in the left upper outer quadrant in Fig. 28.3.

The client in Fig. 28.4 has a distortion at the site of previous surgery. It is important that the practitioner records accurate clinical information and surgical procedures with dates and marks the scars for the image reader. The distortion has similar features to a carcinoma. Previous images are paramount for comparison in such cases.

Technical points to consider,

- It is essential that the practitioner records all scars and takes a brief history so that the image reader is aware of their precise location when reporting the mammogram.
- A thorough explanation of the procedure, particularly compression force, is important as this can reduce anxiety.
- Review previous images, if available.
- If the breast is distorted, a separate projection with the nipple in profile may be required.

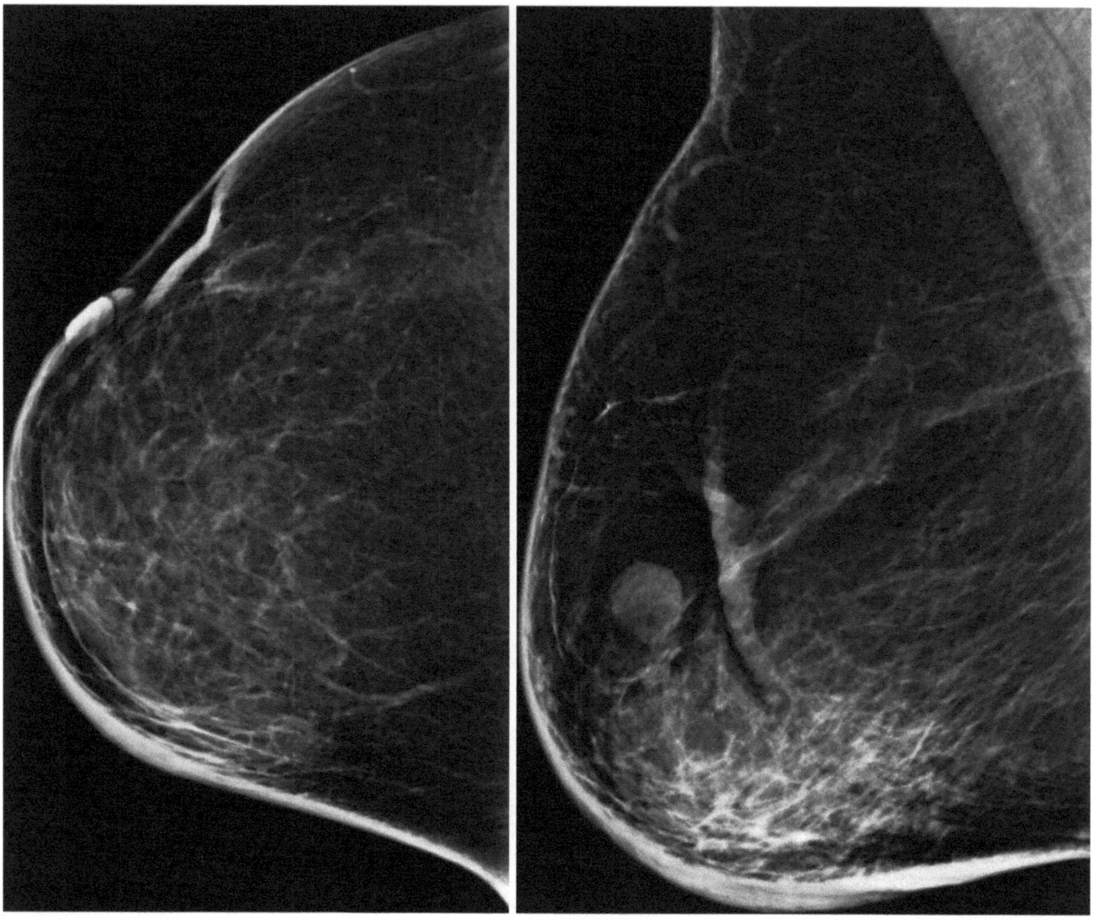

Fig. 28.2 Oedema and skin thickening. The *left* image is a *right* CC the *right* image is a medio lateral oblique

- Some clients experience tenderness and discomfort longer than others so an empathetic and professional manner is important.
- Large posterior seromas can make adequate compression of the breast difficult and additional projections of the anterior of the breast may be required.

Client Care

Clients attending for surveillance mammography often have an increased level of anxiety, particularly for the first annual visit. A brief polite introduction by the practitioner where there is an opportunity for the client to voice concerns or ask questions may help to alleviate this and encourage compliance.

- Any new symptoms/concerns must be recorded.
- If the client requires further tests such as ultrasound, this should preferably be done at the same appointment. If this is not possible the client should be informed of when this will be.
- It is essential that the client leaves the department knowing how and when they will receive their results and when their next surveillance mammogram is due.

Clients with Limited Mobility

A disability can be defined as 'the presence of a limitation in activity or function caused by a biological or psychological condition' [16]. This definition covers a wide spectrum of disabilities.

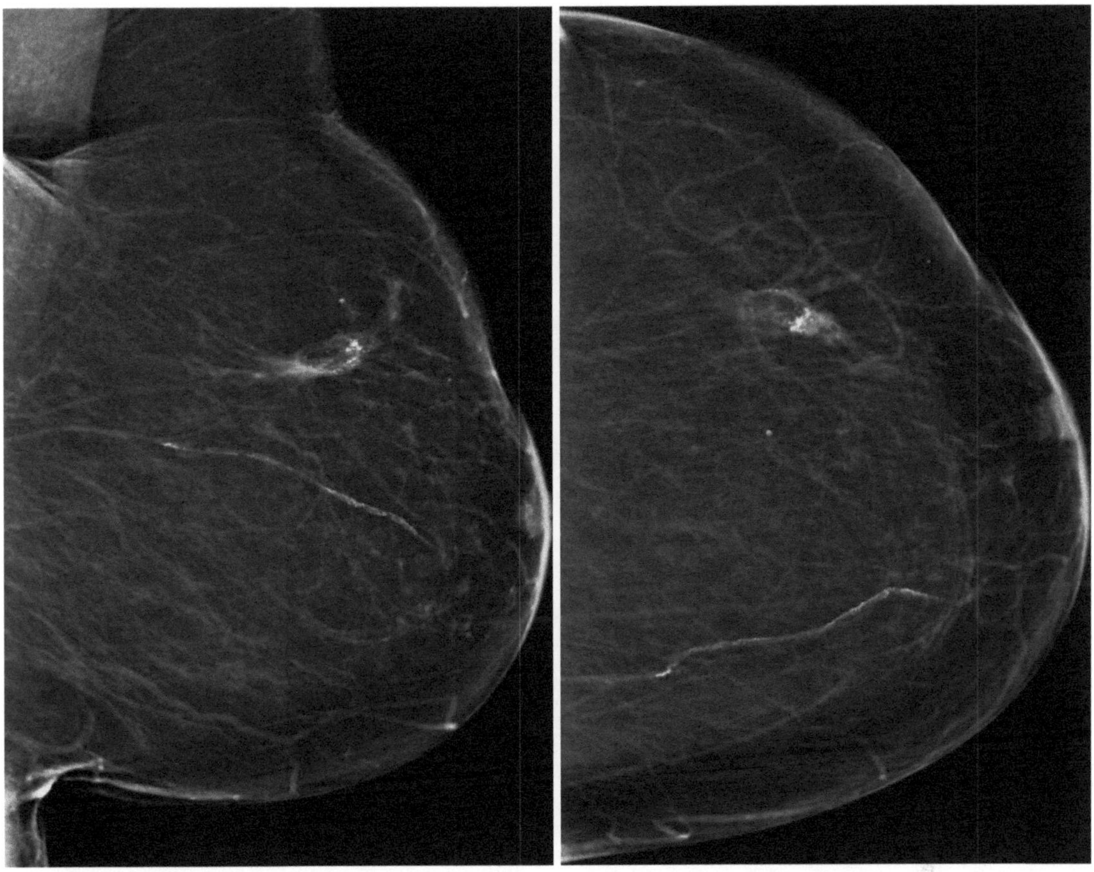

Fig. 28.3 Fat necrosis. The *left* image is a *right* CC the *right* image is a medio lateral oblique

Women with disabilities are at increased risk of breast cancer mortality [17]; there is also low screening uptake amongst clients with limited mobility. Recurring themes that prevent these clients attending breast screening include; previous bad experience, factors related to the environment, finance, lack of knowledge, physical limitations and carers lack of knowledge [18, 19]. Further barriers have been identified as explanation of the procedure, accessible changing facilities and the availability of disabled parking [20].

Producing good quality images whilst ensuring a positive experience for these clients is a challenging task. The procedure itself is physically demanding requiring the practitioner to manipulate the client and often a wheelchair into the correct position. The use of manual handling aids is essential; this can include manual handling slides, cushions and stools. The overall quality of the screening experience is a significant determinant of re-attendance. The interaction between practitioner and client contributes significantly to how the examination is perceived [21–23].

Whilst equal access to services is important for clients with limited mobility, it must also be accepted that breast screening is not possible for all and there is a balance to be found between the potential benefits and harm. Within the UK, there is currently no alternative screening method for those unable to have a mammogram available through National Health Service screening programmes.

Technical points to consider

- Employ safe manual handling techniques at all times with two practitioners in the imaging room.
- Discuss with the client if they are able to stand. It is perfectly acceptable to perform mammography

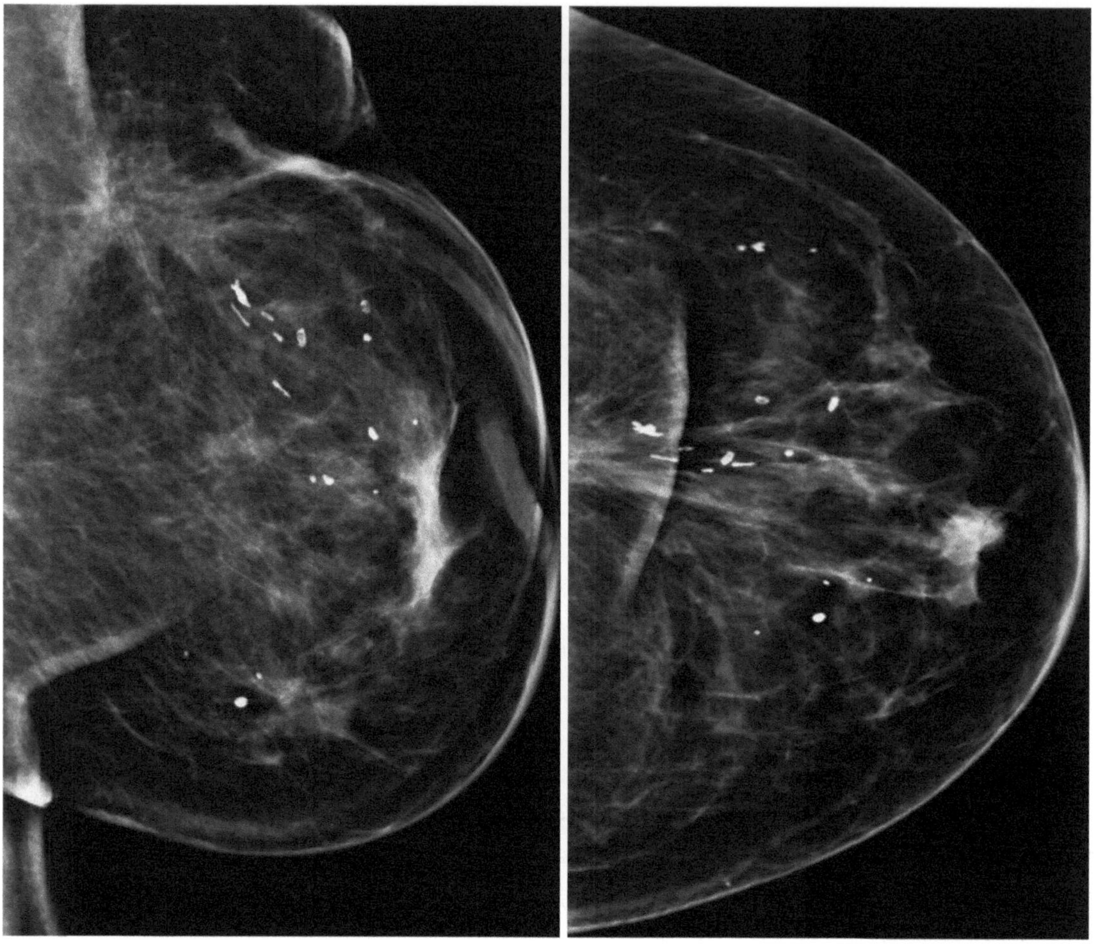

Fig. 28.4 Post surgical changes causing distortion. The *left* picture is a *left* medio lateral oblique the *right* picture is a *left* CC

in an imaging chair or a wheelchair. It is not considered acceptable within the UK or many other countries to permit a supporter in the X-ray field (even with a lead apron.)

- Aim to image as much of the breast as possible in two views. Additional projections may be required to achieve this. Ensure to follow departmental protocol.
- If standard projections are not possible, consider other views such as reverse cranio-caudal (CC) and Latero-medial oblique (LMO). These are described in Chap. 24.
- Be prepared to adapt angles in line with body habitus and ability to move. A shallow angle may help the client feel supported.

Client Care

- If the client is distressed and is unable to cooperate the examination may have to be abandoned.
- Some conditions, such as multiple sclerosis (MS), can have good and bad phases. It could be that the client can be encouraged to re-book an appointment at a better time for themselves.
- A full explanation is essential before the examination. Ensure the examination requirements are fully understood and gain informed consent, their trust and assistance. Give opportunity to ask any questions.

- Use supportive aids such as pads or pillows and avoid any part of the machine digging into the client.
- Ensure that the client knows when and how they will get their results.

References

1. Society of Radiographers code of conduct 2013. 2013. http://www.sor.org/learning/document-library/code-professional-conduct. Accessed 1 Sept 2014.
2. http://www.cancer.gov/cancertopics/pdq/prevention/breast/HealthProfessional#Section_180.
3. Hunt K, Sickles E. Effect of obesity on screening mammography: outcomes analysis of 88,346 consecutive examinations. AJR Am J Roentgenol. 2000;175: 1251–5.
4. Gayde C, Goolam I, Bangash H. Outcome of mammography on women with large breasts. Breast. 2012; 21(4):493–8.
5. Atkins E, Madhavan S, LeMasters T. Are obese women more likely to participate in a mobile mammography program? J Community Health. 2013;38(2):338–48.
6. Friedman A, Hemler J, Rossetti E. Obese women's barriers to mammography and pap smear: the possible role of personality. Obesity. 2012;20(8):1611–7.
7. Maruther N, Bolen S, Brancati F, Clark J. Obesity and mammography: a systematic review and meta-analysis. J Gen Intern Med. 2009;24(5):665–77.
8. Guest A, Helvie M, Chan H, Hadjiiski L, Bailey J, Roubidoux M. Adverse affects of increased body weight on quantitative measures of mammographic image quality. AJR Am J Roentgenol. 2000;173(5):805–10.
9. Mercer C, Hogg P, Lawson R, Diffey J, Denton E. Practitioner compression force variability in mammography: a preliminary study. Br J Radiol. 2013;86:20110596.
10. Department of Health. Ionising radiation (medical exposure) regulations 2000 (IRMER). 2000. https://www.gov.uk/government/publications/the-ionising-radiation-medical-exposure-regulations-2000. Accessed 1 Sept 2014.
11. Robertson C, Arcot Ragupathy S, Boachie C. The clinical effectiveness and cost-effectiveness of different surveillance mammography regimens after the treatment for primary breast cancer: systematic reviews registry database analyses and economic evaluation. Health Technol Assess. 2011;15(34):v–vi–1–322. 1366–5278.
12. McNaul D, Darke M, Garge M, Dale P. An evaluation of post-lumpectomy recurrence rates: is follow up every 6 months for 2 years needed ? J Surg Oncol. 2013;107(6):597–601.
13. Harnett A, Smallwood J, Titshall V, Champion A. Guideline Development Group. Diagnosis and treatment of early breast cancer, including locally advanced disease–summary of NICE guidance. BMJ. 2009;338:b438. doi: 10.1136/bmj.b438.
14. Dershaw D. Mammography in patients with breast cancer treated by breast conservation (lumpectomy with or without radiation). Am J Roentgenol. 1995;164: 309–16.
15. Mendelson E. Evaluation of the post-operative breast. Radiol Clin North Am. 1992;30(1):107–38.
16. Verbrugge L, Jette A. The disablement process. Soc Sci Biol Med. 1994;38:1–14.
17. McCarthy E, Ngo L, Roetzheim R. Disparities in breast cancer treatment and survival for women with disabilities. Annu Int Med. 2006;145:637–45.
18. Todd A, Stuifbergen A. Breast cancer screening barriers and disability. Rehabil Nurs. 2012;37(5):267.
19. Lopez E, Vasudevan V, Lanzone M. Florida mammographer disability training vs needs. Radiol Technol. 2012;83(4):337–48.
20. Jarman M, Bowling J, Dickens P. Factors facilitating acceptable mammography services for women with disabilities. Women's Health Issues. 2012;22(5): 1049–3867.
21. Sze Y, Liu M, Clark M. Breast and cervical cancer screening practices among disabled women aged 40–75: does quality of the experience matter? J Womens Health. 2008;17(8):1321–9.
22. Whelehan P, Evans A, Wells M, Macgillivray S. The effect of mammography pain on repeat participation in breast cancer screening: a systematic review. Breast. 2013;22(4):389–94.
23. Poulos A, Balandin S, Llewellyn G. Women with physical disability and the mammogram: an observational study to identify barriers and facilitators. Radiography. 2010;17:14–9.

29 Male Mammography

Susan E. Garnett

Male breast cancer is rare compared to female breast cancer, with less than 1 % of all breast cancer patients being male [1]. The incidence of male breast cancer is slowly increasing [2]. All breast pathologies found in the female breast may also been seen in the male breast.

Performing male mammography is controversial as cancer can be distinguished from gynaecomastia clinically, and sonography can be performed for confirmation. However research is limited regarding appropriate diagnostic testing [2]. The male breast is undeveloped but is influenced by oestrogen and testosterone affecting the small amount of breast tissue found behind the nipple. This rudimentary breast tissue contains mainly major subareolar ducts and rarely ductal lobular units.

Gynaecomastia

Gynaecomastia is the most common condition in males [1]. An oestrogen surge (in young men), or a drop in testosterone in men older than 60 years can influence development of the rudimentary ducts and lobules behind the nipple producing a symmetrical or asymmetrical lump. This is easily assessed by ultrasound to determine its dendritic nature. More asymmetric and harder masses can also be assessed by ultrasound although mammography is useful for excluding calcifications and secondary lesions.

Doyle et al. [3] in a review study, concluded most male symptoms are benign. However, some radiological features that are considered benign in a female are more uncertain in males, such as well-defined masses or larger rounder and scattered calcifications. In males breast cancer often presents as a firm subareolar mass eccentric to the nipple [1].

Ductal Carcinoma In Situ

Ductal carcinoma in situ (DCIS) has not been well-documented in males, but DCIS can present as a palpable nodularity mimicking gynaecomastia [4]. With continuously improving ultrasound technology calcification can more easily be identified in such rare cases.

Invasive Carcinoma

Invasive ductal carcinoma is the most common breast cancer type. Invasive lobular carcinoma is rarely seen due to few lobule formations [5]. Male breast cancers will rapidly metastase as the breast tissue is minimal and the lymph nodes proximal. Risk factors for breast cancer are similar to female breast cancer but also are gender

S.E. Garnett
Breast Unit, Ground Floor West Wing
University Hospital, Clifford Bridge Road,
Coventry CV2 2DX, UK
e-mail: sue.garnett@uhcw.nhs.uk

P. Hogg et al. (eds.), *Digital Mammography: A Holistic Approach*,
DOI 10.1007/978-3-319-04831-4_29, © Springer International Publishing Switzerland 2015

specific risks including Klinefelters syndrome and oestrogen based drug treatment for prostate cancer. Treatment is identical to female disease, although it is uncertain if risk, genetic and biological characteristics are gender specific [2]. Mastectomy is commonly performed and hormonal treatment given as appropriate.

Mammography

When performing a male mammogram, practitioners must be aware of the sensitivities of the individual in an essentially female environment. Using terms such as 'X-raying the chest wall', giving reassurance and addressing the man's anxiety assists positioning and encourages relaxation. This allows the entire length of the soft tissue region over the muscle down to the lower chest wall to be lifted onto the image receptor.

Mammography in the male is a straightforward procedure because the pectoral muscle is positioned easily in the medio-lateral oblique (MLO) projection. Care must be taken not to work too high into the axilla. The cranio-caudal (CC) projection is more challenging as the soft tissue behind the nipple can slip off the image receptor (IR) before compression force can be applied. This is especially true if the receptor is placed too high up the chest wall. The retro-areolar region must be adequately visualised to assess all the glandular tissue. If the mammography unit can be inverted, a reverse CC view helps to visualise more tissue posteriorly. The mammogram should show the pectoral muscle across two-thirds of the soft tissue image and well below the nipple with a fatty background density. The nipple is easy to image in profile, thereby clearly demonstrating the rudimentary ductal system in the sub areolar region.

Tall men can present difficulties for the female operator. Seating the client will help positioning of the upper chest wall across the IR. X-raying a man is no more challenging than a small breasted woman. In fact the better developed pectoral muscle aids imaging of the overlying soft tissue.

Key Points

- Mammography **is straightforward**, the MLO is easily performed. The CC needs care to perform especially if the breast tissue is limited.
- Practitioners need to consider male sensitivity when performing a mammogram
- Male breast tissue consists of rudimentary ducts and lobules
- Gynaecomastia is the most common condition and imaging is not always required.
- Male breast cancer is rare and treatment is currently equivalent to female disease. Mastectomy is most commonly performed

References

1. Charlot M, Béatrix O, Chateau F, Dubuisson J, Golfier F, Valette PJ, Réty F. Pathologies of the male breast. Diagn Interv Imaging. 2013;94:26–37.
2. Ruddy KJ, Winer EP. Male breast cancer: risk factors, biology, diagnosis, treatment, and survivorship. Ann Oncol. 2013;24(6):1434–43.
3. Doyle S, Steel J, Porter G. Imaging male breast cancer. Clin Radiol. 2011;66(11):1079–85.
4. Noor L, McGovern P, Bhaskar P, Lowe JW. Bilateral DCIS following gynaecomastia surgery. Role of nipple sparing mastectomy. A case report and review of the literature. Int J Surg Case Rep. 2011;2:106–8.
5. Briest S, Vang R, Terell K, Emens L, Lange JR. Invasive lobular carcinoma of the male breast: a rare histology in an uncommon disease. Breast Care (Basel). 2009; 4(1):36–8.

30 Digital Breast Tomosynthesis

Yit Y. Lim and Anthony J. Maxwell

Technological advances have resulted in the replacement of traditional film-screen mammography with digital mammography, which has been shown to be more accurate in younger women, in those with dense breasts and in pre- and peri-menopausal women [1]. However, one of the major limitations of mammography remains, that is the issue of overlapping breast tissue mimicking or obscuring a lesion. This leads to women receiving unnecessary recalls for further tests (and the associated adverse psychological effects) and to cancers being missed. The introduction of digital mammography has allowed the development of new image acquisition and processing techniques, such as digital breast tomosynthesis (DBT), which promises to overcome some of the limitations of conventional 2D mammography. DBT minimises the effect of tissue superimposition and allows better visualisation of the internal structure of the breast by displaying the tissues in a series of thin contiguous slices. An example is shown in Fig. 30.1a, b.

Y.Y. Lim (✉) • A.J. Maxwell
Consultant Academic Breast Radiologist,
The Nightingale Centre and Genesis Prevention Centre,
University Hospital of South Manchester,
Southmoor Road, Manchester M23 9LT, UK
e-mail: yit.lim@uhsm.nhs.uk;
anthony.maxwell@manchester.ac.uk

Techniques

The basic principle of DBT is the acquisition of a three-dimensional block of data by taking a number of images of the breast at slightly different angles. This is achieved by moving the X-ray tube and detector in an arc whilst making a series of exposures. The dose for each exposure is relatively small, such that the overall dose is comparable to that from a conventional mammogram.

Each manufacturer has a slightly different approach to the actual method of acquisition. The number of exposures taken per view ranges from 9 to 25, taken over an arc of between 11° and 50°. The acquisitions may be either continuous or "step and shoot". The continuous method, as the name implies, involves a smooth continuous movement of the tube and detector during image acquisition. This is faster than the "step and shoot" method but results in slightly lower image resolution due to an element of motion blurring. The "step and shoot" method involves multiple pauses during image acquisition and is more time-consuming but results in sharper images. However, as with conventional mammography, the longer the acquisition time, the greater the opportunity for blurring due to patient or equipment movement. The image acquisition time varies from 3 to 25 s per view. This will have to be taken into account when considering the throughput of patients, especially if DBT is to be used in large population screening programmes.

P. Hogg et al. (eds.), *Digital Mammography: A Holistic Approach*,
DOI 10.1007/978-3-319-04831-4_30, © Springer International Publishing Switzerland 2015

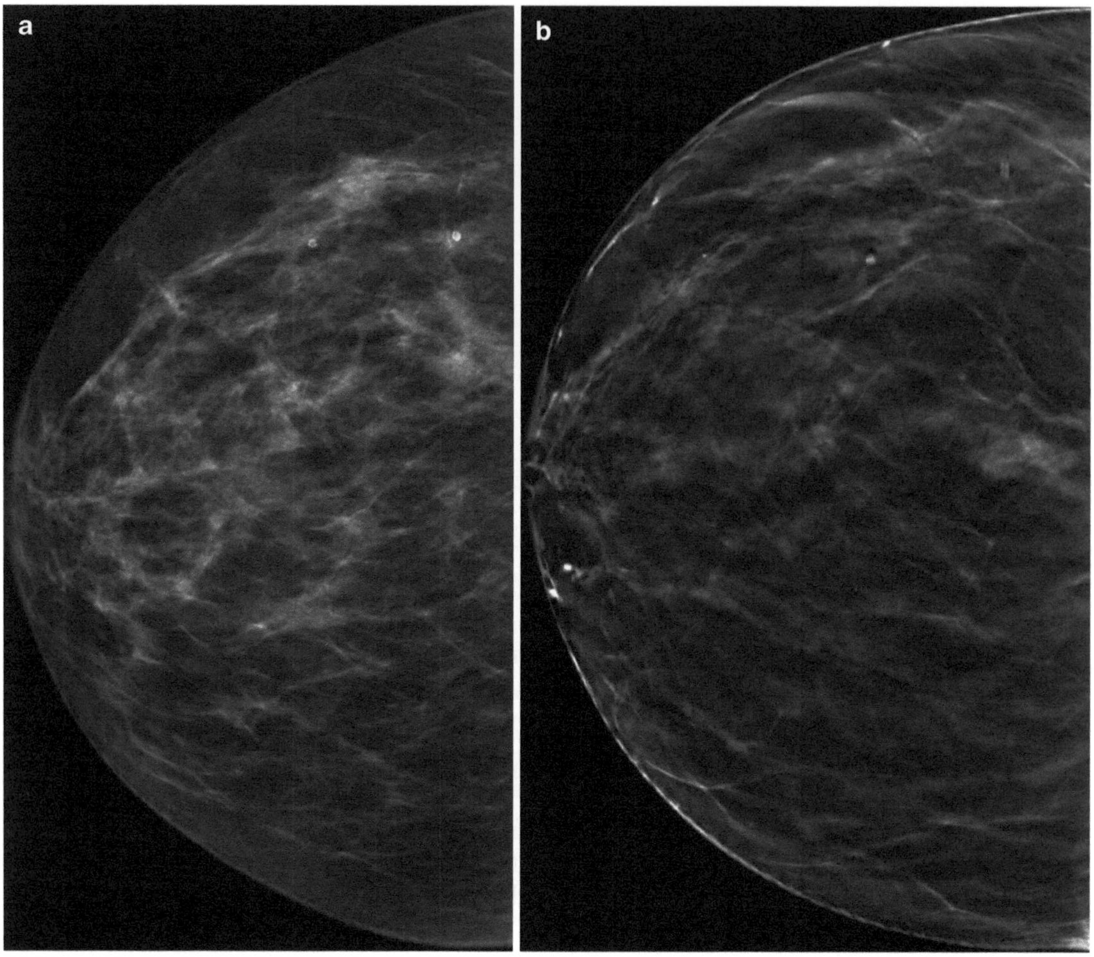

Fig. 30.1 (**a**) Right CC view shows an asymmetrical density in the outer half. (**b**) Representative slice from a tomosynthesis series shows normal glandular tissue with no underlying abnormality

Once acquired, the images are processed prior to display. The commonly used reconstruction algorithms are filtered back projection and iterative reconstruction. Filtered back projection is normally used in CT scanning and is faster as it calculates the image in a single reconstruction step but is more susceptible to noise. Iterative reconstruction is more complex, but the additional processing time is of little significance with modern computer technology. It has the advantage of being less sensitive to noise and streak artefact.

Indications

As a Primary Screening Tool

A number of population-based screening studies have demonstrated excellent results with the use of tomosynthesis in combination with digital mammography. These studies have shown an increase in cancer detection rate of 9.5–40 % [2–4] with a significant reduction in false positive rates. Other studies [5, 6] have also shown that DBT plus digital mammography has higher

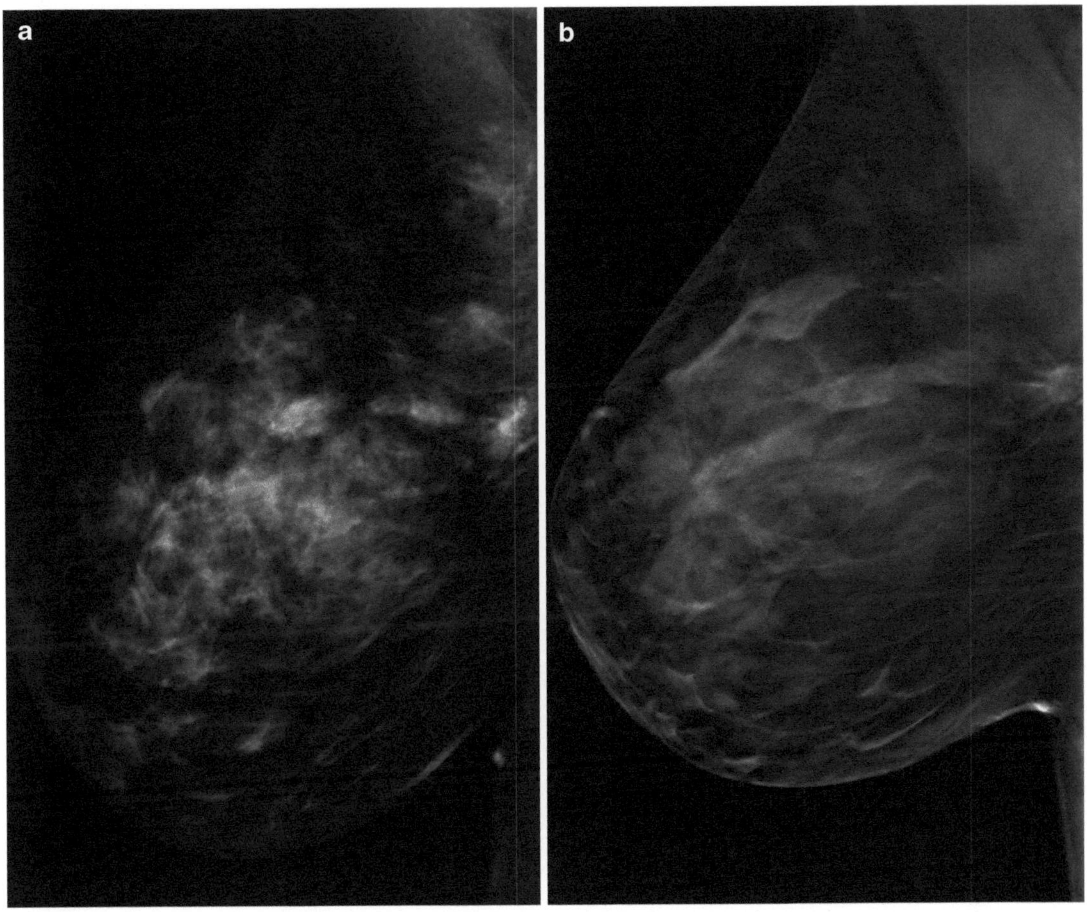

Fig. 30.2 (**a**) Right MLO view demonstrates a large area of architectural distortion in the retroareolar region which is confirmed to be an invasive ductal carcinoma on core biopsy. (**b**) Representative slice from a tomosynthesis series demonstrating spiculated masses in the retroareolar region and overlying the pectoralis muscle in keeping with multifocal carcinoma

diagnostic accuracy than digital mammography alone. Figure 30.2a, b show an example of cancer seen on digital mammography and DBT. It is worth reading the next Chap. 31, as two practitioners and a radiologist reflect on their experiences of using DBT in screening.

Although these results [2–6] support the use of tomosynthesis as a primary screening tool, there are a number of other factors to consider:

1. Cost. In countries with a national screening programme, such as the United Kingdom, replacement or conversion of all the mammography machines to systems with tomosynthesis capability would require considerable investment. Although competition between manufacturers may result in some price reduction, cost is likely to remain a significant factor for the foreseeable future. Furthermore, the large amount of digital data generated by DBT will take up a considerable volume of storage space on PACS, in many cases necessitating the purchase of additional capacity.
2. Image interpretation time. Studies have demonstrated a significant increase in image

interpretation time with the addition of tomosynthesis to digital mammography compared to conventional digital mammography alone (91 s vs. 45 s per case in the Oslo Tomosynthesis Screening Trial [2]). Another study reported an average increase of 47 % in the image interpretation time with the addition of tomosynthesis, although the additional reading time was less for those with greater reading experience [7]. However, there is a limit to how much the image interpretation time can be reduced owing to the number of images that must be viewed, even for those readers with considerable experience. This has to be taken into account when planning workload and staffing requirements.

3. Dose. Most of the published research has focused on the advantages of using DBT in addition to conventional digital mammography. However, this approximately doubles the radiation dose compared to digital mammography alone. The dose varies slightly between the different manufacturers [8, 9] but the total mean glandular dose remains within the UK diagnostic reference level of 3.5 mSv per view. This is regarded as acceptable, given the benefits of increased cancer detection rates and reduction in recall rates, although a lower dose would be preferable. Software is now available which will synthetically reconstruct the projection images to create a 2D image from the tomosynthesis dataset, thereby avoiding the need for a separate 2D exposure. The overall dose is therefore comparable to conventional mammograms. Although earlier studies have shown a slight reduction in sensitivity, a recent study in a large population group has shown that DBT plus synthetic 2D images are comparable to DBT plus conventional digital mammograms [10]. Another large study is currently in progress to evaluate another strategy to reduce dose. The Malmo Breast Tomosynthesis Screening Trial aims to compare DBT with digital mammography but women in the trial will undergo two-view mammography and single-view DBT in the MLO projection. A similar study comparing one-view DBT plus one-view digital mammography to two-view digital mammography has shown better lesion characterisation with one-view DBT in combination with one-view digital mammography [11]. One-view DBT has also been shown to have better sensitivity and negative predictive value than digital mammography in women recalled from screening [12]. Based on current evidence, the UK National Health Service Breast Screening Programme (NHSBSP) guidelines recommend the use of two-view DBT in screening assessment women [13].

For Further Assessment of Mammographic Abnormalities

Assessment of Asymmetry, Distortions or Masses

The current recommendation from the UK NHSBSP is that DBT can be used for further assessment of women with screen-detected asymmetry, distortions or masses. The Hologic Dimensions is the only DBT system currently approved for this within the United Kingdom [13]. Other manufacturers' systems are currently being evaluated. A study by Michell et al. has shown that the addition of DBT increases the diagnostic accuracy in the assessment of screen-detected soft tissue abnormalities [14]. Other studies have demonstrated that DBT is at least as accurate as spot compression view in the assessment of non-calcified abnormalities [15, 16]. Zuley et al. demonstrated that DBT significantly improves diagnostic accuracy by better characterisation of the lesions in comparison to supplemental mammographic views [17]. DBT has also been shown to be superior to digital mammography in estimating tumour size [18, 19]. Although there are no clear guidelines for its use in symptomatic patients, it is expected that further assessment of indeterminate or suspicious mammographic abnormalities with DBT is likely to have the same benefits as in screening patients.

Assessment of Microcalcification

Most published studies have shown that DBT has an equivalent performance to digital mammography in the assessment of microcalcification, although overall it appears to offer no particular advantages. Furthermore, in the population-based Oslo Tomosynthesis Screening Trial by Skaane et al. [2], there was no increase in the detection rate of ductal carcinoma in situ. In view of its higher dose, therefore, the UK NHSBSP [13] has advised that DBT should not be routinely used for the assessment of calcification. This advice may change with further improvements in technology.

Potential Future Application

Women with very dense breasts have a four- to six-fold increased risk of developing breast cancer in comparison with women with little or no dense tissue [20–22]. These women are further disadvantaged by the significantly reduced sensitivity of digital mammography due to the masking effect of the dense breast tissue [20, 23]. The combination of DBT and digital mammography offers the potential to increase cancer detection rates [24, 25] and reduce recall rates [25] in such women. Further research is being undertaken, and DBT may well play a major role in the personalised screening of higher risk women in the future, particularly in those with dense breasts.

References

1. Pisano ED, Gatsonis C, Hendrick E, Yaffe M, Baum JK, Acharyya S, Conant EF, Fajardo LL, Bassett L, D'Orsi C, Jong R, Rebner M, Digital Mammographic Imaging Screening Trial (DMIST) Investigators Group. Diagnostic performance of digital versus film mammography breast-cancer screening. N Engl J Med. 2005;353(17):1773–83. Epub 2005 Sep 16.
2. Skaane P, Bandos AI, Gullien R, Eben EB, Ekseth U, Haakenaasen U, Izadi M, Jebsen IN, Jahr G, Krager M, Niklason LT, Hofvind S, Gur D. Comparison of digital mammography alone and digital mammography plus tomosynthesis in a population-based screening program. Radiology. 2013;267(1):47–56. doi:10.1148/radiol.12121373. Epub 2013 Jan 7.
3. Ciatto S, Houssami N, Bernardi D, Caumo F, Pellegrini M, Brunelli S, Tuttobene P, Bricolo P, Fanto C, Valentini M, Montemezzi S, Macaskill P. Integration of 3D digital mammography with tomosynthesis for population breast-cancer screening (STORM): a prospective comparison study. Lancet Oncol. 2013;14(7):583–9. doi:10.1016/S1470-2045(13)70134-7. Epub 2013 Apr 25.
4. Haas BM, Kalra V, Geisel J, Raghu M, Durand M, Philpotts LE. Comparison of tomosynthesis plus digital mammography and digital mammography alone for breast cancer screening. Radiology. 2013;269(3):694–700. doi:10.1148/radiol.13130307. Epub 2013 Oct 28.
5. Rafferty EA, Park JM, Philpotts LE, Poplack SP, Sumkin JH, Halpern EF, Niklason LT. Assessing Radiologist performance using combined digital mammography and breast tomosynthesis compared with digital mammography alone: results of a multicenter, multireader trial. Radiology. 2013;266(1):104–13. doi:10.1148/radiol.12120674. Epub 2012 Nov 20.
6. Svahn TN, Chakraborty DP, Ikeda D, Zackrisson S, Do Y, Mattsson S, Andersson I. Breast tomosynthesis and digital mammography: a comparison of diagnostic accuracy. Br J Radiol. 2012;85(1019):e1074–82. doi:10.1259/bjr/53282892. Epub 2012 Jun 6.
7. Dang PA, Freer PE, Humphrey KL, Halpern EF, Rafferty EA. Addition of tomosynthesis to conventional digital mammography: effect on image interpretation time of screening examinations. Radiology. 2014;270(1):49–56. doi:10.1148/radiol.13130765.
8. Technical evaluation of Hologic Selenia Dimensions digital breast tomosynthesis system. NHSBSP equipment report 1307. http://www.cancerscreening.nhs.uk/breastscreen/publications/nhsbsp-equipment-report-1307.pdf.
9. Technical evaluation of Siemens Mammomat Inspiration digital breast tomosynthesis system. NHSBSP equipment report 1306. http://www.cancerscreening.nhs.uk/breastscreen/publications/nhsbsp-equipment-report-1306.pdf.
10. Skaane P, Bandos AI, Eben EB, Jebsen IN, Krager M, Haakenaasen U, Ekseth U, Izadi M, Hofvind S, Gullien R. Two-view digital breast tomosynthesis screening with synthetically reconstructed projection images: comparison with digital breast tomosynthesis with full-field digital mammographic images. Radiology. 2014;271(3):655–63.
11. Gennaro G, Hendrick RE, Toledano A, Paquelet JR, Bezzon E, Chersevani R, di Maggio C, La Grassa M, Pescarini L, Polico I, Proietti A, Baldan E, Pomerri F, Muzzio PC. Combination of one-view digital breast tomosynthesis with one-view digital mammography versus standard two-view digital mammography: per lesion analysis. Eur Radiol. 2013;23(8):2087–94. doi:10.1007/s00330-013-2831-0. Epub 2013 Apr 26.
12. Waldherr C, Cerny P, Altermatt HJ, Berclaz G, Ciriolo M, Buser K, Sonnenschein MJ. Value of one-view breast tomosynthesis versus two-view mammography in diagnostic workup of women with clinical signs and symptoms and in women recalled from screening. AJR Am J Roentgenol. 2013;200(1):226–31. doi:10.2214/AJR.11.8202.
13. Current position on use of tomosynthesis (DBT) in the NHS Breast Screening Programme. http://www.cancerscreening.nhs.uk/breastscreen/publications/current-position-tomosynthesis.pdf.
14. Michell M, Iqbal A, Wasan RK, Evans DR, Peacock C, Lawinski CP, Douiri A, Wilson R, Whelehan P. A com-

parison of the accuracy of film-screen mammography, full-field digital mammography, and digital breast tomosynthesis. Clin Radiol. 2012;67(10):976–81. doi:10.1016/j.crad.2012.03.009. Epub 2012 May 23.
15. Tagliafico A, Astengo D, Cavagnetto F, Rosasco R, Rescinito G, Monetti F, Calabrese M. One-to-one comparison between digital spot compression view and digital breast tomosynthesis. Eur Radiol. 2012;22(3):539–44. doi:10.1007/s00330-011-2305-1. Epub 2011 Oct 11.
16. Brandt KR, Craig DA, Hoskins TL, Henrichsen TL, Bendel EC, Brandt SR, Mandrekar J. Can digital breast tomosynthesis replace conventional diagnostic mammography views for screening recalls without calcifications? A comparison study in a simulated clinical setting. AJR Am J Roentgenol. 2013; 200(2):291–8. doi:10.2214/AJR.12.8881.
17. Zuley ML, Bandos AI, Ganott MA, Sumkin JH, Kelly AE, Catullo VJ, Rathfon GY, Lu AH, Gur D. Digital breast tomosynthesis versus supplemental diagnostic mammographic views for evaluation of noncalcified breast lesions. Radiology. 2013;266(1):89–95. doi:10.1148/radiol.12120552. Epub 2012 Nov 9.
18. Fornvik D, Zackrisson S, Ljungberg O, Svahn T, Timberg P, Tingberg A, Andersson I. Breast tomosynthesis: accuracy of tumor measurement compared with digital mammography and ultrasonography. Acta Radiol. 2010;51(3):240–7. doi:10.3109/02841850903524447.
19. Mun HS, Kim HH, Shin HJ, Cha JH, Ruppel PL, Oh MY, Chae EY. Assessment of extent of breast cancer: comparison between digital breast tomosynthesis and full-filed digital mammography. Clin Radiol. 2013;68(12):1254–9. doi:10.1016/j.crad.2013.07.006. Epub 2013 Aug 19.
20. Boyd NF, Guo H, Martin LJ, Sun L, Stone J, Fishell E, Jong RA, Hislop G, Chiarelli A, Minkin S, Yaffe MJ. Mammographic density and the risk and detection of breast cancer. N Engl J Med. 2007;356(3): 227–36.
21. Wolfe JN, Saftlas AF, Salane M. Mammographic parenchymal patterns and quantitative evaluation of mammographic densities: a case-control study. AJR Am J Roentgenol. 1987;148(6):1087–92.
22. Harvey JA, Bovbjerg VE. Quantitative assessment of mammographic breast density: relationship with breast cancer risk. Radiology. 2004;230(1):29–41. Epub 2003 Nov 14.
23. Whitehead J, Carlile T, Kpoecky KJ, Thompson DJ, Gilbert Jr F, Present AJ, Threatt BA, Krook P, Hadaway E. Wolfe mammographic parenchymal patterns. A study of the masking hypothesis of Egan and Mosteller. Cancer. 1985;56(6):1280–6.
24. Seo N, Kim HH, Shin HJ, Cha JH, Kim H, Moon JH, Gong G, Ahn SH, Son BH. Digital breast tomosynthesis versus full-field digital mammography: comparison of the accuracy of lesion measurement and characterization using specimens. Acta Radiol. 2014; 55(6):661–7.
25. Rafferty E, Niklason L. FFDM vs FFDM with Tomosynthesis for Women with Radiographically Dense Breasts: An Enriched Retrospective Reader Study. Radiological Society of North America 2011 Scientific Assembly and Annual Meeting, November 26 – December 2, 2011, Chicago IL. http://archive.rsna.org/2011/11016626.html. Accessed November 19, 2014.

31 Reflection on the Oslo Tomosynthesis Screening Trial

Robin Lee Hammond, Randi Gullien, and Per Skaane

Introduction

Digital Breast Tomosynthesis (DBT) is a new promising technique for breast imaging based on the FFDM platform. In this narrative we share our experience of using it within a breast screening trial. The chapter commences by giving context, to understand the setting in which the trial took place. Then we reflect on the trial from a radiographer's perspective. Finally we reflect on the trial from a radiologist's perspective. Further information about DBT can be found in the previous Chap. 30, and also in Chap. 16.

R.L. Hammond, R.T.(R)(M)(ARRT) (✉)
Lead Mammographer, Mammography Screening, Department of Radiology and Nuclear Medicine, Breast Imaging Centre, Oslo University Hospital, Kirkeveien 166, Oslo N-0407, Norway
e-mail: robham@ous-hf.no

R. Gullien, MSc
Senior Radiographer, Department of Radiology and Nuclear Medicine, Breast Imaging Centre, Oslo University Hospital, Kirkeveien 166, Oslo N-0407, Norway
e-mail: uxraul@ous-hf.no

P. Skaane, PhD
Professor, Department of Radiology and Nuclear Medicine, Breast Imaging Centre, Oslo University Hospital, Kirkeveien 166, Oslo N-0407, Norway
e-mail: perska@ous-hf.no

Context

In December 2012, Oslo University Hospital completed The Oslo Tomosynthesis Screening Trial (OTST), a large-scale prospective 2-year study evaluating DBT in a high volume screening setting. It was conducted within the Norwegian Breast Cancer Screening Program (NBCSP). The trial focused mainly on cancer detection, comparing the combination of DBT plus FFDM with conventional full field digital imaging (FFDM) [1]. DBT (together with FFDM) was offered to all women attending the screening centre in Oslo County. Participation was voluntary.

The NBCSP is a population based breast cancer screening programme organised by the Cancer Registry of Norway and assures that all women between the ages of 50 and 69, every second year, receive an invitation to attend their local screening centre. Each centre follows the National Quality Assurance Manual (QAM); this document contains guidelines for various professions, including radiographers and others working within the screening programme.

Mammography screening in Oslo County is a continuous workflow performed by a team of three radiographers per screening lab. Each lab in the centre is designed with an adjacent interview room and two changing rooms. One radiographer interviews the women, the second is able to position women for imaging, and the third makes the exposures and assesses the quality of the images. Images are evaluated immediately on

P. Hogg et al. (eds.), *Digital Mammography: A Holistic Approach*,
DOI 10.1007/978-3-319-04831-4_31, © Springer International Publishing Switzerland 2015

a 3-mega-pixel monitor before the woman leaves the screening centre. All images are sent to the picture archiving and communication system (PACS), prior to the woman leaving. This quality process reduces the number of women that need to return for follow-up due to poor images or for technical reasons when the images are interpreted independently by two radiologists at later date. For FFDM, approximately 5 min per mammography examination is allocated, a maximum of 12 women per hour; for DBT combined with FFDM, 10 women per hour.

Radiographer Reflections on the Oslo Tomosynthesis Screening Trial

The client schedule at the start of OTST was reduced, knowing that time could be a problem when incorporating DBT into our workflow. This workload reduction was necessary to allow the radiographers more time to adapt to the new equipment, listen to what the women were concerned about and know how to respond to women's questions. Common questions asked by women about DBT included:

- Will it take longer?
- Will it be even more painful or involve more squeezing?
- Is it similar to MRI or CT?
- How much radiation exposure is involved, compared with standard mammography?

Most women did not ask about technical differences between FFDM and DBT. The most common observation from a woman after DBT was, "is it over, already?" As part of the trial we also received ethical approval to investigate women's attitudes and perceptions about DBT. We found the majority of women had a low level of anxiety for adverse radiation health effects, and they believed they received a better examination. They didn't perceive DBT to be more painful or longer than FFDM.

One of the most common questions we have been asked about DBT, by radiographers in other screening centres, relates to the use of compression force. In our DBT trial we used the same compression force as for FFDM. The reason for this comes down to the OTST research protocol - it was designed to compare FFDM and DBT images [2]. To do this, it was necessary to control confounding variables and consequently we compressed breasts to the same levels for FFDM and DBT, as recommended in the QAM, before the OTST. Our trail did not attempt to optimise compression force for DBT; we anticipate work will be done in this area in the future.

We found our DBT equipment to be user friendly and fast. The feature allowing for review of the tomo reconstructions immediately after each acquisition was helpful. One of our initial concerns surrounded the C-arm movement during tomo sweeps, however it was apparent that the gantry sweep was far enough away from a woman and presented no risk.

To achieve high quality mammograms, radiographers need good technical skills to position a woman, as well as knowledge to critically evaluate the images to determine if their quality is adequate for diagnostic purposes. Therefore, during OTST we conducted periodic evaluations to assess client positioning and image quality; the latter was assessed using the PGMI (Perfect, Good, Moderately, Good, Inadequate) classification system. We used the same PGMI criteria for DBT, as recommended in the QAM for FFDM images. However, we remain open for discussion as to whether additional PGMI criteria should be added for the evaluation of DBT images. With this in mind we draw the reader's attention to Chap. 36, *Observer Studies in Mammography*, for further information on image quality and visual grading, and critique of PGMI.

Most positioning errors were caused by not including all the breast tissue on the lateral aspect of the image. We found that DBT requires a little more room to accommodate the wide-angle tomo sweep needed to produce images. Evaluation of images resulted in our positioning technique being modified – this involved leaving a little more room on both sides of the breast, a slightly larger radiation field than we were used to, so as not to exclude breast tissue from being imaged. Selecting the correct size of compression paddle was also important in avoiding this problem.

Client-related artefacts tended to arise from client motion or shoulders being in the field of view. Client immobilisation was paramount and discouraging them from talking during the image acquisition process is essential. We never asked clients to hold their breath while imaging.

It is worth noting that the Norwegian Radiation Protection Authority developed a trial protocol for DBT quality control. Using this it became clear that the daily quality control test is extremely valuable for identifying problems [3].

Implementation of Tomosynthesis

From the onset, it was important to take the opportunity to learn as much as possible and incorporate best practices. We commenced implementation with assistance from the manufacture's application specialist. Familiarisation with the equipment occurred quickly, this took into account quality testing, use of computer software and using the technology in practice.

The training process was relatively straight forward, as it allowed the radiographers to build on skill and knowledge they already possessed. Developing DBT clinical skills for radiographers commenced with practice on a phantom, enabling understanding to be gained on how it is performed. Radiographers all received technical information, as well as demonstrations and practice in positioning techniques. Software and hardware familiarity was gained through experiential learning and reading user manuals; particular attention was paid to overcoming error messages. Interpersonal skills were further enhanced by considering the new types of questions being asked by clients and how they might be addressed.

The radiographers were encouraged to share their experiences and opinions, and this allowed for good learning opportunities to occur. Overall it was a steep learning curve, but not an insurmountable one. Once radiographer confidence was established it became clear that tomosynthesis examinations alone do not take any more time than a conventional FFDM. This observation might be important to a service considering implementation of a DBT practice.

Radiologist Reflections on the Oslo Tomosynthesis Screening Trial

DBT has the potential to overcome some major limitations of conventional mammography, including false positive interpretations and the poor sensitivity of mammography in women with dense breast parenchyma. The great advantage of DBT is the elimination of superimposed tissue and consequently the improved detection and interpretation of lesions otherwise hidden by overlapping dense breast parenchyma. Our experience is concordant with the literature; there is a reduction in recall rates with the potential for increased cancer detection. Architectural distortions and small spiculated masses are more easily identified on the thin 1 mm DBT slices, as compared to FFDM 2D projection images [4].

The potential of DBT to improve sensitivity as well as specificity is of great interest for breast cancer screening. It has been an open question whether tomosynthesis should be performed in one or in both (CC and MLO) standard views. Experience so far indicates that improved diagnostic performance is more substantial when 2D are combined with tomosynthesis in both views. The consequence of two-view FFDM plus two-view tomosynthesis would, however, be a doubling of the radiation dose, which would not be acceptable in most screening programmes. A solution to this challenge is synthetic 2D images reconstructed from the 3D dataset of DBT. The synthesised images are created by summing and filtering the stack of reconstructed DBT slices. Thus, an image comparable to a maximum intensity projection (MIP) image is created. Synthetic 2D instead of conventional 2D images allows combined 2D plus 3D (DBT) to be implemented in breast cancer screening with approximately the same radiation dose as for conventional FFDM.

Results on DBT in breast cancer screening are promising, showing significantly lower recalls and significantly higher cancer detection [1]. Different study designs may explain the great variations reported so far. The longer interpretation time must be weighted against the significant improved diagnostic performance when considering implementation of DBT in a breast cancer screening service.

References

1. Skaane P, Bandos AI, Gullien R, Eben EB, Ekseth U, Haakenaasen U, et al. Comparison of digital mammography alone and digital mammography plus tomosynthesis in a population-based screening program. Radiology. 2013;267(1):47–56.
2. Houssami N, Skaane P. Overview of the evidence on digital breast tomosynthesis in breast cancer detection. Breast. 2013;22(2):101–8.
3. Pedersen K, Hammond R, Østerås B. Application of a protocol for constancy control of digital breast tomosynthesis systems: results and experiences. In: Maidment AA, Bakic P, Gavenonis S, editors. Breast imaging. Berlin/Heidelberg: Springer; 2012. p. 635–41.
4. Skaane P, Bandos AI, Gullien R, Eben EB, Ekseth U, Haakenaasen U, et al. Prospective trial comparing full-field digital mammography (FFDM) versus combined FFDM and tomosynthesis in a population-based screening programme using independent double reading with arbitration. Eur Radiol. 2013;23(8):2061–71.

32 Purpose of Interventional Procedures

Susan E. Garnett

Interventional procedures are an increasing workload of the breast diagnosis unit. They include digital stereotactic devices and also sophisticated biopsy systems to either sample a lesion or remove it entirely. In some circumstances this negates open surgery and its co morbidities. Interventional procedures include the methods listed in Table 32.1.

Biopsy Diagnosis

A stereotactic mammography biopsy system is a method of locating impalpable, non sonographic lesions for harvesting a tissue sample. It is an accurate means of locating and demonstrating the biopsy site. It requires a co operative client to remain still throughout the procedure who is assisted by skilled empathetic practitioners working as a team and include the patient in the process.

Principle of Stereotaxis

Stereotaxis works on the principle of parallax; that is the distance of shift of a lesion relative to a fixed point. It allows calculation of the depth or distance from that fixed point. A computer is used to calculate this depth using two 2D images taken at the same angulation (15°) each side of the vertical plane.

Table 32.1 List of interventional procedures

Interventional procedures
Ultrasound
Guided various biopsy types, clip and wire placement
Upright stereotactic biopsy,
14 g or 10 g vacuum assisted systems
Clip placement
Wire marker placement
Small lesion removal
Lateral arm attachments
Prone table stereotactic biopsy
14 g or vacuum assisted systems
Clip placement
Small lesion removal
Cut out or fenestrated paddle
And cross wire system for marker wire placement
MRI guided procedures
14 g or vacuum assisted systems
Clip placement
Wire marker placement
Small lesion removal
Tomosynthesis guided procedures
14 g or vacuum assisted systems
Clip placement
Wire marker placement
Small lesion removal

S.E. Garnett
Breast Unit, Ground Floor West Wing
University Hospital, Clifford Bridge Road,
Coventry CV2 2DX, UK
e-mail: sue.garnett@uhcw.nhs.uk

P. Hogg et al. (eds.), *Digital Mammography: A Holistic Approach*,
DOI 10.1007/978-3-319-04831-4_32, © Springer International Publishing Switzerland 2015

Diagram

Calcification is the main type of lesion to require this procedure as these are not easily identified sonographically. However ultrasound technology is improving and more elements of calcium are identified with higher frequency probes. Sonolucent clips are often deployed at the end of a stereotactic procedure to aid visualisation by ultrasound for further biopsies or to subsequently localise pre operatively. Clips are also used if there is doubt about lesion visibility or the total removal of calcification post biopsy. The area is then clearly identified for pre-operative localisation.

3D Perception

Practitioners are required to perform stereotactic procedures efficiently and precisely. The area to be biopsied needs locating accurately to ensure the radiation dose is minimal. Developing a perception of the three dimensional appearance of the mass or cluster of calcification by calculating its shape from two orthogonal projections will aid effective positioning and targeting of the lesion.

A co-ordinate system of x, y, and z is used to describe the position of the lesion. Although the computer system calculates where the lesion is within the field of view the mammographer must understand how the unit is acquiring the image and be able to make adjustments to enable accurate targeting.

All breast types, size, shape and breast density are encountered and challenge the mammographers skills of positioning whilst maintaining patient acceptance and comfort. Small breasts with limited depth of breast tissue are positioned with a standoff device to protect the receptor surface and provide patient comfort. Large breasts will require accurate location and positioning on the image receptor to reach the lesion for adequate biopsy.

Localisation Procedures

Localisation procedures are done pre operatively to achieve complete resection of the impalpable mass. Ultrasound is the method of choice if visualised or premarked with a clip at biopsy.

Two radiographic methods of localisation are currently used in the UK.

- Cut out paddle and cross hair wire grid
- Stereotaxis

Both are efficient when trained practitioners are undertaking the chosen procedure. Increasingly marker clips are deployed at the site of biopsy, both sonographically and stereotactically which acts as a beacon for the lesion and enables ultrasound to be used as the preferred localisation method which is more comfortable for the patient.

With the onset of the screening programme more impalpable lesions require a biopsy and then a pre operative localisation procedure. Devices were invented based on the tomographic principle of parallax shift. These were stand alone units (prone tables) or add-ons to the mammographic unit (upright unit). Stereography has advanced with the invention of tomosynthesis and better imaging of subtle lesions whilst removing background information to focus on the lesion characteristics. Tomographic biopsy is now done to accurately target smaller and more subtle lesions. This reduces the number of more involved and less tolerated MRI biopsies.

Indications for Stereotaxis

- Indeterminate calcification not visualised on ultrasound
- Lesions demonstrated in only one mammographic view
- Lesion in the posterior aspect of the breast or deep in the breast at ultrasound

Contraindications

- Ultrasound identified lesions
- Claustrophobic clients
- Patients unable to be immobilised or keep still

Key Points

- Stereotaxis is used if the lesion is not visible on ultrasound e.g. fine calcification
- Stereotaxis uses two 30° angled 2D images to calculate the position of a lesion from its shift
- Mammographers need to perceive the 3D appearance of a lesion in the stereotactic process
- Stereotaxis is used for biopsy and localisation procedures
- Localisation procedures uses either stereotaxis or cross wire techniques
- Stereotaxis uses either dedicated prone table or upright add on devises
- Lateral arm devices are useful for lesions deep in the breast which cannot be reached from above or if the breast is too thin to allow biopsy from above

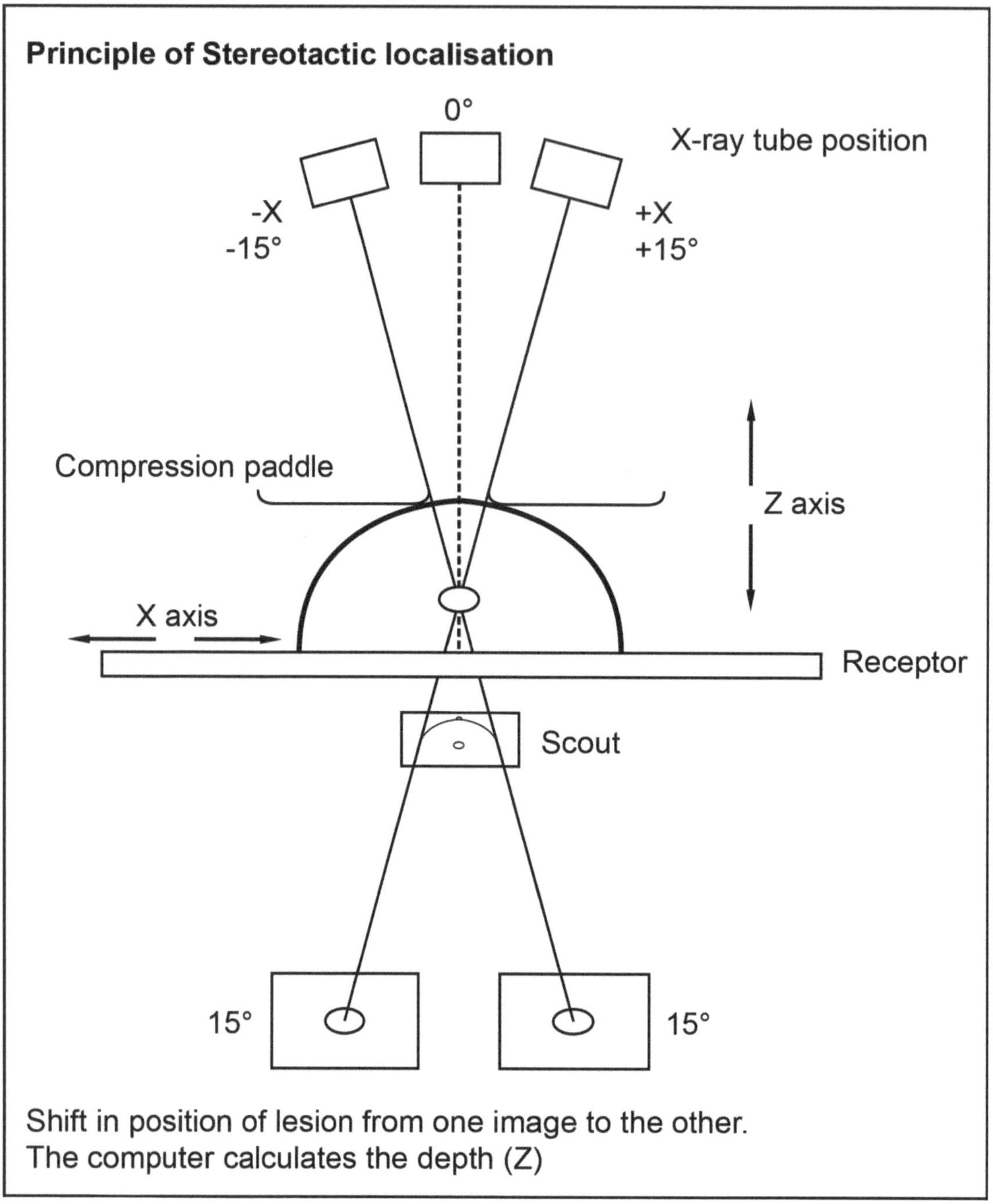

Suggested Reading

1. Andolina VF, Lillé SL. Mammographic imaging: a practical guide. 3rd ed. Baltimore: Wolters Kluwer Health/ Lippincott Williams & Wilkins Baltimore; 2011.
2. Smetherman DH. Screening, imaging and image-guided biopsy techniques for breast cancer. Surg Clin North Am. 2013;93(2):309–27.

33 Stereotactic Image Guided Interventional Techniques

Rita M. Borgen

Introduction

Stereotactic image guided interventional techniques are well established procedures incorporated as part of the diagnosis and treatment of breast disease. These techniques offer high levels of diagnostic accuracy in a timely manner providing a definitive diagnosis in the majority of cases.

The primary use of stereotaxis is the location of non palpable lesions to aid intervention. Areas of calcification, deep lesions and lesions in mammographically demonstrated abnormalities not seen on ultrasound are ideal for stereotactic mammographic guidance [1]. The design of stereotactic equipment utilises a pair of angled images to triangulate the position of a lesion within a three dimensional plane. This triangulation accurately locates the abnormality from co-ordinates, which calculate the horizontal and vertical planes and the true depth of the lesion in the breast. All co-ordinates are determined from measurements based on reference points, which are set by the operator [2]. The following will outline the available techniques utilised in current clinical practice to provide stereotactic image guided intervention. These techniques will include:

- Stereotactic Core Biopsy (SCB)
- Vacuum Assisted Biopsy (VAB)
- Needle Localisation (NL)

Stereotactic Core Biopsy

Image guided breast SCB became well established into clinical practices from the early 1990s [3, 4] and became the primary method used to sample mammographically impalpable breast lesions and areas of micro calcification. SCB has been described as relatively non-invasive and accurate [3], yet more recently SCB has been highlighted as being technically challenging [5, 6]. Failure rates of calcium retrieval following SCB have been reported as high as 7.5 % [6]. However, a number of studies have indicated that the presence of an invasive component may be underestimated by needle core biopsy with a diagnosis of pure DCIS in 15–20 % of cases which may be reduced by the utilisation of a vacuum assisted biopsy [7].

Ultimately the success of SCB is multi-factorial with equal weight given to planning both before and during the procedure. Pre SCB all patients should undergo a thorough evaluation which should include clinical examination and additional imaging [8]. Additional imaging techniques including coned/focal compression views, magnification techniques and ultrasound evaluation will aid the practitioner to a full lesion evaluation prior to the core biopsy.

R.M. Borgen
Breast Screening Service, East Lancashire Hospitals NHS Trust, Casterton Avenue, Burnley BB10 2PQ, UK
e-mail: Rita.borgen@elht.nhs.uk

P. Hogg et al. (eds.), *Digital Mammography: A Holistic Approach*,
DOI 10.1007/978-3-319-04831-4_33,

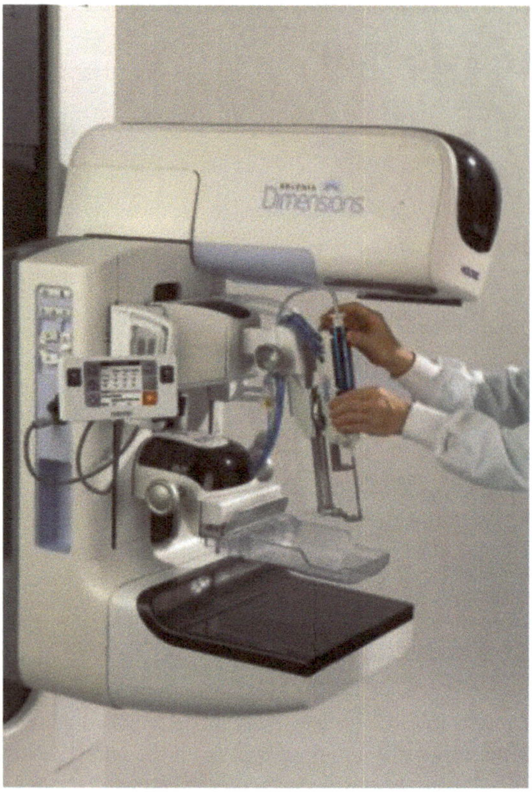

Fig. 33.1 Image provided courtesy of Hologic

The majority of SCB procedures are undertaken using a conventional upright digital stereotactic add on device. An example is demonstrated in Fig. 33.1.

An alternative to the upright stereotactic system is the prone biopsy system. This incorporates all the components of the upright unit with the addition of a support table with a circular aperture onto which the client lies. The breast is positioned through the aperture and accessed from beneath the table. The prone biopsy approach is well documented in the published literature [2].

Explanation of the Procedure

Prior to the commencement of the SCB it is important that a full explanation is given to the client including a description of any likely risks associated with the procedure; these may include bleeding, haematoma and pain. All staff in attendance should be introduced to the client and consent for the procedure should be gained. Informed consent is required for any procedure, but written consent is not essential for image guided core biopsy within the UK. Policies regarding obtaining written consent for breast interventional procedures are produced locally in accordance with hospital policy [9]. Obtaining medical history and other contraindications, for example anticoagulation, is essential prior to carrying out the procedure [10].

Client and Breast Positioning

Prior to the commencement of an SCB a full discussion is undertaken between practitioners, regarding the position of the client, to facilitate the most effective plane of approach. The approach should enable the practitioner to easily position the client and facilitate accurate lesion targeting within the parameters of the stereotactic device. Appropriate positioning should ensure the shortest distance to the lesion is achieved by the biopsy needle. In general most stereotactic units require a minimum amount of tissue beneath the lesion to accommodate the firing mechanism of the biopsy device and prevent damage to the image receptor. If the breast thickness is found to be insufficient for SCB to be undertaken, methods to increase the thickness of the breast can be carefully attempted. This is usually undertaken by the addition of a spacer bar or platform sited between the breast and the support plate artificially increasing the breast thickness. Alternatively the procedure may be performed via the horizontal approach [11]. This is achieved with the addition of a lateral arm to the stereo unit.

Appropriate client positioning prior to biopsy is determined by the position of the lesion within the breast. In an upright stereo device clients with lesions within the upper half of the breast should be positioned in the cranio caudal position. Lesions in the lower inner quadrant are positioned medio-laterally and lesions identified in the lower outer quadrant positioned latero-medially. An illustration of this is can be visualised in the diagram above (Fig. 33.2).

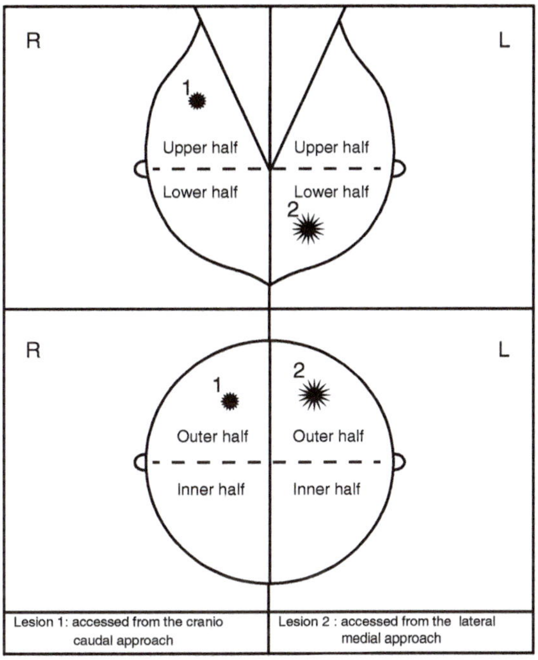

Fig. 33.2 Illustration of lesion accessability in relation to location within the breast

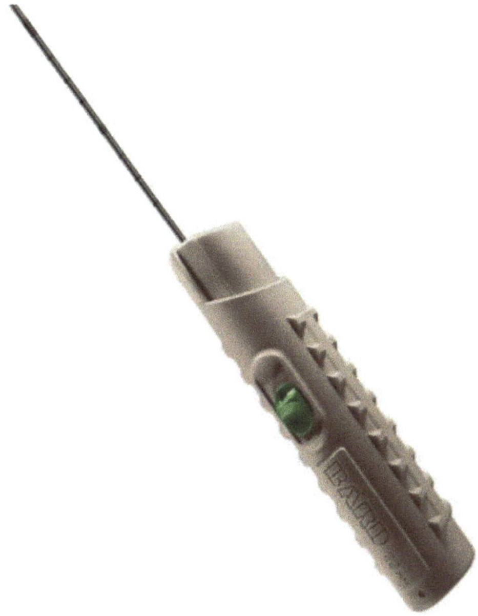

Fig. 33.3 Image provided courtesy of C.R. Bard Inc

Technique

Following client positioning a scout image is taken. This will aid positioning of the lesion within the digital window and provide a visual reference throughout the procedure; the stereo pair is then acquired. The X-ray tube is moved in the horizontal plane to different positions either side of the vertical axis, this generates two images forming the stereo pair. In most cases the fixed angulation is ±15° [2], and is determined by the manufacturer. The combination of the degree of tube angulation and the position of the lesion within the breast will influence the degree of shift seen in the resultant stereo pair. It is important that the practitioner is familiar with this concept therefore it is advisable to study the characteristics associated with lesion shift by practice with a dedicated biopsy phantom.

Once the appropriate stereotactic images have been acquired biopsy targets are set. The rationale for targeting small lesions, areas of distortion and clusters of calcification may differ from unit to unit and will usually be defined within local protocols. Following targeting the skin is prepared and local anaesthesia administered. Again the choice of anaesthesia is decided locally but in many units a local anaesthesia combined with adrenaline is used. The addition of adrenaline acts locally as a vasoconstrictor reducing bleeding and systemic absorption. The lasting action of the anaesthetic is also prolonged with the addition of adrenaline.

Prior to the insertion of the biopsy needle a small cut is made into the skin allowing access for the biopsy needle and minimise the possibility of skin tearing.

Currently there are a number of spring loaded automated core biopsy devices available for purchase. These comprise of either a fully or part disposable system available in a range of needle lengths, 10–16 cm and gauges 14–18, 14 gauge being the most commonly used in stereotactic biopsy.

For the majority of lesions the choice of a 10 cm biopsy needle is adequate (Fig. 33.3). However when a large compressed thicknesses is achieved and the lesion appears to be deep within the breast it is advisable to use a 13 cm needle to reach the lesion [12].

It is usual for between 5 and 10 core samples to be taken. The exact number of samples retrieved will be guided by local sampling regimes, the type of lesion to be sampled, and in some cases client compliance.

The optimum number of samples required to achieve a reliable histological diagnosis varies, with fewer samples required for mass lesions than areas of microcalcification [9]. For adequate sampling of microcalcification an optimum of either three or more cores containing calcium or five or more flecks of calcium in total should be retrieved [13]. As such, specimen imaging of the core samples is essential to demonstrate the removal of a representative sample of calcification [13]. During specimen imaging the breast should remain in compression because if further sampling is required then the procedure can immediately recommence.

Once the required number of samples has been obtained a gel based marker may be placed into the biopsy site. Studies have shown the placement of gel based markers following SCB can facilitate post operative ultrasound localisation at a later date [14]; they can also assist the multidisciplinary team discussion in cases of non-concordant results. The placement of gel based markers following biopsy may be routine practice in many units however the decision to deploy markers varies and may often be directed by a 'marker placement protocol' outlining to the practitioner the situations where a marker may be deployed.

Following the procedure the application of a constant amount of pressure to the wound site for approximately 5 minutes is advised. This will achieve haemostasis and minimise the risk of haematoma formation. When bleeding has ceased a simple pressure dressing should be placed to cover the wound. The client should be issued with appropriate after care instructions including a follow-up appointment to obtain results of the biopsy.

Vacuum Assisted Biopsy (VAB)

The development of VAB in the late 1990s provided an invaluable addition to achieving accurate pre-operative diagnosis. VAB rapidly overcame the limitations of SCB particularly in diagnosing small lesions and areas of microcalcification where under sampling may have underestimated disease [15].

Currently, The UK National Institute for Clinical Health and Care Excellence (NICE) and the UK National Health Breast Screening Programme (NHSBSP) have validated the use of VAB in both the diagnostic and therapeutic setting. The indications for use of VAB include:

- Failed conventional core biopsy
- Indeterminate pathology diagnosed at core biopsy
- Small clusters of calcification which may be difficult to sample with conventional 14 g SBC
- Discordant imaging/pathological correlation
- Small lesions and clusters of calcification in difficult to access areas of the breast
- Complete excision of benign breast lesions

There are many examples in the literature outlining the benefits for VAB, highlighting its association with increased rates of calcium retrieval and lower rates of under diagnosis in both in-situ and invasive disease [8].

Currently there are four VAB systems available commercially. Three of these comprise of a single entry operating system while the fourth, Vacora ® (BARD®), utilises a multiple entry approach. Two examples of the single entry systems (i.e. the ATEC® (HOLOGIC®) and the EnCore Enspire® (BARD®)) are represented in Figs. 33.4 and 33.5, the third being Mammotome®, Breast Care, Ethicon Endo-Surgery®. A comprehensive comparative review of all four VAB systems has been undertaken by Wilson et al. (2009) and is recommended reading for the practitioner [16].

VAB can be incorporated with both upright and prone stereotactic systems with initial imaging and client positioning being similar to that undertaken prior to SCB. It requires a single insertion of the biopsy probe and thereafter contiguous samples of tissue are acquired with vacuum assistance. VAB incorporates the use of a range of probes from 7 to 12 gauge, the larger gauge probes being mostly used for therapeutic excisions. Suction is applied to the sampling chamber to draw in the lesion to be sampled. The integrated rotating cutter advances across the sampling chamber separating the breast tissue. The resultant specimen is then transported into the specimen collection area. The VAB also has

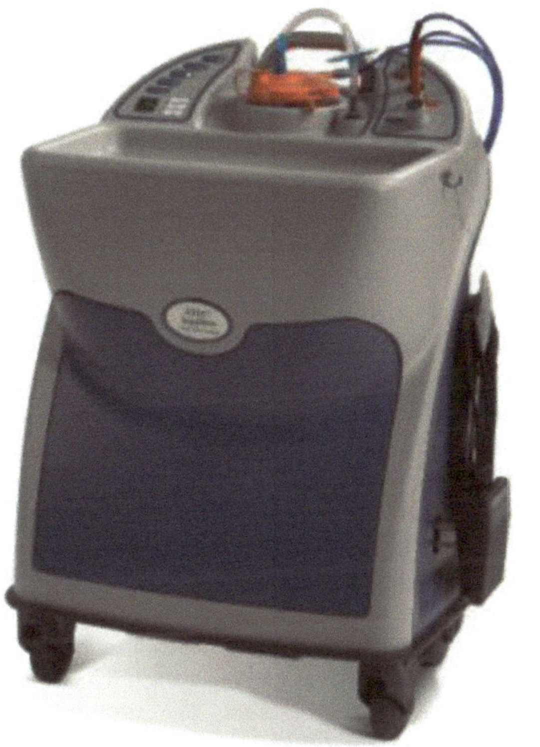

Fig. 33.4 ATEC® (HOLOGIC®) Image provided courtesy of Hologic

the facility to wash out the biopsy site via an integrated saline flush, this aims to reduce and evacuate any haematoma formation.

A lateral arm available with some VAB systems (Fig. 33.6) allows for small previously inaccessible lesions close to the chest wall and lesions in clients with limited breast tissue to be adequately sampled in the upright position.

It is usual for a minimum of 12 samples to be taken throughout the procedure during which the probe is rotated through 360° [14]; an example of the sample size is demonstrated in Fig. 33.7. However the number of samples required to optimally evaluate a lesion has initiated much debate and may be in part attributed to a number of variable parameters which include mammographic appearance and operator preference [17].

As the volume of tissue retrieved during the VAB is much larger than that sampled during conventional SCB it is necessary to administer a larger amount of local anaesthesia to the biopsy site. The amount of local anaesthesia required to adequately anaesthetise the site has been widely discussed in

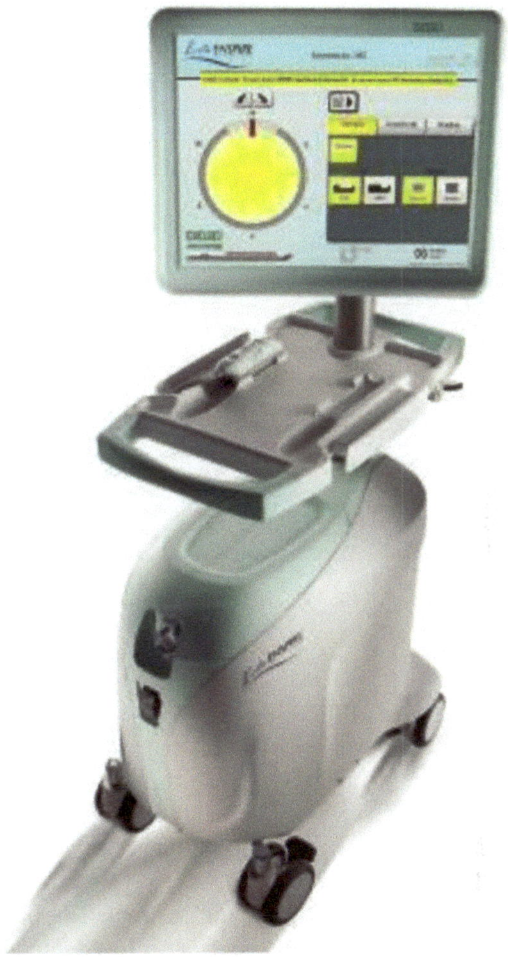

Fig. 33.5 EnCoreEnspire® (BARD®) Image provided courtesy of C.R. Bard Inc

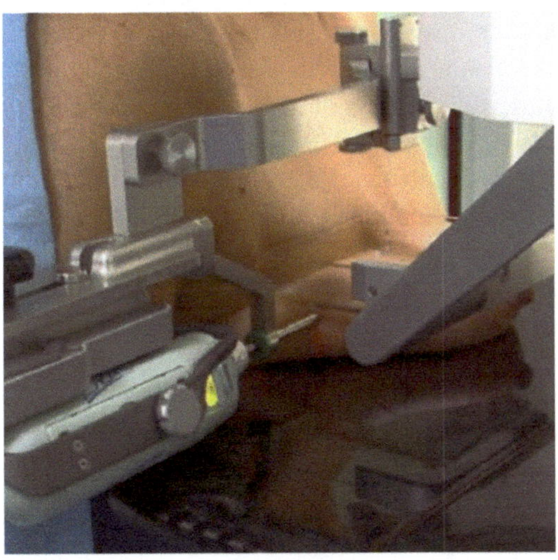

Fig. 33.6 VAB: Upright Stereotactic System incorporating the use of a 'Lateral Arm' (Image provided courtesy of C.R. Bard Inc)

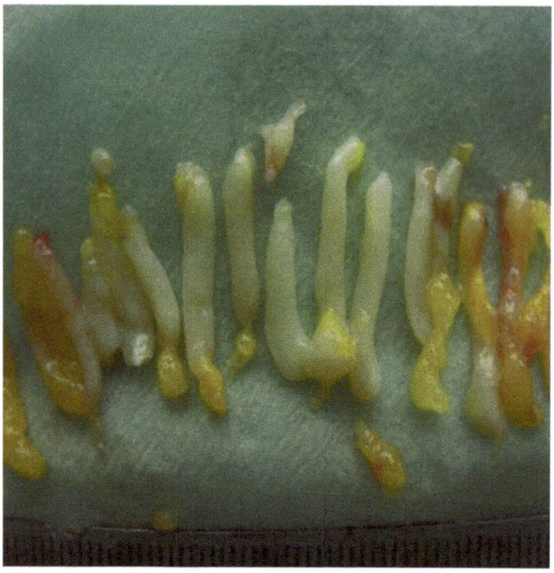

Fig. 33.7 VAB; Biopsy sample (Image provided courtesy of C.R. Bard Inc)

the literature [18]. However, within the UK, the administration of approximately 10–12 ml with infiltration of additional anaesthesia during the procedure if necessary is common practice. The strength of the anaesthesia used may vary and be will usually be determined locally.

Once the required amount of tissue has been retrieved a biopsy marker clip is deployed into the biopsy site. VAB may remove the vast majority of the lesion and in some cases the entire lesion. Marker deployment facilitates correct localisation of the biopsy site if further surgery is necessary wherein the marker clip will be removed [19, 20]. However migration of marker clips has been indicated in case reports [21] and other studies [22]. It is advisable to image the client whilst still in compression post clip insertion.

Overall VAB is well tolerated and popular with clients. It provides an alternative to surgical excision as it is carried out under local anaesthesia. Post procedural complications are low showing no significant differences to those attributed to SCB [15]. The use of VAB has become established in many UK breast units as part of the management pathway in clients who have previously required surgical excision biopsy, an example of such a pathway is well described by Rajan et al. [23].

VAB may also be utilised in conjunction with both ultrasound and magnetic resonance imaging modalities.

Pre-operative Needle Localisation

Stereotactic pre-operative needle localisation is primarily used to localise impalpable lesions, areas of architectural distortion and clusters of microcalcification prior to surgery. The aim of the procedure is to facilitate the removal of the lesion at the first surgical operation [12]. It requires placement of the wire into, but no further than 10 mm beyond the lesion [24]. The wire is housed within an introducing needle which is directed to the lesion via stereotactic or ultrasound guidance. A number of localisation wires are available in the marketplace each with a varying shaped stabilising hook. The most common shapes being curved, single or multiple barbed.

The shape of the hook in some cases affects the stability of the wire, a double barbed localisation wire being described as the most commonly used in the UK whilst remaining stable in the breast [25]. The curved shaped hook is less stable but has the facility to be repositioned prior to wire deployment if required [12].

Patient preparation prior to localisation is not dissimilar to that undertaken prior to SCB. Previous images must be evaluated to determine optimum patient positioning, this is especially important as the localisation wire and the mammogram together form the sole mechanism of guidance for the surgeon to undertake accurate excision [26].

Once the patient has been positioned and the optimum scout image produced the stereo pair images are taken. It is generally accepted that a combination of the shortest route and the lesion visibility partly determine the most accurate approach to the lesion.

Following target acquisition the skin is prepared and local anaesthesia is administered. The localising needle is placed in the breast and the central wire deployed into the target area. Once the needle has been withdrawn the residual wire can be seen protruding from the skin. It is necessary for this to be coiled, covered with a dressing and taped to the breast, the wire within the breast will not move as it is anchored by the localising barbs.

Final check images should be taken to aid the surgical team in theatre. The optimum position is achieved if the wire has transected the lesion and lies within a distance of 10 mms. This position will facilitate optimum surgical excision (Fig. 33.8).

When larger areas of microcalcification require localisation the insertion of bracketing wires can be considered. This method was first described by Silverstein et al. in 1987 [27]. The insertion of bracketing wires has been attributed to a reduction in the need for re-excision when large areas of microcalcification are localised [28].

Radio-Guided Occult Lesion Localisation (ROLL)

Introduced in 1996 the technique of ROLL offers an alternative to conventional wire guided stereotactic and/or ultrasound localisation. The technique involves a direct injection of Technetium 99m labelled colloid human albumin into the lesion via image guidance.

The procedure is performed up to 5 h prior to surgery whereupon the surgical excision is performed guided by a gamma probe. This facilitates a skin excision close to the site of greatest radioactivity enabling the surgeon to excise the lesion achieving the best possible cosmesis. Once the lesion has been removed the excision cavity can be checked for residual tumour [12].

As sentinel node biopsy (SNB) is the operation of choice in patients where normal axillary lymph nodes are identified ROLL may be performed along with SNB. Firstly the ROLL isotope injected into the lesion and the second injected around the areola which will be absorbed by the lymphatic chain and directed to the sentinel lymph node.

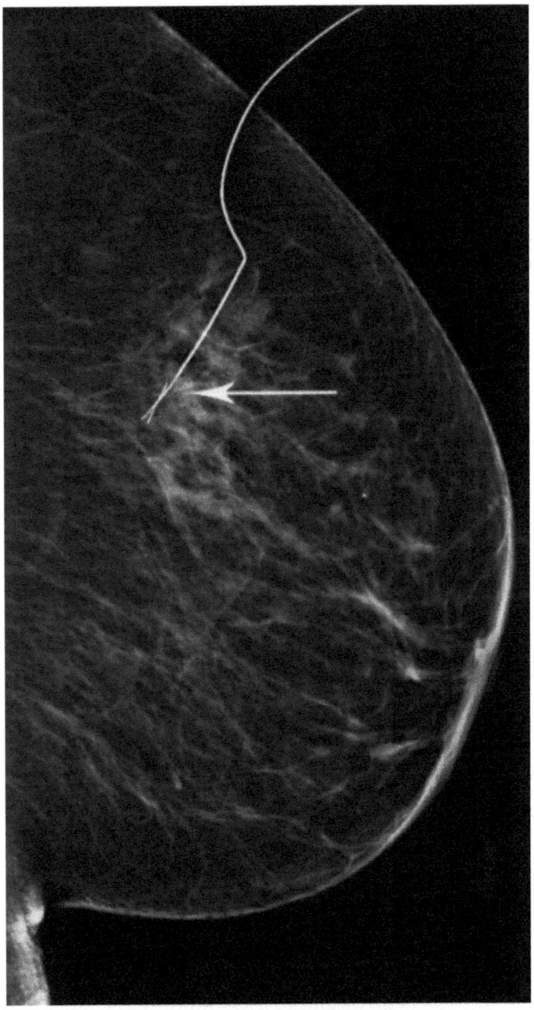

Fig. 33.8 Accurate positioning of localisation wire

The introduction of ROLL has been shown to be associated with a faster, more accurate technique which provides better cosmetic results and a higher incidence of tumour free margins, ensuring complete excision [29, 30].

References

1. Peart O. Mammography and breast imaging: just the facts. New York: McGraw-Hill Companies; 2005.
2. Willison KM. Fundamentals of stereotactic breast biopsy. In: Fajardo LL, Willison KM, Pizzutiello RJ, editors. Comprehensive approach to stereotactic breast biopsy. Boston: Wiley-Blackwell; 1996.

3. Parker SH, Lovin JD, Jobe WE, et al. Non palpable breast lesions: stereotactic automated large core biopsies. Radiology. 1991;180:403–7.
4. Parker SH, Jobe WE, Dennis MA, et al. Non palpable breast lesions: ultrasound guided automated large core biopsies. Radiology. 1993;187:506–11.
5. Brenner RJ, Bassett LW, Fajardo LL, et al. Stereotactic core needle breast biopsy; a multi institutional prospective trial. Radiology. 2001;218:866–72.
6. Rakha EA, Ellis IO. An overview of assessment of prognostic and predictive factors in breast cancer needle core biopsy specimens. J Clin Pathol. 2007;60(12):1300–6.
7. Kwok KMK, Lui CY, Fung PYE, Chan LK, Lam HS. Incidence, causes and implications of unsuccessful calcification retrieval at stereotactic breast biopsy – 5 years' experience. J Hong Kong Coll Radiol. 2009;11:154–60.
8. Wallis M, Tarvidon A, Helbich T, Schreer I. Guidelines from the European Society of Breast Imaging for diagnostic interventional breast procedures. Eur Radiol. 2007;17:581–8.
9. O'Flynn EAM, Wilson ARM, Michell MJ. Image guided breast biopsy: state of the art. Clin Radiol. 2010;65(4):259–70.
10. British Society of Breast Radiology. Protocol for breast biopsy in patients taking anticoagulants and antiplatelet therapy. 2012.
11. Chan T, Wong KW, Tsui KW, Lau HY, Au Yeung MC. Breast thickness and lesion depth measurement using conventional stereotactic biopsy systems. J Hong Kong Coll Radiol. 2003;6:28–9.
12. Evans A, Pinder S, Wilson R, Eliis I. Breast calcification, a diagnostic manual. London: Greenwich Medical Media; 2002.
13. Bagnall MJC, Evans AJ, Wilson ARM, et al. When have mammographic calcifications been adequately sampled at needle core biopsy? Clin Radiol. 2000;55: 548–53.
14. McMahon MA, James JJ, Cornforth EJ, et al. Does the insertion of a gel-based marker at stereotactic breast biopsy allow subsequent wire localisation to be carried out under ultrasound guidance? Clin Radiol. 2011;66:840–4.
15. Ramachandran N. Breast intervention: current and future roles. Imaging. 2008;20:176–84.
16. Wilson R, Kavia S. Comparison of large-core vacuum assisted breast biopsy and excision systems. In: Brun del Re R, editor. Minimally invasive breast biopsies, Recent results in breast cancer research, vol. 173. Berlin/Heidelberg: Springer; 2009.
17. Lomoschitz FM, Helbich TH, Rudas M, et al. Stereotactic 11 -gauge vacuum-assisted breast biopsy: influence of number of specimens on diagnostic accuracy. Radiology. 2004;232:897–903.
18. Brem RF, Schoonjans JM. Local anaesthesia in stereotactic vacuum assisted breast biopsy. Breast. 2001;7:72–3.
19. Rosen EL, Vo TT. Metallic clip deployment during stereotactic breast biopsy; retrospective analysis. Radiology. 2001;218:510–6.
20. Burbank F, Forcier N. Tissue marking clip for stereotactic breast biopsy; initial placement accuracy, long term stability, and usefulness as a guide for wire localisation. Radiology. 1997;205:407–15.
21. Burnside ES, Sohlich RE, Sickles EA. Movement of a biopsy –site marker clip after completion of stereotactic directional vacuum –assisted breast biopsy: case report 1. Radiology. 2001;221:504–7.
22. Parikh JR. Clip migration within 15 days of 11 gauge vacuum assisted stereotactic breast biopsy. Am J Roentgenol. 2005;184 Suppl 3:S43–6.
23. Rajan S, Shaaban AM, Dall BJG, Sharma N. New patient pathway using vacuum assisted biopsy reduces diagnostic surgery for B3 lesions. Clin Radiol. 2012;67: 244–9.
24. ABS at BASO. The association of breast surgeons at the British Association of Surgical Oncology. Guidelines for the management of symptomatic breast disease. Eur J Surg Oncol. 2005;31:S1–21.
25. Chaudary MA, Reidy JF, Chaudhuri R, Mills RR, Hayward JL, et al. Localisation of impalpable breast lesions; a new device. Br J Surg. 1990;77: 1191–2.
26. Saarela AO, Rissanem TJ, Lähteenmäki KM, Soini K, et al. Wire –guided excision of non palpable breast cancer; determinants and correlation between radiologic and histologic margins and residual disease in re-excision. Breast. 2001;18:28–34.
27. Silverstein MJ, Gamagami P, Rosser RJ, et al. Hooked-wire directed breast biopsy and over penetrated mammography. Cancer. 1987;59:715–22.
28. Cordiner CM, Litherland JC, Young IE. Does the insertion of more than one wire allow successful excision of large clusters of malignant calcification. Clin Radiol. 2006;61:686–90.
29. Ramesh HSJ, Anguille S, Chagla LS, Harris O, et al. Recurrence after ROLL lumpectomy for invasive breast cancer. Breast. 2008;17:637–9.
30. Van der Ploeg IM, Hobbelink M, Van den Bosch M, Mali WP, et al. Radio guided occult lesion localisation (ROLL) for non palpable breast lesions; a review of the relevant literature. Eur J Surg Oncol. 2008; 34:1–5.

Contrast Enhanced Investigations

34

Eva M. Fallenberg

Introduction

Sensitivity of mammography is limited especially in dense breasts [1]. Additional imaging modalities have been developed to compensate for some of the technical limitations of conventional mammography, such as lack of contrast and superimposing tissue.

Initial approaches assessing contrast uptake of the breast were made in the 1980s using CT scanning. Whilst this technique was useful in the detection of breast cancer, it resulted in very high radiation doses to the breast, thyroid and the chest wall [2]. Presently, breast MRI with high spatial resolution using gadolinium containing contrast agents is considered the most sensitive imaging method overall, but there remains some concerns regarding specificity particularly with inexperienced readers and lack of widespread availability with biopsy facilities and costs. The introduction of digital mammography around 2,000 enabled further developments like contrast enhanced digital mammography and tomosynthesis [3–5].

Contrast enhanced digital mammography (CEDM) demonstrates contrast uptake of breast cancers. When a malignant tumour is still small, it is nourished and oxygenated by diffusion, but as the tumour grows the diffusion process becomes insufficient for its requirements. If the tumour grows larger than 2 mm, there will be a lack of oxygen and nutrients. By releasing vascular endothelial growth factor, the tumour induces vessel growth from the surrounding vessels towards the tumour. This is called neoangiogenesis.

The new tumour feeding vessels are poor quality and have leaky walls which results in contrast material being deposited in the tumour interstitial spaces. This process enables contrast enhancement of the tumour.

Encouraging clinical results of examinations with CEDM with different examination protocols have been published in the past few years, all of them acquired on a prototype of a commercially available full-field digital silicon based flat panel system [6–15]. The initial studies could demonstrate, that due to the contrast uptake of the lesion the technique is feasible. The resulting dynamic curves have been comparable to MRI [6, 7]. An increase in the detection rate of breast lesions up to 17.5 % by using contrast enhanced mammography could be demonstrated in the more recent studies [7–15].

This chapter describes: different examination protocols of CEDM; the clinical indications of this technique; important issues about contrast administration and contraindications and side effects of contrast agents.

E.M. Fallenberg
Clinic of Radiology, Charite-Universitätsmedizin
Berlin, Campus Virchow-Klinikum, Berlin, Germany
e-mail: eva.fallenberg@charite.de

P. Hogg et al. (eds.), *Digital Mammography: A Holistic Approach*,
DOI 10.1007/978-3-319-04831-4_34, © Springer International Publishing Switzerland 2015

Basic Principle of Contrast Mammography Technique

In CEDM the different X-ray attenuation characteristics of various composites of the breast, especially the glandular tissue, fat and iodine based contrast agents are demonstrated. However, the exposure parameters used in conventional mammography are not optimal to visualise the low concentration contrast uptake. Consequently the technique had to be adapted to enable visualisation.

To demonstrate iodine uptake in the breast, it has to be imaged with an X-ray spectrum above and below the so called K-edge of iodine located at 33.2 kVp. If the breast is imaged after contrast injection with a kVp-spectrum below this value, (which is equivalent to the normal spectrum of about 26–32 kVp used in conventional digital mammography) the iodine in the breast does not cause a significant visible increased absorption of X-rays. The resulting image is comparable to a normal mammogram demonstrating the usual features being looked for when searching for possible breast cancer such as masses, densities, architectural distortions and microcalcifications.

If the kVp is increased to a higher energy level output above the k-edge of iodine at 33.2 kVp, it is possible to visualise low concentrations of Iodine without significantly increasing patient dose. To do so, the energy level needs to be raised to 45–47 kVp combined with an additional filtering of the X-ray-spectrum with a copper filter to obtain an X-ray spectrum with a peak above the k-edge. This will be absorbed by iodine, if it is enriched in the tissue. The beam is filtered to reduce the lower energy parts of the spectrum and therefore avoid image noise induced by these photons. The resulting image is called a high energy image [13, 14].

These low and high energy images are then combined to produce an image demonstrating the iodine uptake only. The background tissue is removed.

The low energy image, with all the anatomical information and the recombined image showing areas with increased iodine concentration are used together to obtain diagnostic information. Anatomical structures and mammographically demonstrated abnormalities such as masses, architectural distortions, microcalcifications and densities maybe visualised. Additional contrast uptake is often an indication of malignant change.

Temporal Subtraction Technique

Due to the experiences with contrast enhanced breast MRI and technical limitations, a temporal subtraction approach was initially used in CEDM. In this procedure, the patient is positioned seated in front of the mammography system, the breast is compressed either in the CC, the MLO or the ML view. First a standard high energy image is obtained. The breast remains compressed and the contrast agent is injected intravenously. After the contrast agent injection repeated exposures of the same breast are performed over a time of 2–10 min. This results in a series of one pre contrast and several post contrast high energy images of the same breast in one view only with some dynamic information. In most studies the CC view is preferred, as it is more tolerable for the patient than other projections. The advantage of this approach is the ability to obtain dynamic information comparable to breast MRI. Disadvantages of this approach are: there is no image containing anatomical information; it is very sensitive to movement artefact; it can be uncomfortable for the patient due to the long breast compression time (up to 10 min depending on the chosen number of repetitions). Motion can result in artefacts and problems with orientation of the images due to slight differences in breast position. This might degrade the quality of the images and their diagnostic accuracy. Also only one view of one breast is acquirable and no information of the contralateral breast is obtained.

The resulting dose levels are dependent on breast composition and thickness as well as the number of images of the sequence. One high energy image requires approximately 20 % of a normal mammography image.

Bilateral Dual-Energy Technique

Currently the most widely accepted approach is the bilateral two-view contrast enhanced spectral mammography (CESM). The contrast agent is injected through an intravenous line which is usually within the anticubital vein. After injection the patient is disconnected from the injector. Two minutes after the start of the injection the patient is positioned as for a normal two view mammogram. The system program results in a double exposure, with one high and one low kVp image per projection. The system switches automatically from the low to the high energy mode. Depending on the exposure time an additional time of 1–2 s for the switch from low to high energy mode is required. Within approximately 5 min CC and MLO bilateral images can be performed in the same way as conventional mammography. With this approach it is possible to acquire several bilateral images with a single contrast injection. Assessment of the locality and extent of the lesion is much more accurate with the two view approach.

The dose of CESM also depends on the breast thickness and composition and results in approximately 1.2 times of the conventional digital mammography dose. Nevertheless the resulting dose of CESM is below the recommended dose levels of the EUREF guidelines for mammography screening. (http://www.euref.org/european-guidelines/5th-edition)

Several studies have demonstrated the increased sensitivity of CESM compared to mammography without a decrease in specificity [8, 9]. Also the initial experiences comparing bilateral CESM with MRI showed nearly equal results [10, 11].

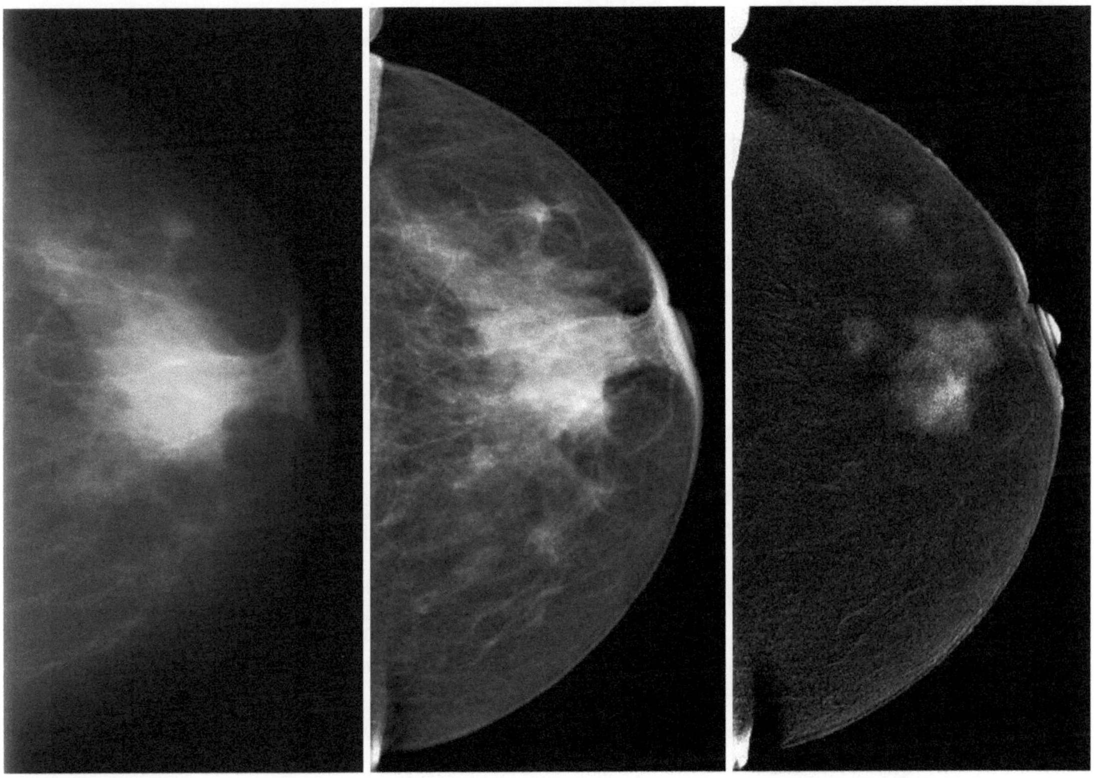

Fig. 34.1 Example of an analog mammography and the low energy and recombined CESM image (CC-view) showing a 6 cm mucinous carcinoma in a 75 year old woman with a palpable mass in the left breast. CESM images have been aquired on an a-Si based full field digital mammography Prototype CESM (GE Senographe DS, Chalfont St. Giles, UK). Now a FDA approved product (Senobright) for additional workup of inconclusive MX and US

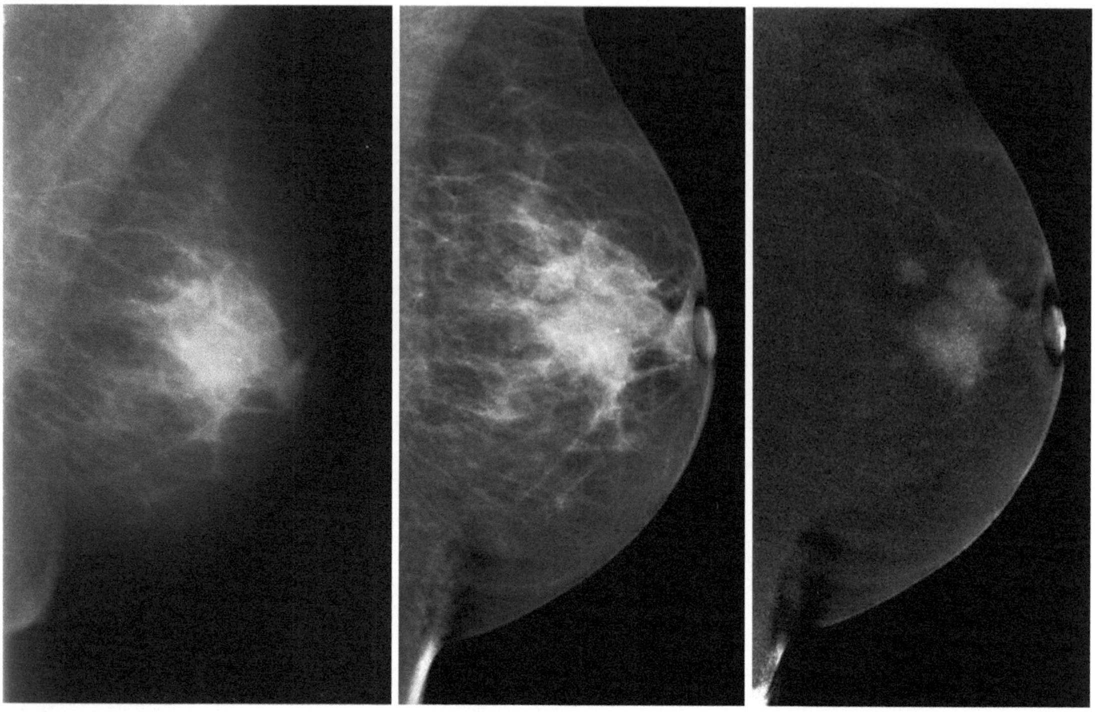

Fig. 34.2 MLO view of the same example as in Fig. 34.1

Figures 34.1 and 34.2 clearly demonstrate the presence of a 6 cm mucinous carcinoma in the recombined CESM image.

Contrast Agent Administration

For contrast enhanced mammography iodinated X-ray contrast agents are used. Usually a concentration of 300 mg/ml Iodine and a dose of 1.5 ml/kg body weight (minimum 50 ml, maximum 120 ml) is sufficient.

The patient should be consented for the injection according to local protocols which include informing her about the possible side effects and asking about her medical history to identify possible contraindications. If there is no contraindication an intravenous line should be inserted, preferably into the anticubital vein. It is recommended to test this line with about 10 ml sodium chloride injected manually for confirming correct placement and flow. If the line is working well, this cannula will be connected to an automatic injector ideally.

The contrast agent is injected with a flow rate of about 3 ml/s. If the vessel is noted to be very small or the injection is difficult when testing the venous access before the contrast injection, the injection speed may need to be adapted. A saline flush of 20–30 ml can be considered after contrast medium injection, but it is not mandatory.

Iodinated contrast agents are used frequently in clinical practice and are generally considered safe. Nevertheless there are some contraindications and side effects the patient has to be informed about or they have to be ruled out before doing the examination. Low and iso-osmolar, non-ionic contrast agents are preferable as they tend to have fewer side effects.

Table 34.1 Commonly used iodinated contrast agents

Compound	Name	Type	Iodine content	Osmolality	
Ionic	Iothalamate meglumine (Conray) Mallinckrodt	Monomer	325 mg/ml	1,843	High
Ionic	Ioxaglate (Hexabrix) Guerbet	Dimer	320 mgI/ml	580	Low
Non-ionic	Iopamidol (Isovue 300) Bracco	Monomer	300 mgI/ml	616	Low
Non-ionic	Iohexol (Omnipaque 350) GE	Monomer	350 mgI/ml	884	Low
Non-ionic	Ioversol (Optiray) Guerbet	Monomer	300	651	Low
Non-ionic	Ioxilan (Oxilan 300) Guerbet	Monomer	300 mgI/ml	610	Low
Non-ionic	Iopromide (Ultravist 300–370) Bayer	Monomer	300–370 mgI/ml	610–774	Low
Non-ionic	Iodixanol (Visipaque 320) GE	Dimer	320 mgI/ml	290	Low
Non-ionic	Iobitridol (Xenetix 300) Guerbet	Monomer	300 mgI/ml	695	Low

There are several contrast agents with different iodine concentrations available on the market. An overview is displayed in Table 34.1.

Contrast Agent Side Effects

Contrast Medium Nephrotoxicity

Administration of contrast agents to patients suffering from Kidney dysfunction can result in kidney failure. The patient should be asked about any known kidney disease and the kidney function should be tested with a blood test before doing the examination, especially if the patient is elderly or has any history of kidney disease or elevated serum-creatinine levels especially related to diabetic nephropathy. Also dehydration, age over 70 years, congestive heart failure and concurrent administration of nephrotoxic drugs like non-steroid anti-inflammatory medicine can increase the risk [16].

If the creatinine levels are acceptable but the patient has risk factors, the patient should be well hydrated. Nephrotoxic drugs should be stopped for 24 h and alternative imaging modalities should be considered.

If the kidney function is less than <45 ml/min/1.73 m^2 eGFR, patients are at elevated risk for contrast agent induced nephropathy and administration of contrast agent should be avoided.

Interaction with the Thyroid Gland

The iodine injection can also induce a severe hyper thyreosis with a thyreotoxic crisis in patients with occult hyper thyreosis or thyroid nodules. Also any radioiodine therapy of thyroid nodules is not possible for about 6 months, after applying contrast agents, so this should be checked by a detailed patient anamnesis and thyroid function blood test [17].

Allergic Reactions

Like all contrast agents and pharmaceutical drugs acute mild, moderate or severe allergic reactions with a rush, itching, exanthema, urticaria, nausea, vomiting, difficulty to breathe or shock including respiratory and cardiac arrest can occur.

The risk for these reactions is increased in patients with a previous history of reactions to iodine-based contrast agents, known asthma or allergy to some medicines.

To reduce the risk of any allergic reaction, non-ionic contrast agents are preferable, and the patient should be monitored for 30 min in the department.

Drugs and equipment for resuscitation should be readily available.

In patients with known reaction or elevated risk, an alternative test should be considered, if that is not possible, a suitable alternative contrast agent should be used and a premedication should be considered [18].

Extravasation

If the intravenous access is not placed correctly or at a less optimal injection side, like the lower limb or small distal veins, extravasation of the contrast agent can occur. It is important to ensure good intravenous access. This can be tested by injecting sodium chloride manually in order to observe correct placement. Adjust the flow rate if the injection is difficult or the vessel is small, provided there is no extravasation when testing.

Common Side Effects and Reactions

A feeling of ascending heat in the whole body, a feeling of needing to urinate and a metallic taste in the mouth are normal, but can cause alarm and therefore the patient should be informed about these possibilities prior to commencing the examination. They may also feel the contrast agent flowing into the vein, as the agent is usually slightly colder than the human body.

Further information on these contrast issues can be found in European society of urology. http://www.esur.org/guidelines/

Clinical Applications

As contrast enhanced digital mammography is invasive and requires intravenous administration of contrast agents it is mainly a tool for the non screening setting. As such, indications for CESM are in the assessment of inconclusive findings in conventional mammography, work up of equivocal lesions in dense breasts and staging patients with newly diagnosed breast cancer. It may also have a role as a first line assessment tool in some symptomatic cases. As the indications for CESM are similar to those for MRI, it may be considered as an alternative to MRI in women with contraindications to MRI such as metallic implants, cochlea implants or claustrophobia. Further indications include situations where MRI is unavailable or not reimbursed and a preoperative assessment of disease extent is required. Exclusion of recurrence in follow up cases and detection of mammographically occult cancers in women with proven axillary metastasis may also benefit from CESM.

Conclusion

Contrast enhanced mammography is a very promising, widely available technique, able to improve the diagnostic performance of mammography. It is relatively simple to perform.

References

1. Pisano ED, Gatsonis C, Hendrick E, et al. Diagnostic performance of digital versus film mammography for breast-cancer screening. N Engl J Med. 2005;353:1773–83.
2. Chang CH, Nesbit DE, Fisher DR, et al. Computed tomographic mammography using a conventional body scanner. AJR Am J Roentgenol. 1982;138:553–8.
3. Diekmann F, Diekmann S, Taupitz M, et al. Use of iodine-based contrast media in digital full-field mammography–initial experience. Rofo. 2003;175:342–5.
4. Smith AP, Hall PA, Marcello DM. Emerging technologies in breast cancer detection. Radiol Manage. 2004;26:16–24; quiz 25–27.
5. Lewin JM, Niklason L. Advanced applications of digital mammography: tomosynthesis and contrast-enhanced digital mammography. Semin Roentgenol. 2007;42:243–52.
6. Diekmann F, Diekmann S, Jeunehomme F, Muller S, Hamm B, Bick U. Digital mammography using iodine-based contrast media: initial clinical experience with dynamic contrast medium enhancement. Invest Radiol. 2005;40:397–404.
7. Dromain C, Balleyguier C, Muller S, et al. Evaluation of tumor angiogenesis of breast carcinoma using contrast-enhanced digital mammography. AJR Am J Roentgenol. 2006;187:W528–37.
8. Dromain C, Thibault F, Muller S, et al. Dual-energy contrast-enhanced digital mammography: initial clinical results. Eur Radiol. 2011;21:565–74.
9. Dromain C, Thibault F, Diekmann F, et al. Dual-energy contrast-enhanced digital mammography: initial clinical results of a multireader, multicase study. Breast Cancer Res. 2012;14:R94.
10. Fallenberg EM, Dromain C, Diekmann F, et al. Contrast-enhanced spectral mammography versus MRI: initial results in the detection of breast cancer and assessment of tumour size. Eur Radiol. 2014;24:256–64.

11. Jochelson MS, Dershaw DD, Sung JS, et al. Bilateral contrast-enhanced dual-energy digital mammography: feasibility and comparison with conventional digital mammography and MR imaging in women with known breast carcinoma. Radiology. 2013;266:743–51.
12. Lobbes MB, Lalji U, Houwers J, et al. Contrast-enhanced spectral mammography in patients referred from the breast cancer screening programme. Eur Radiol. 2014. doi:10.1007/s00330-014-3154-5.
13. Lewin JM, Isaacs PK, Vance V, Larke FJ. Dual-energy contrast-enhanced digital subtraction mammography: feasibility. Radiology. 2003;229:261–8.
14. Puong S, Bouchevreau X, Patoureaux F, Iordache R, Muller S. Dual-energy contrast enhanced digital mammography using a new approach for breast tissue cancelling. Proc SPIE Med Imaging. 2007;6510:65102H.
15. Diekmann F, Freyer M, Diekmann S, et al. Evaluation of contrast-enhanced digital mammography. Eur J Radiol. 2011;78:112–21.
16. Stacul F, van der Molen AJ, Reimer P, et al. Contrast induced nephropathy: updated ESUR Contrast Media Safety Committee guidelines. Eur Radiol. 2011;21:2527–41.
17. van der Molen AJ, Thomsen HS, Morcos SK, Contrast Media Safety Committee ESoUR. Effect of iodinated contrast media on thyroid function in adults. Eur Radiol. 2004;14:902–7.
18. Bellin MF, Stacul F, Webb JA, et al. Late adverse reactions to intravascular iodine based contrast media: an update. Eur Radiol. 2011;21:2305–10.

Part V

Service Quality Assurance

Radiographic Service Quality

35

Caroline J. Dobson and Clare S. Alison

Introduction

The success of breast cancer diagnosis requires consistent production of high quality mammograms to allow optimal visualisation of breast tissue. It is internationally recognised that the standards required in both screening programmes and symptomatic services need to be regularly monitored and audited. Individual practitioners are also required to regularly monitor and audit their work in order to maintain production of high quality images and allow improved performance of the imaging service [1].

This chapter is a practical guide for image quality evaluation and an evaluation of mammography standards. Within this chapter, these will be defined by The Quality Assurance Guidelines for Mammography, NHSBSP publication No. 63 [2] and Breast Screen Australia, National Accreditation Standards 2001 [3].

C.J. Dobson (✉)
Superintendent Radiographer, Breast Imaging, Thirlestaine Breast Centre, Thirlestaine Road, Cheltenham GL53 7AS, UK
e-mail: Caroline.dobson@glos.nhs.uk

C.S. Alison
Clinical Instructor, Breast Imaging, Thirlestaine Breast Centre, Thirlestaine Road, Cheltenham GL53 7AS, UK
e-mail: Clare.alison@glos.nhs.uk

Why Do Practitioners Require Service Quality Standards?

Standards are required to maintain a high quality service and not allow individual interpretation to lower that standard. They are also required to ensure maximum benefit and minimal harm to clients, whilst maximising cancer detection. Both physical and psychological needs of the client need to be observed (see Chaps. 9, 10, 11, 12, 13 and 14), to minimise discomfort, while still achieving the high standard required.

How Do Practitioners Ensure They Are Working to the Required Standards?

Practitioners should regularly measure and evaluate their performance using a grading system; for example Perfect, Good, Moderate, Inadequate (PGMI). Other systems that have been used are Good, Diagnostic, Un-diagnostic (GDU), and Excellent, Adequate, Repeat (EAR). The value of using grading systems have been criticised in the past, but, until such time as a suitable alternative is found, PGMI continues to be used in many mammography departments [4]. Chapter 36 considers these scales and observer studies in more detail.

The PGMI system was introduced to the National Health Service Breast Screening Program (NHSBSP) in 1993 and was quickly adopted by Australia, New Zealand and Norway

P. Hogg et al. (eds.), *Digital Mammography: A Holistic Approach*,
DOI 10.1007/978-3-319-04831-4_35,

Breast Screening Programs [4]. It is now widely recognised internationally for critically evaluating mammograms. It is used to provide a standardisation of image reviewing and for setting guidance rules for use by both individual practitioners and reviewers assessing images.

Peer review and formal appraisal are other useful tools for ensuring the standard is maintained. These too should take place on a regular basis. These will be expanded upon later on in the chapter.

The criteria for critically evaluating the mammogram are detailed in The Quality Assurance Guidelines for Mammography, NHSBSP publication No. 63 [2]. Please refer to Chap. 36 for more information on evaluating mammogram image quality.

Technical Repeats (TP) and Technical Recall (TC)

A qualified practitioner will be able to critically appraise the technique and diagnostic quality of the mammographic images they have acquired and justify appropriate repeats. With the introduction of digital x-ray systems the practitioner has to utilise their expertise for instant decision making. Digital imaging has the advantage of generating an image instantly after exposure thus providing rapid feedback to the practitioner if the image is suboptimal [5]. Judgement on whether a repeat is required can be made while the client is present thus avoiding a recall for further imaging due to a technical error (TC) and unnecessary anxiety for the client.

A technical repeat (TP) is when a practitioner makes the decision to repeat the same projection after identifying an error [2]. Assistant Practitioners (AP) working should agree with their supervising practitioner (qualified radiographer) as to whether a TP is justifiable [6].

Technical acceptability of an image may not always be adequately judged by the practitioner at time of acquisition. As an example, the acquisition stations utilised are not of the same high specification as the reporting monitors. Often image blur is unable to be detected until the point of image reading on the reporting workstation, thus subjecting the client to a possible technical recall (TC).

(Applies to both CC and MLO images)

- Significant part of breast not imaged
- Incomplete or incorrect identification
- Incorrect exposure
- Inadequate compression hindering diagnosis
- Blurred images
- Overlying skin folds obscuring image
- Overlying artefact obscuring image

Fig. 35.1 Reasons for repeat images

Reasons for Repeat Images

Local protocols have been successfully implemented in many breast departments, indicating to practitioners the reasons to repeat an image. The professional decision to repeat must remain with the justifying qualified practitioner.

An example of a local protocol is that any image falling into the inadequate category, as detailed in Fig. 35.1 should be repeated. This protocol is though subjective and open to interpretation.

It is regarded as good practice for a department to audit and review TP and TC rates and the reasons for them, as they can provide evidence of both equipment and practitioner performance. This enables good management of underperformance in both areas.

Peer Review

The reliability of PGMI can be further improved by peer review. Practitioners should be aware of their own proficiency but also how they compare to those of their peer group. Implementation of an organised peer review system with structured feedback and records should aim to maintain high standards and disseminate good practice within the department [7]. If underperformance is identified an action plan should be agreed. This may include additional training and a review of working practice to ensure practitioners maintain the necessary expertise to reach the standard required, thus providing a service acceptable to the general public.

QA Role and Visits

Peer review also takes place during a formal visit to the unit by the regional QA Radiographer during a QA visit within the U.K. screening service. During this visit the standard of mammography will be assessed using a Mammographic Image Assessment form (Fig. 35.2). The aim of the QA visit is to confirm that the radiographic quality of the unit conforms to expected standards and to identify areas of underperformance. Recommendations will be made where improvement is required.

Auditing Clinical Practice

Each practitioner should review and reflect on their clinical practice as part of regular personal performance monitoring and continuous professional development (CPD). Regular review of professional performance is essential and each practitioner should receive feedback on their performance. Breast Screening Programmes are responsible for recording, collecting and monitoring repeat examination data. All practitioners have a responsibility to regularly audit their number of repeat examinations against local protocols and national standards.

The NHSBSP guidance on collecting, monitoring and reporting repeat examinations, Publication No. 4, version 2 [8], gives very clear guidance on the collecting of data and this guidance should be used when monitoring performance of the mammographic team and equipment.

Training needs can be identified from monitoring performance using the information from PGMI and TP, TC records. If underperformance is identified an action plan should be agreed. This

MAMMOGRAPHIC IMAGE ASSESSMENT

Dates of Assessment: | Static/ Mobile

Assessor(s): | Clinic Code | Date Taken | Mammographer

Case No.	View	Correct patient ID & Markers		Appropriate exposure		Adequate compression to hold breast firmly - no movement		Image sharp		No artefacts obscuring image		No obscuring skin folds		Nipple in profile		MLO's: Pectoral muscle to nipple level		MLO's: Pectoral muscle at appropriate angle		MLO's: IMF shown clearly		CCs: Medial border demonstrated		CCs: Back of breast clearly shown with some medial central & lateral		CCs: Some axillary tail shown		Symmetrical Images	whole breast imaged	Comments
		R	L	R	L	R	L	R	L	R	L	R	L	R	L	R	L	R	L	R	L	R	L	R	L	R	L			
1	MLO																													
	CC																													
2	MLO																													
	CC																													
3	MLO																													
	CC																													
4	MLO																													
	CC																													
5	MLO																													
	CC																													
6	MLO																													
	CC																													
7	MLO																													
	CC																													
8	MLO																													
	CC																													
9	MLO																													
	CC																													
10	MLO																													
	CC																													

Notes:No less than 20 exams should be reviewed, more if problems/trends are highlighted. No patient identifying numbers should be used. To view trends easily only place an X in boxes where criteria are NOT met

Fig. 35.2 A mammographic image assessment form

MAMMOGRAPHIC IMAGE ASSESSMENT

Dates of Assessment: **Static/ Mobile**

Assessor(s): **Clinic Code** **Date Taken** **Mammographer**

Case No.	View	Correct patient ID & Markers		Appropriate exposure		Adequate compression to hold breast firmly - no movement		Image sharp		No artefacts obscuring image		No obscuring skin folds		Nipple in profile		MLO's: Pectoral muscle to nipple level		MLO's: Pectoral muscle at appropriate angle		MLO's: IMF shown clearly		CCs: Medial border demonstrated		CCs: Back of breast clearly shown with some medial central & lateral		CCs: Some axillary tail shown		Symmetrical Images	whole breast imaged	Comments
		R	L	R	L	R	L	R	L	R	L	R	L	R	L	R	L	R	L	R	L	R	L	R	L	R	L			
11	MLO																					X	X	X	X	X	X			
	CC															X	X	X	X	X	X									
12	MLO																					X	X	X	X	X	X			
	CC															X	X	X	X	X	X									
13	MLO																					X	X	X	X	X	X			
	CC															X	X	X	X	X	X									
14	MLO																					X	X	X	X	X	X			
	CC															X	X	X	X	X	X									
15	MLO																					X	X	X	X	X	X			
	CC															X	X	X	X	X	X									
16	MLO																					X	X	X	X	X	X			
	CC															X	X	X	X	X	X									
17	MLO																					X	X	X	X	X	X			
	CC															X	X	X	X	X	X									
18	MLO																					X	X	X	X	X	X			
	CC															X	X	X	X	X	X									
19	MLO																					X	X	X	X	X	X			
	CC															X	X	X	X	X	X									
20	MLO																					X	X	X	X	X	X			
	CC															X	X	X	X	X	X									

Notes:No less than 20 exams should be reviewed, more if problems/trends are highlighted. No patient identifying numbers should be used. To view trends easily only place an X in boxes where criteria are NOT met

Fig. 35.2 (continued)

may include additional training and a review of working practice to ensure practitioners maintain the necessary expertise to reach the standard required, thus providing a service acceptable to the general public.

To support the individuals audit their clinical practice, the radiography manager should regularly collect data from **all** repeat examinations (TR = TP + TC). The information collected should be:

- The number and percentage of TRs, TPs and TCs for each practitioner in the unit.
- The number and percentage of TRs, TPs and TCs by reason code.
- The number and percentage of TRs, TPs and TCs by practitioner and reason.

This data should be monitored locally and the outcome of the audit should be available for feedback to the practitioners.

If a problem is identified a clear action plan, with time scales should be agreed.

Continuous Professional Development (CPD)

All professional staff have a duty to continuously develop and improve themselves as a professional. CPD includes work based learning, professional activities and formal, educational learning. Evidence of CPD should be promoted and meet the learning requirements of the practitioner and should have at its focus the delivery of a high quality mammography service.

Figures 35.3, 35.4, 35.5, 35.6, 35.7, 35.8, 35.9, 35.10, 35.11, 35.12, 35.13, 35.14, 35.15 and 35.16, demonstrate examples of Perfect, Good, Moderate and Inadequate images, with and without artefacts.

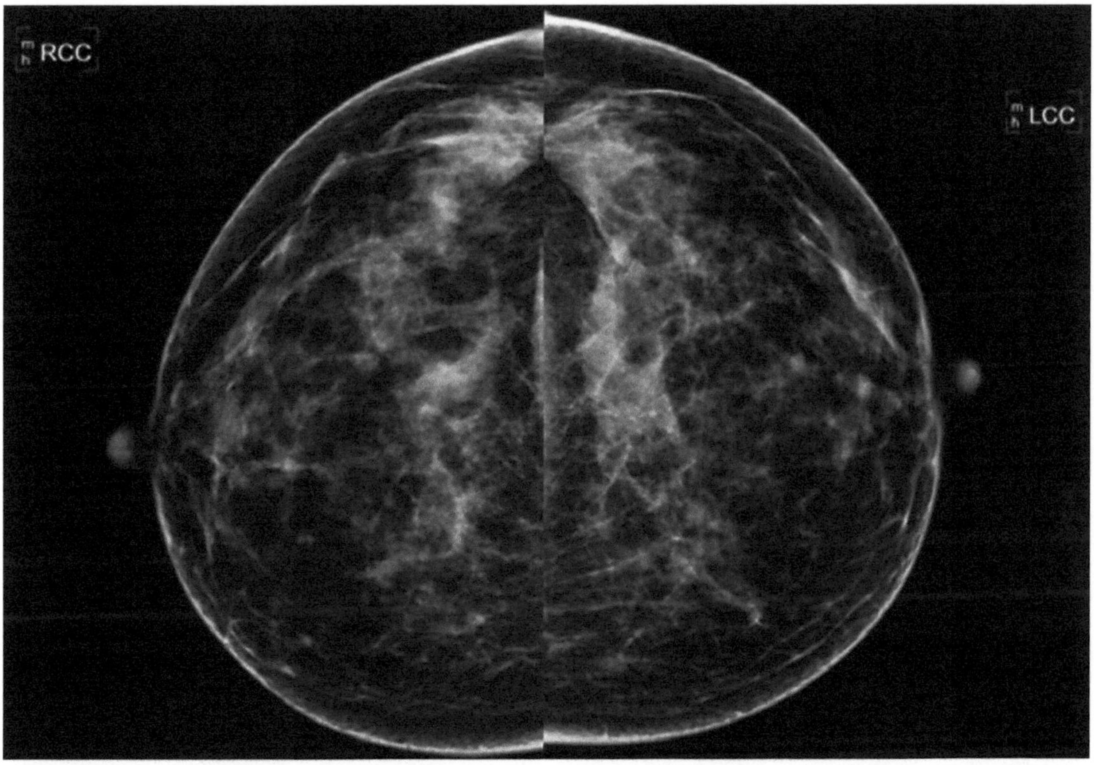

Fig. 35.3 Perfect CC images matching all criteria

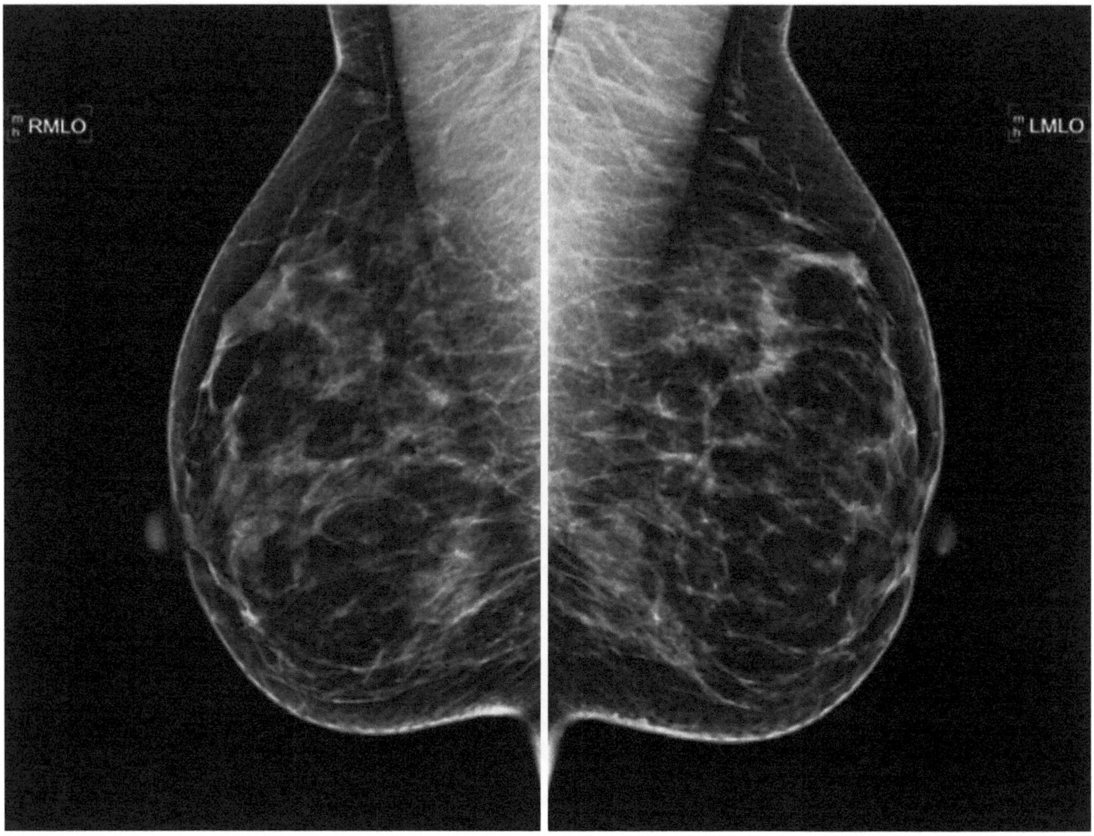

Fig. 35.4 Perfect MLO images matching all criteria

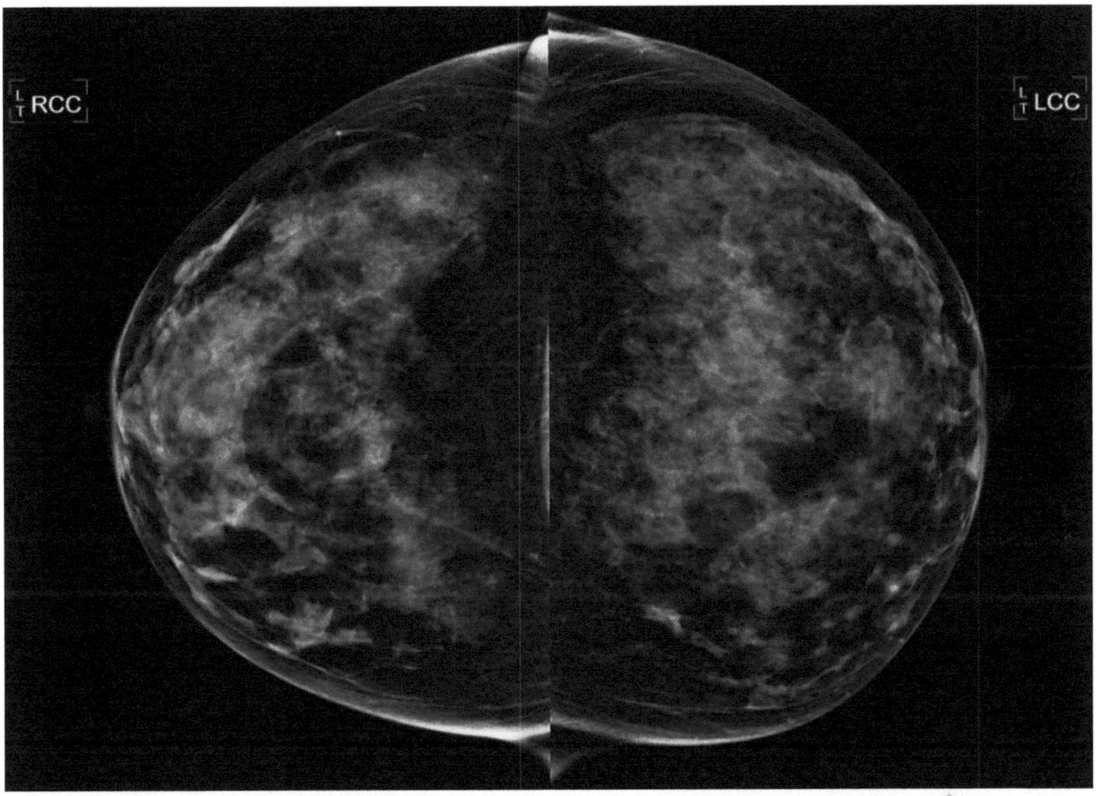

Fig. 35.5 Good CC images. There is a minor crease over the postero- lateral edge of the Right CC. It is not obscuring any breast tissue, therefore, this image does not need to be repeated. **Learning points**: check the lateral side of the breast under the paddle and the underside in contact with the detector for creases, smooth skin if necessary before imaging

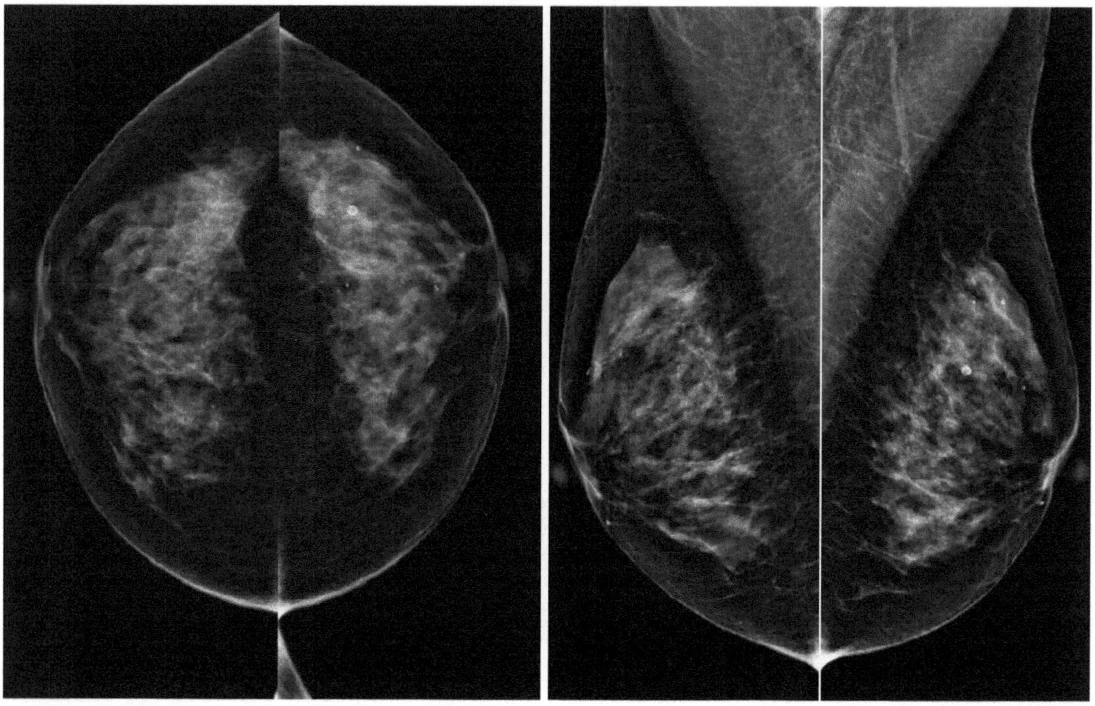

Fig. 35.6 Good images. The nipple on the Left CC is slightly laterally rotated, losing a little breast tissue at the back of the breast. However, the breast tissue is within 1 cm of that on the Left MLO, therefore, this image does not need to be repeated. **Learning points**: ensure the nipple is at 90° from the chest wall and optimal amount of breast tissue is pulled on to the detector before imaging

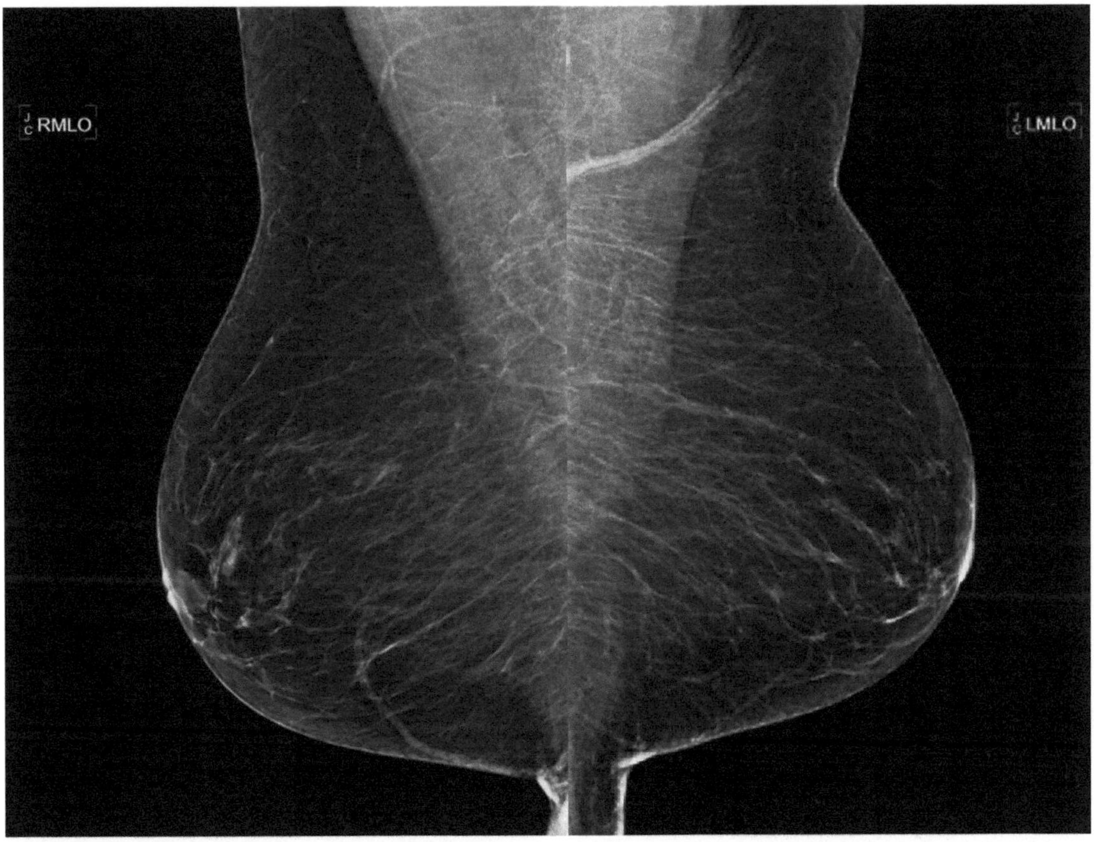

Fig. 35.7 Good MLO images. There is a minor crease in the Left axilla. This is not obscuring any breast tissue therefore is not a repeatable image. **Learning point**: lift the shoulder and smooth the axilla before applying compression

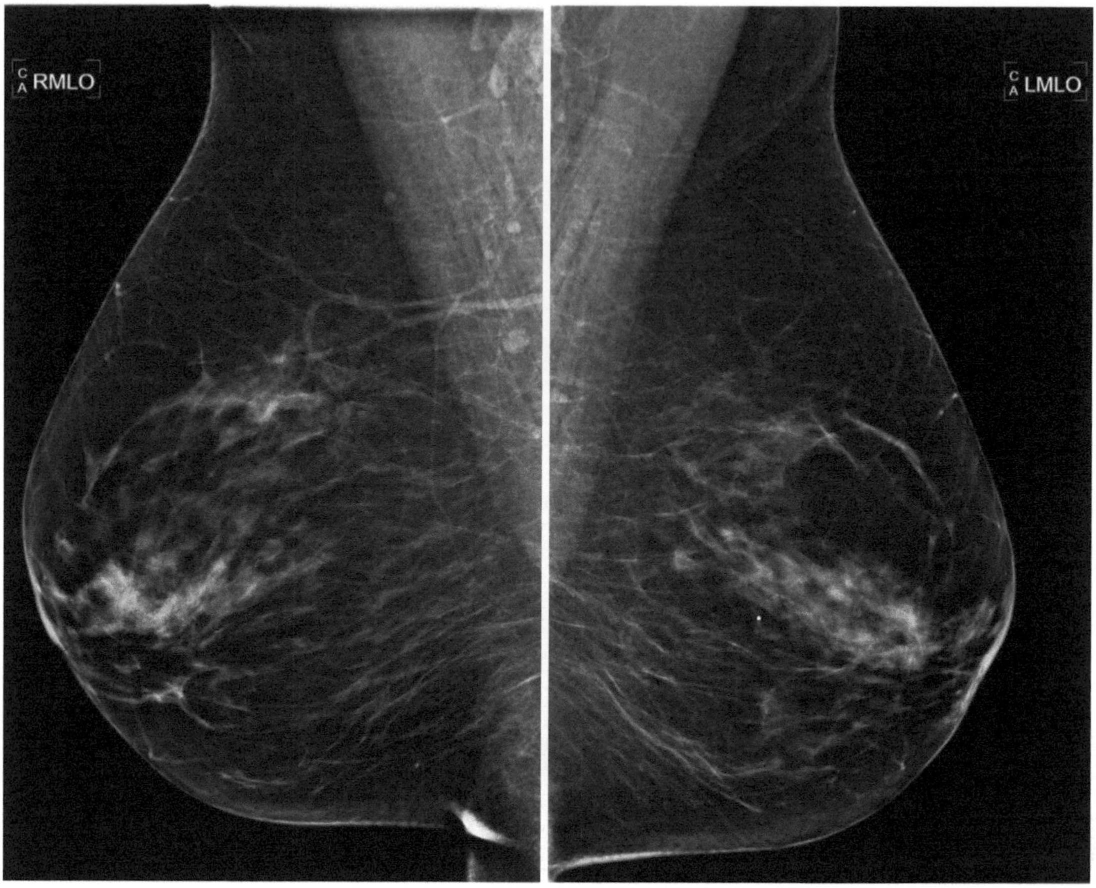

Fig. 35.8 Good MLO images. There is a minor crease in the Right infra-mammary fold (IMF). This is not obscuring any breast tissue therefore is not a repeatable image. **Learning point**: smooth the IMF downwards towards the feet before applying compression

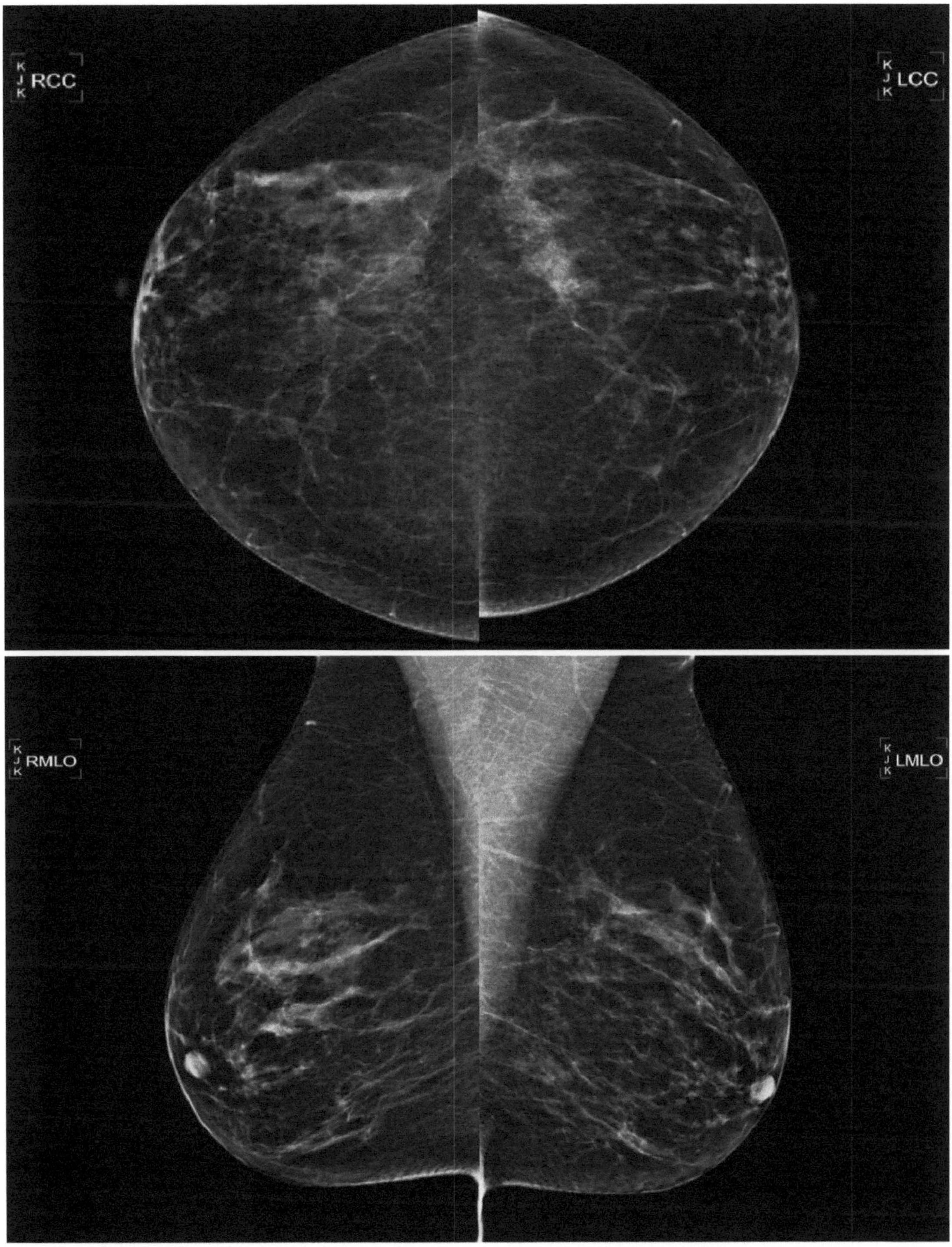

Fig. 35.9 Moderate images. Nipples are not in profile on the MLO views but are distinguishable from the retro-areolar tissue. There is slight asymmetry and the pectoral muscle is not at the correct angle, or down to nipple level, on the Right MLO. Most of the breast tissue is imaged, the IMFs are clearly demonstrated and, as the nipples are in profile on the CC images, these images do not need to be repeated. **Learning points**: check that the nipples are in profile before compression, if they are not reposition to bring more breast tissue onto the detector plate, either laterally or medially, depending on which way the nipples are turning. This will also ensure the pectoral muscle is down to nipple level. The uppermost corner of the detector plate must be placed at the back of the axilla to ensure the pectoral muscle is imaged at the correct angle

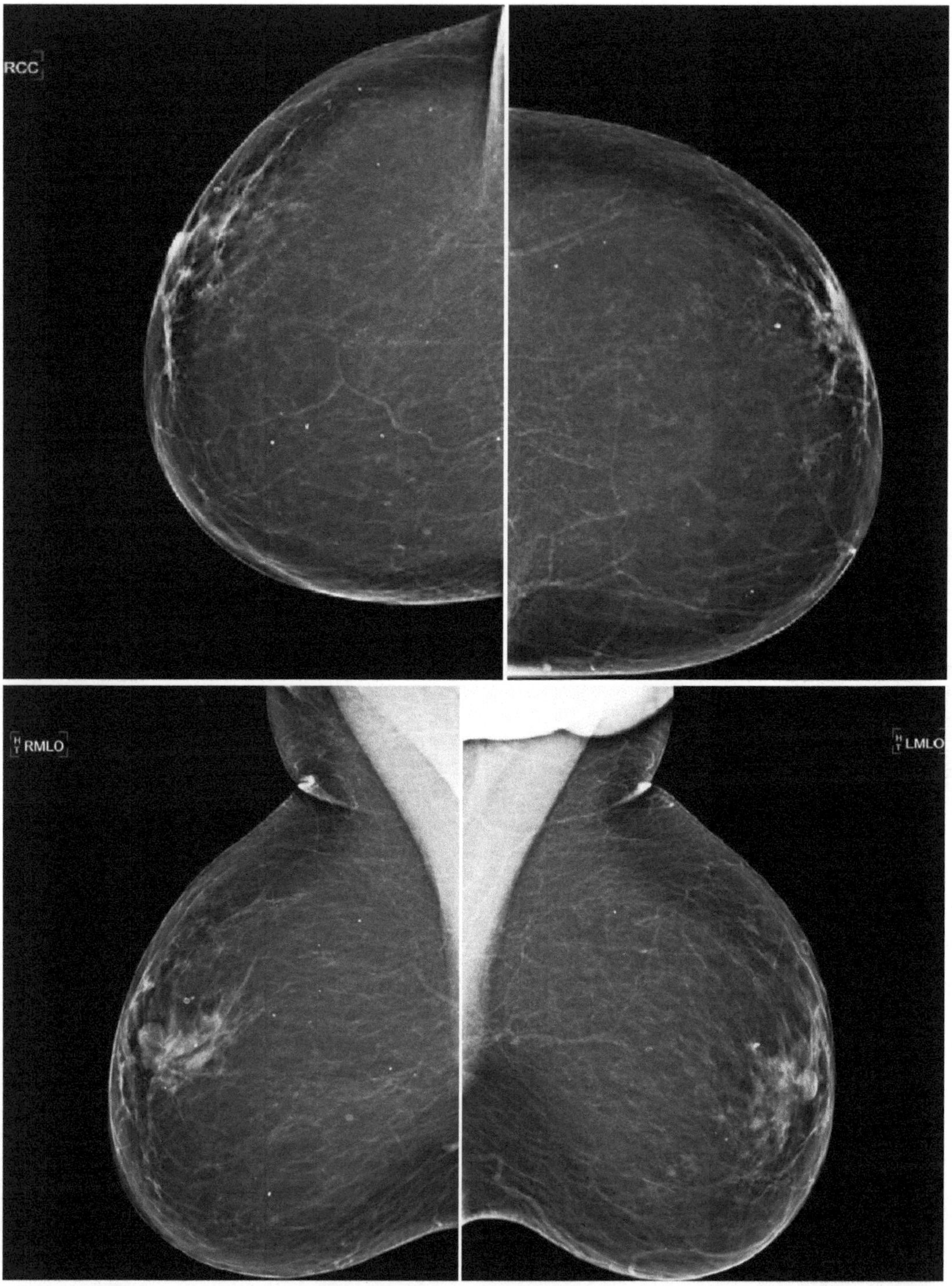

Fig. 35.10 Moderate images. The nipples are not in profile on the MLO views but distinguishable from retroareolar tissue and are in profile on the CC views. Nipples are not at 90° from chest wall on the CC views and the images are not asymmetric. The crease on the lateral aspect of the right CC is obscuring a little breast tissue as is the artefact across the top of the left MLO. The creases in both axillas are minor. The IMF on the right is not clearly demonstrated. Most of the breast tissue is imaged therefore, these images do not need to be repeated. **Learning points**: ensure the position of the breast for the CC's is central to the field of view to avoid asymmetry. Smooth crease as described in Figs. 35.5 and 35.7 above. If nipples are not in profile and IMF's are not clearly demonstrated the patient may be standing too close to the detector plate. A small side step away from the plate and a little back will enable positioning for the MLO's easier. Ensure the patients chin is held up out of the field of view

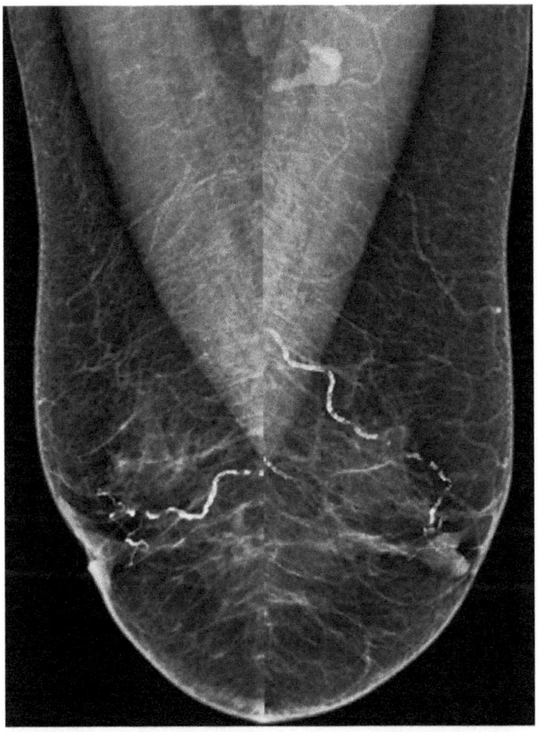

Fig. 35.11 Moderate MLO images. The IMF on both MLO are not clearly demonstrated. The nipple is not in profile on the left and the pectoral muscles are not down to nipple level in both MLO however, there is too much pectoral muscle imaged at the top. Most of the breast tissue is imaged therefore, these images do not need to be repeated. **Learning points**: The detector plate is too high thus causing the patient to be stretched up and standing too close to the plate. This has caused the loss of the IMF. The position of the patients feet is paramount for positioning the MLO views. A small side step away from the plate and lowering of the detector will enable good positioning. The nipple must be in profile on the CC view in this case

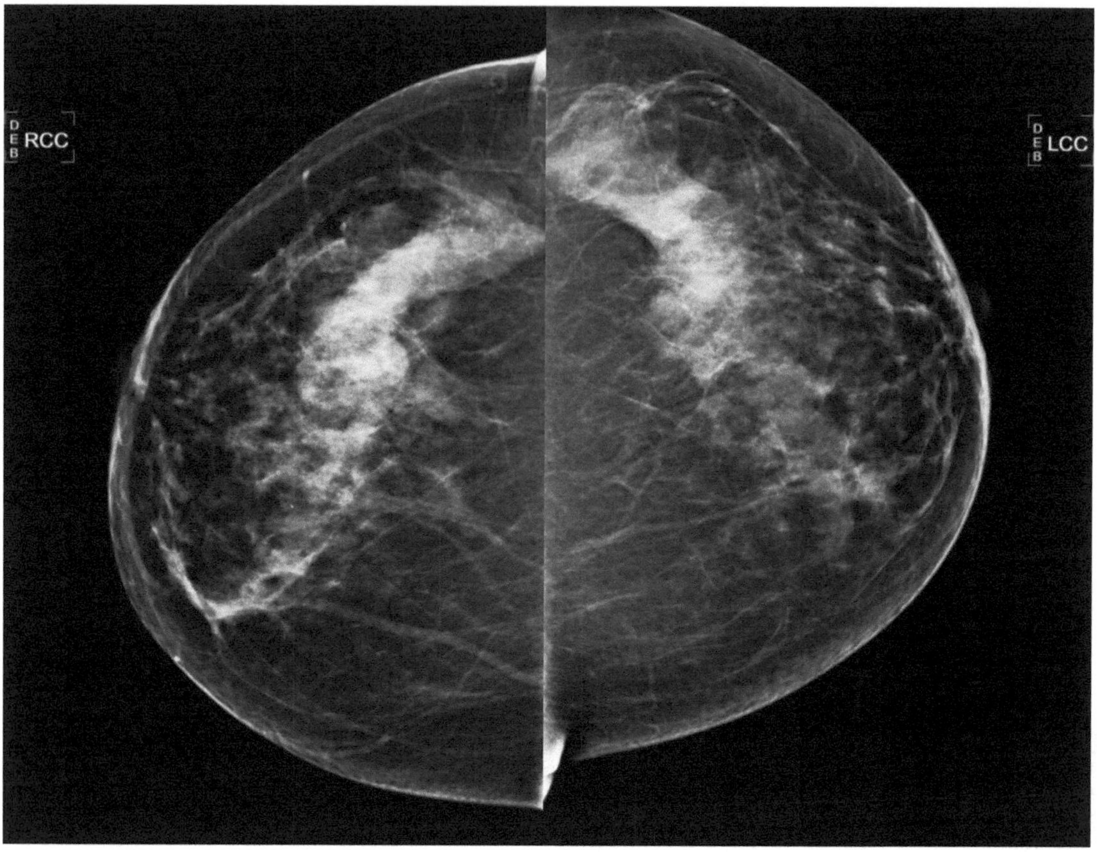

Fig. 35.12 Moderate CC images. A minor amount of breast tissue is missing from the lateral edge of the left CC. This part of the breast will be clearly demonstrated on a good MLO view and therefore does not need to be repeated. **Learning point**: position the breast centrally within the field of view

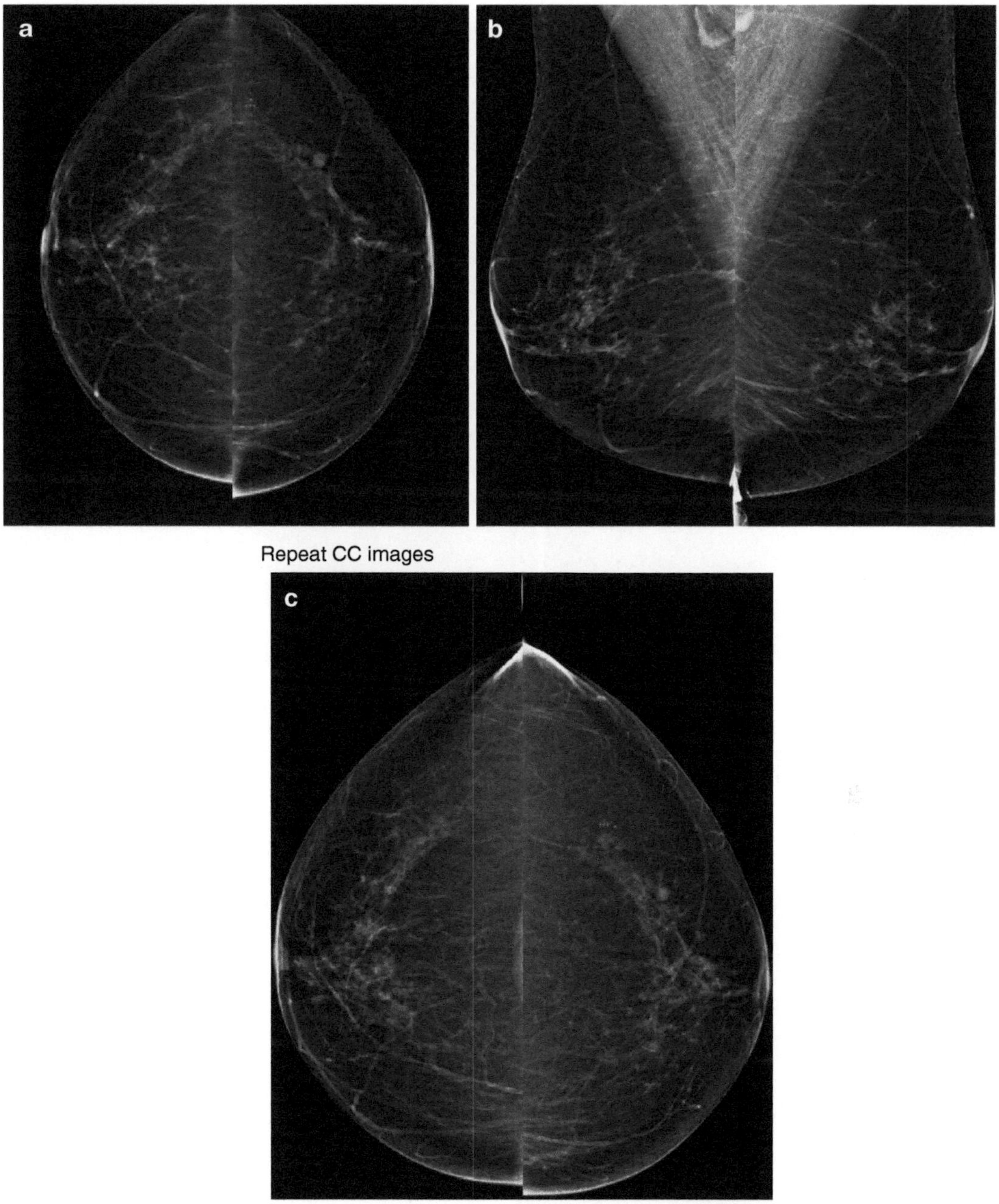

Fig. 35.13 (a–c) Inadequate images. Both of the CC images have breast tissue missing off the back. The right MLO is blurred. Some lesions can only be seen in one view and blurring could obscure small abnormalities such as micro-calcifications therefore these images are inadequate and need repeating. The repeat CC images above demonstrate how much breast tissue was missing from the initial ones

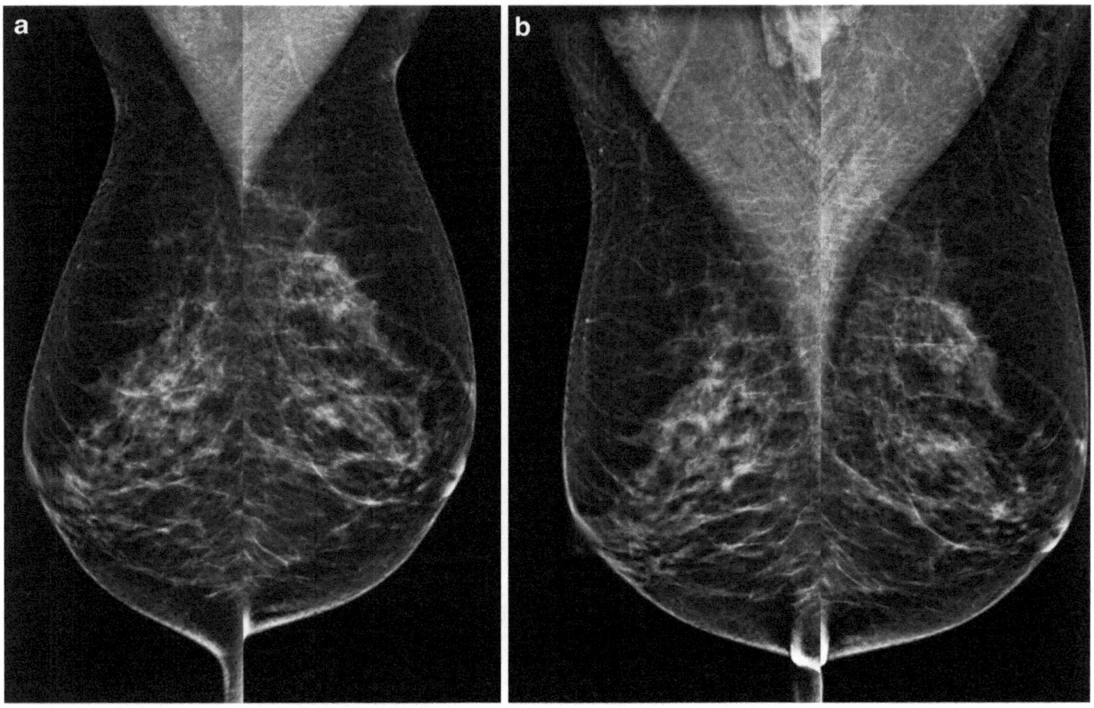

Fig. 35.14 (**a**, **b**) Inadequate MLO Images. The pectoral muscles are not down to nipple level therefore breast is missing from the back on both views. The repeat images (**b**) demonstrate how much tissue was missing from the initial images. **Learning point**: ensure the shoulder is pulled over adequately and the uppermost corner of the detector plate is positioned at the back of the axilla

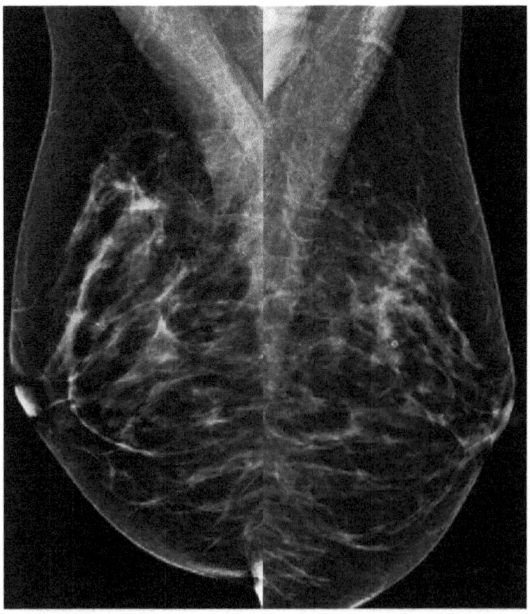

Fig. 35.15 Inadequate MLO images. The images are asymmetrical with breast missing from the bottom of the left MLO thus not demonstrating the left IMF. This image could be repeated. **Learning point**: ensure the feet are in the correct position for both views and that the detector plate is at the correct height. Check that the bottom of the breast is included in the field of view using the light beam. Lowering the lighting in the x-ray room may help

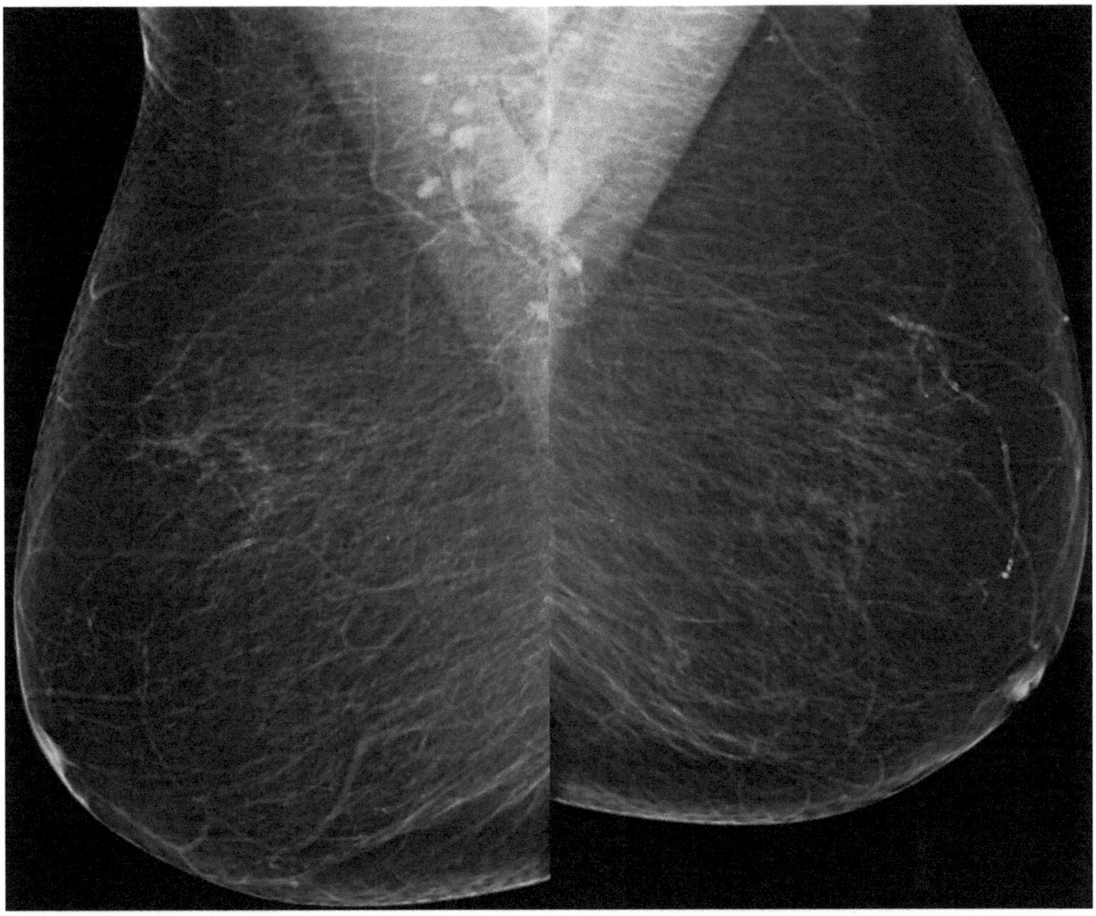

Fig. 35.16 Inadequate MLO images. There is breast missing from the top of both MLO's, particularly the left. The IMF's are not demonstrated and the pectoral muscles are not down to nipple level. There is a significant amount of breast missing from these images therefore these should be repeated. **Learning points**: ensure the detector plate is at the correct height, higher up in this case, and the patient has taken a side step away from the plate. Lift the breast more onto the plate to bring the IMF's into the field of view

References

1. Moreira C, Svoboda K, Poulos A, Taylor R, Page A, Rickard M. Comparison of the validity and reliability of two image classification systems for the assessment of mammogram quality. J Med Screen. 2005;12:38–42.
2. The National Health Service Breast Screening Programme. Quality assurance guidelines for mammography, vol. 63. Sheffield: NHSBSP Publication; 2006.
3. The National Quality Management Committee of Breast Screen Australia. National Accreditation Standards: BreastScreen Australia Quality Improvement Programme, Canberra, 2001.
4. Lee L, Stickland V, Wilson R, Evans A. Fundamentals of mammography. London: Churchill Livingston; 2003. p. 108–9.
5. Hashimoto BE. Practical digital mammography. New York: Thieme; 2008. p. 9.
6. The Society of Radiographers. The scope of practice for assistant practitioners in clinical imaging. London: The Society of Radiographers; 2012.
7. Starr L, Mercer C. Peer review – an essential part of learning and development. Symposium Mammographicum, Bournemouth 2014. The Nightingale Centre, University Hospital of South Manchester, 2013.
8. The National Health Service Breast Screening Programme. Collecting, monitoring and reporting repeat examinations, vol. 4. Sheffield: NHSBSP Publication No. 4, version 2; 2006. p. 10.

Observer Studies in Mammography

36

Peter Hogg, Sara Millington, David Manning, and Hussien Mraity

Introduction

Mammography is a special imaging technique and is unusual in a number of ways: some of these are technical because of the type of tissue under investigation and some apply to the distinctive nature of the client group. But in one important aspect mammography is like all other medical imaging: it requires a decision-making process. All meaningful decisions are made in conditions where information is imperfect or uncertain and mammographic interpretation is no exception to this general rule.

Factors that contribute to this uncertainty can be divided into those that are *image dependent* and relate to the visual clarity (conspicuity) of various features which inform the characterisation of lesions and those that are *image independent*; and relate to what the observer knows about the image information. Quality control tests provide a range of physical procedures that measure presentation of image features. Some of the tests are phantom-based, designed to measure parameters to assess the equipment is functioning to the desired specifications. However, observers interpreting patients' images in radiology sometimes disagree with each other (inter-observer variance) and with themselves (intra-observer variation) on the significance of image features. So a complete appraisal of the clinical quality of a mammogram should include the reader's diagnostic decision in the process.

A clearer understanding of these human factors has evolved through the development of medical imaging observer studies. These are now an important part of assessing technology, imaging methods and reader performance. In this chapter we will look at some characteristics of reliable quality assurance tests using human observers.

What Type of Observer Study to Use?

Before setting out on an observer study it is important to consider first what goals you want your study to achieve. This is in the interests of

P. Hogg (✉)
School of Health Sciences, University of Salford, Allerton Building, Salford M5 4WT, UK
e-mail: P.Hogg@salford.ac.uk

S. Millington
Countess of Chester Hospital NHS Trust, Chester, UK
e-mail: saramillington@nhs.net

D. Manning
Department of Radiography, Lancaster Medical School, Faculty of Health & Medicine, Furness College, Lancaster University, Lancaster LA1 4YG, UK
e-mail: d.manning@lancaster.ac.uk

H. Mraity
Department of Physics, College of Science, University of Kufa, Kufa, Iraq

School of Health Sciences, Allerton Building, University of Salford, Salford M5 4WT, UK
e-mail: hussein.mraity@uokufa.edu.iq; h.a.a.mraity@edu.salford.ac.uk

P. Hogg et al. (eds.), *Digital Mammography: A Holistic Approach*,
DOI 10.1007/978-3-319-04831-4_36, © Springer International Publishing Switzerland 2015

economy because some methods are more complex and time-consuming than others and depend on what question is being posed. We can take examples of some practical questions to indicate appropriate types of study:

1. *You want to know if a brand new, untried imaging method has promise.*

   In this case a simple study using test patterns or phantoms can generate plenty of images quite easily. Three or four non-expert observers can then give a subjective opinion on some aspect of the image that you define such as the resolution or contrast. This can be compared with similar images produced using an established technique to see if there is an agreed, observable difference. The test will show if there is an effect and its magnitude.

2. *You want to know which of several methods of (say) image processing is preferred.*

   Here, clinical images are needed and expert observers to view them. Potentially, many images may be required and, because the method is a subjective assessment, more than one observer is needed. Just how many is a practical as well as a statistical question because in this case skilled judgement and image knowledge is a requirement. Between three and five observers are considered acceptable, each viewing about ten images for each processing condition. Viewing the unmarked, randomly presented images can be quick and subjects are asked to simply state a single preference or to rank them in order. It can be taken a quantitative step further by using a scoring system through visual grading analysis (VGA) of anatomical features.

Assessing Image Quality in the Clinical Setting

Now we will consider how images are appraised visually in the clinical setting, this takes into account anatomical features and visual grading analysis tools. Building on this we critique the current approaches and introduce the notion of validated criteria and validated visual grading analysis scales.

High image quality is critical for the early detection of breast cancer. The subjective nature of some measures of image quality makes a definition difficult unless the diagnostic objective of the examination is clearly specified. However image quality may be evaluated in terms of positioning, adequacy of compression force application, exposure, contrast, sharpness and noise [1–3]. Good radiographic technique is essential to ensure that as much breast tissue as possible is included on the image. Sufficient compression force should be applied in order to spread out the glandular tissue. Optimal exposure factors are important to obtain sufficient image contrast, so producing a suitably noise-limited image. Sharpness is related to a number of factors, including positioning, adequacy of compression force application exposure and an absence of client/equipment motion.

Image Quality Criteria

The UK National Health Service Breast Screening Programme (NHSBSP) suggests the following image quality criteria should be used when assessing medio-lateral oblique (MLO) images [4]

- Whole breast should be imaged
- Nipple in profile
- Correct annotations
- Appropriate exposure
- Appropriate compression force
- Absence of movement
- Skin fold free
- Absence of artefacts
- Symmetrical images (R (right) MLO versus L (left) MLO)

Using the above criteria, Fig. 36.1 illustrates diagnostic quality RMLO and LMLO mammogram images.

Similarly, the NHSBSP advise the following image quality criteria for cranio-caudal (CC) images

- Medial border should be imaged
- Some axillary tail should be present
- Pectoral muscle shadow may be shown
- Nipple in profile
- Correct annotations
- Appropriate exposure

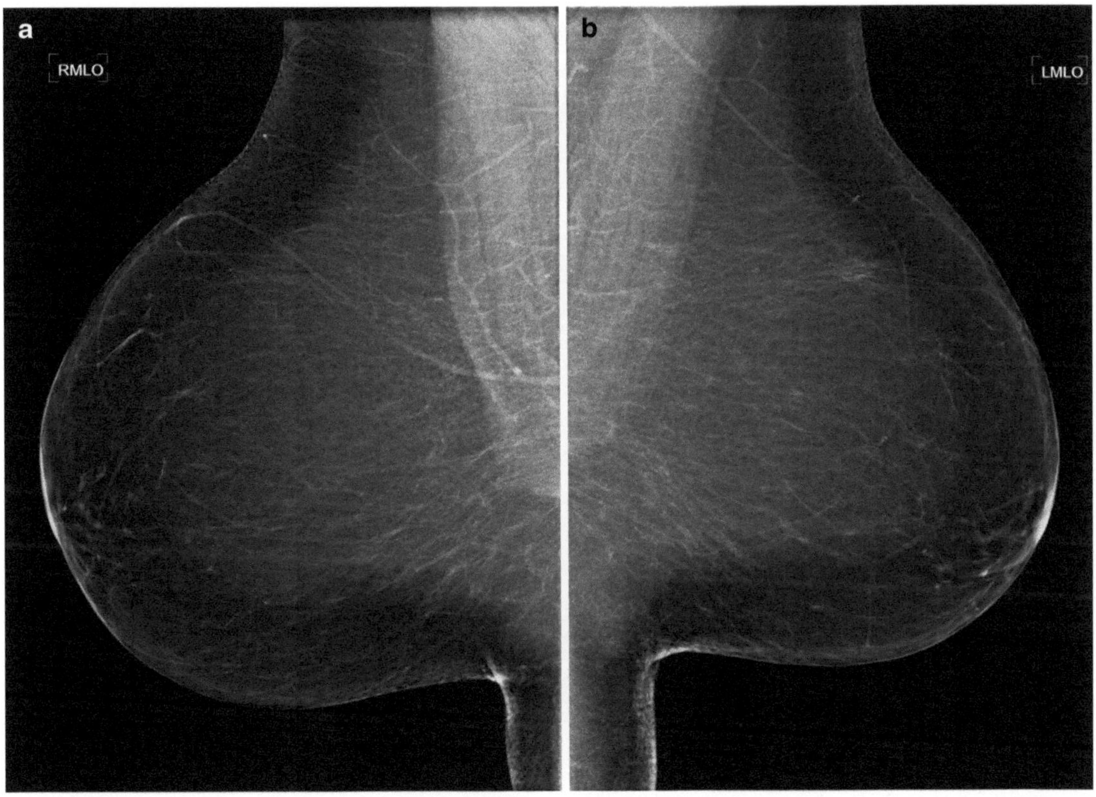

Fig. 36.1 High quality diagnostic medio-lateral oblique images

- Appropriate compression force
- Absence of movement
- Skin fold free
- Absence of artefacts
- Symmetrical images (RCC versus LCC)

Using the above criteria, Fig. 36.2 illustrates diagnostic quality images of RCC and LCC mammograms.

Positioning

Using these image quality criteria, for serial studies (such as in screening), it is advantageous to review previous images, when available, prior to imaging the client. This practice allows previous areas of difficulty to be identified (e.g. thin pectoral muscle or lack of infra mammary angle); furthermore comparison between current and previous mammograms enables the observer to check whether the entire breast has been included. Detailed information on client positioning can be found in Chaps. 21, 22 and 23.

Compression Force

Compression force should be sufficient to separate the overlying structures in the breast, to create a uniform and reduced tissue thickness and to immobilise the breast - thereby minimising the potential of motion unsharpness [5, 6]. The reduced tissue thickness minimises geometric unsharpness and scatter, both of which should enhance image quality. Further discussion on compression force application can be found in Chap. 22.

Exposure Factors

Exposure factors normally determined by the imaging equipment. These are optimised to enable detail in both dense glandular and less dense fatty tissues to be demonstrated, breast tissue to be seen through the pectoral muscle on the MLO projection and the skin edge to be visualised.

See Chap. 16 for further information on exposure factors.

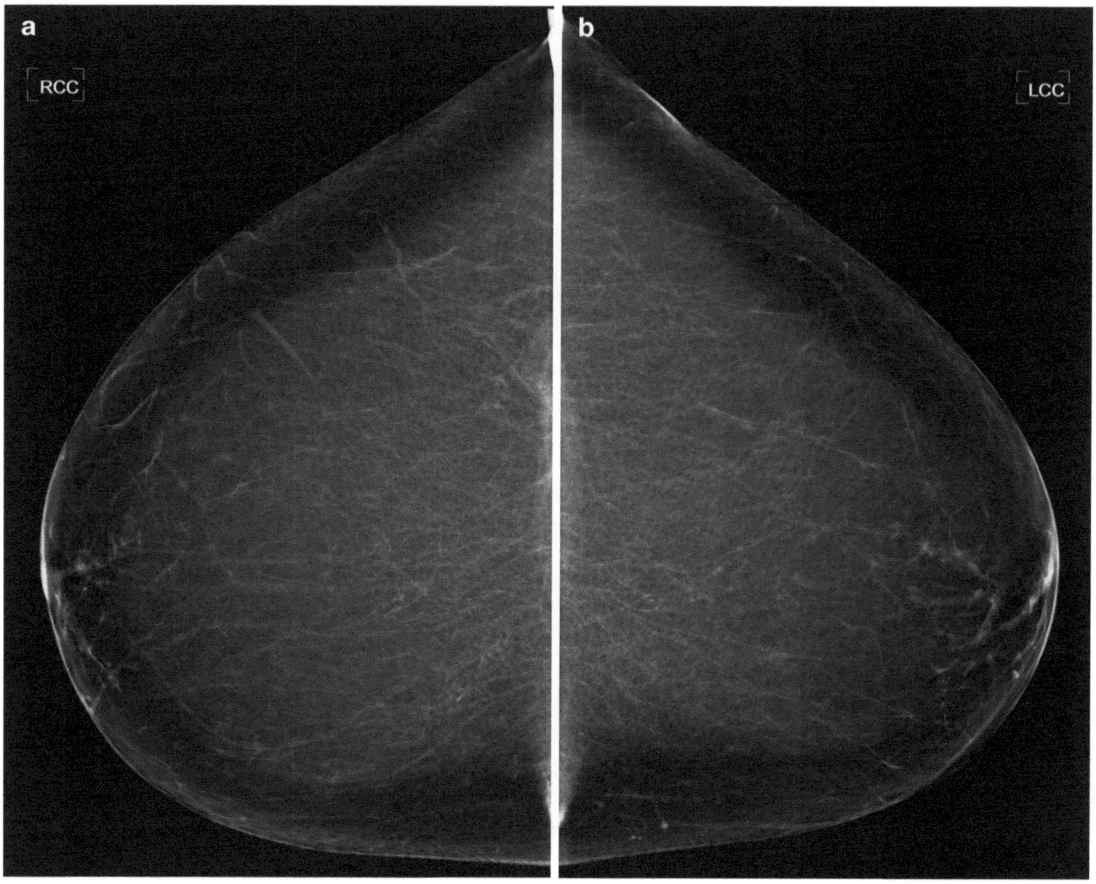

Fig. 36.2 High quality diagnostic cranio-caudal images

Contrast

As developing cancers can have similar density to glandular breast tissue, high contrast is essential to differentiate suspicious features from normal appearances. There are many variables which affect contrast between lesions and surrounding tissue, these include exposure factor optimisation, use of compression force and breast position. Good technique is therefore necessary for adequate lesion visibility.

Sharpness

In the clinical setting, sharpness is related to displaying distinct anatomical features with clear edges. Lack of sharpness increases the risk of low density lesions being missed and some features being incorrectly characterised. The sharpness of an image is related to all of the following: [7, 8]

- Client motion
- Contrast
- Physical characteristics of the image detector

Noise

Noise gives the image a grainy, mottled appearance and can obscure or even mimic small lesions. If noise is present then the perception of microcalcifications can be challenging. Further information about noise can be found in Chap. 16.

Visual Grading Analysis Tools in Mammography

PGMI

Possibly the most well-known visual grading analysis tool is PGMI [9] (Perfect, Good, Moderate, Inadequate). The tool comprises a set of criteria (see below); each criterion is judged as perfect, good, moderate or inadequate. As demonstrated, the criteria consider a broad range of areas which go well beyond the image itself (eg date of examination). Some clinical departments have adapted this tool to allow a numeric visual quality score to be assigned to mammography images, where perfect, good, moderate and inadequate are translated to numbers (eg 4 = perfect; 1 = inadequate). Many journal papers have used adaptations of this scale to visually judge image quality.

1. All breast tissue imaged (fat tissue visualised posterior to glandular tissue)
2. Correct image identification clearly shown
   - date of examination
   - client identification—name and number and/or date of birth
   - side markers
   - positional markers
   - radiographer identification
3. Correct exposure according to workplace requirements
4. Good compression force
5. Absence of movement
6. Absence of artefacts
7. Absence of skin folds
8. Symmetrical images.

Further clarification of point 1 is given for the CC and MLO views: on the CC projection the posterior nipple line (PNL) must be within 1 cm of the PNL on the MLO view the medial border of the breast should be demonstrated, with the nipple in profile and in the midline of the breast. For the MLO projection the pectoral muscle should be a sufficient width and reach nipple level, the infra-mammary fold should be well demonstrated with the nipple in profile and the posterior nipple line (PNL) should be within 1 cm of the PNL on the CC view.

- For an image to be classed as perfect criteria 1–8 must be met.
- Good images meet criteria 1–5 with minor degrees of variation for criteria 6–8
- Moderate images will have most of the breast tissue imaged, the nipple may not be in profile and for the CC images the nipple not in the midline. The MLO images may not have the pectoral muscle down to nipple level but the posterior breast tissue must be demonstrated and the IMF may not be well demonstrated. Criteria 2–5 must be met, artefacts and skin folds which do not obscure the breast tissue fall into the moderate category along with asymmetrical images.
- Inadequate images may have a significant part of the breast not imaged; incorrect identification; incorrect exposure; inadequate compression; blurring: artefacts or skin folds obscuring the breast tissue.

EAR

EAR (Excellent, Acceptable, Repeat) is another visual grading analysis tool. The criteria are very similar to PGMI, with the addition of 'correct number of images taken'.

All practitioners should regularly review their images both individually and along with their peers as part of Quality Assurance. Self-assessment tools help to ensure that the review is a standardised process.

Many publications have commented on the subjective nature of EAR and PGMI [10, 11], and their usefulness has been questioned. Although countries such as Norway and Australia use PGMI [12], many breast imaging centres in the UK have ceased to use it except in NHSBSP training centres to assess the standards of trainee practitioners. Self-assessment and peer reviewing of images is more routinely used for qualified practitioners. Currently within the UK there is no nationally agreed visual grading analysis tool, however the National Breast Screening QA Centre is in the process of developing a new self- assessment tool to be used with digital images.

Viewing Conditions

Image display devices are addressed in Chap. 16 but it is important to mention them here in the context of viewing conditions. Image quality should be assessed on monitors that are fit for purpose. The NHSBSP recommend that image display devices capable of at least 5MP (megapixel) resolution should be used when reporting digital mammography images [13]. One area worthy of consideration is within the clinical imaging room, as these acquisition monitors are often used for checking image quality prior to a client leaving the department. They have lower MP values and are not designed to be used for reporting. Importantly, whatever monitor quality is used it is crucial that they are fit for purpose. Ambient room lighting should be dimmed to a consistent value for viewing images.

A Critical Reflection on Image Quality Criteria and Visual Grading Analysis Tools Used in Mammography

An assumption of the ability to detect features representing pathology in radiology is that it is related to image quality - if quality increases then pathology detection should, generally, increase too. Assessment of quality by visual means is clinically realistic and if done adequately it will have valuable implications for the imaging service. However, assessing image quality by visual means can be hard to achieve, if the assessment is to give accurate and repeatable results and if it is going to predict diagnostic performance.

Radiology and radiography literature is plagued with poorly designed and poorly implemented methods of visually assessing image quality. For many imaging procedures European quality criteria highlighting specific anatomical structures have been defined and these are often referred to for research and clinical purposes. Attempts have been made to update and translate these into visual grading criteria suitable for digital imaging. Unfortunately the original European quality criteria can only give an assessment of how well an image will perform for very general clinical tasks and they may be inadequate at predicting diagnostic performance for specific pathologies. Mammography is no different to the rest of radiology and radiography, since more rigorously validated image quality criteria which can be more task specific do not exist.

As we have already seen, within mammography, various clinically important anatomical structures for the mammogram have been identified that carry information concerning the presence of pathology; the ability to visualise these structures is used as a basis for visual image quality assessment. The important underlying assumption with this is the detection of pathology correlates well with the visibility of this normal anatomy.

Building on the criteria, visual grading analysis tools (eg PGMI and EAR) have been created and they remain in common use. The use of such tools, it was hoped, would minimise subjectivity and also offer the potential to provide a numeric value of visual image quality that would correlate with cancer detection. However, similar to the criteria, none of the visual grading analysis tools used in mammography have been validated. For clinical and research purposes there is a need for robust visual grading *scales* to be created and validated. Below we explain one approach on how this might be achieved.

Bandura's [14] theory provides a suitable theoretical basis for visual grading *scale* development and validation [15, 16]. This is because visual image quality evaluation requires interaction between human attitude/perception and physical attributes in an image. Psychometrics, a branch of psychology, deals with measuring human attributes that cannot be measured directly. In this context, the [psychometric] visual grading scale would comprise a set of statements (items) that attempt to measure perception of visual image quality in a valid and consistent fashion. Using Bandura's theory, visual grading scale development and validation comprises several steps.

First, a draft set of quality statements (scale items) is created using generic [17] and mammography specific literature. They would include essential visual anatomical characteristics that should reflect mammographic image quality. Second, a focus group of clinical mammography experts would review and, if required, modify the items. The items are then worded positively (50 %) and negatively (50 %), to minimise affirmation bias. Then, a Likert scale is included for scoring. A Likert scale of 1–5 is suitable, where 1 would be strongly disagree with the item; 5 would be strongly agree with the item. Second, a set of approximately 7 FFDM mammographic image sets, with qualities varying from poor to excellent, are identified through consensus by a panel of experts. Physical measures, such as signal to noise ratio, could be included to assist the selection process. Third, the draft scale is pilot tested with a small number of clinical mammography professionals to identify and correct any ambiguity associated with item wording. Fourth, the scale is used to assess visual quality of the 7 mammographic image sets by suitably trained clinical mammography professionals. To reduce error, at least 150 professionals should do this, resulting in 7×150 completed visual grading scales. Fifth, the data should be analysed statistically to validate the visual grading scale [18, 19]. This analysis can result in several scales being produced, examples could include: 1. Full scale to assess left or right CC/MLO image sets; 2. Full scale for CC only and full scale for MLO only; 2. Shorter scales (with fewer scale items) for '1' and '2'.

Assuming validity and reliability are acceptable then the scale should be published along with its validation data. At this stage the visual grading scale would be ready for clinical and research applications. It is normal practice in psychometrics that further research is conducted on the scale. In the case of mammography, this could include assessing validity/reliability on larger and more diverse mammography image sets. Also the scale could be administered on larger and more diverse groups of observers (e.g. practitioners with differing levels of experience). It is worth noting that the scale may be valuable for assessing trainee radiologists and radiographers, as well as qualified practitioners, in their ability to differentiate between adequate and inadequate image qualities under examination and clinical conditions.

Data arising from visual grading scale points can be plotted on a graph and the area under the curve can be considered as the measure of image quality difference between two (or more) options which are being compared. Data for the two options can then be analysed in a manner similar to that used in receiver operating characteristics (ROC) analysis [20]. ROC will be considered in the next section.

Reader Performance

So far we have considered two potential questions (ie 'you want to know which brand new, untried imaging method has promise'; 'you want to know which of several methods of (say) image processing is preferred'). Now we move to the third and final question in this chapter.

3. *You want to know if changing one aspect of the mammography procedure affects diagnostic performance.*

This is a higher order question and could be applied to a change in the image acquisition method, such as altering the compression force; or it could question the effects of changing the image readers. Regarding reader performance, it can also be applied to monitoring the diagnostic rate of individuals. This has been put into practice in the UK National Health Service Breast Screening Service (UKNHSBSS) through the PERFORMS system of quality assurance [21]. Such an observer study needs to be clear what it is comparing and to make sure the study is as objective as possible. This means that the study design and method is more complex and time-consuming than the previous examples. Real images are needed and the test-set must be rigorously selected to contain a sample representing the range of cases, normal and abnormal, seen in practice. As a rider to this, it would be unwise to have a normal to abnormal ratio in the test set that simulates screening populations. This would have so few positive cases (low prevalence) that it would give poor statistical power to the study in measuring the sensitivity or true positive detection-rate. Observers must be readers with appropriate training and skills to carry out clinical mammography reporting and they are asked to decide whether pathology is present or not in each image in a test set.

Observer Studies: The Basic Paradigm

Observer tests work through the following steps: (1) show images with known truth to observers, (2) record their decisions as correct or incorrect. (3) calculate a chosen figure of merit (FOM) that appropriately credits or penalises observer decisions and (4) the condition with greater FOM is superior. But there are some important features of image and observer selection that should be understood.

Observers

If a study is aimed at determining the diagnostic performance of an individual then the question of how many observers are required is, of course one. But if the question centres on the diagnostic effects of a change in protocol, then the number required for adequate statistical power and minimum bias is greater. About five observers are considered adequate but this value is derived with consideration of the number of images that will be read. Tables have been published for image sample sizes for numbers of observers ranging from four to ten with the corresponding expected statistical power and accuracy [22].

Images

The test set must be made up of a sample of images that fully represent the range of normal and abnormal appearances seen in practice. Ideally, there should be roughly equal numbers of each state and it is important to have subtle pathology as well as more obvious lesions in the set. There must be confirmed certainty of the diagnostic state so that all observer decisions can be measured against the 'ground truth' or gold standard. This is often a challenging task and it is helpful to define beforehand exactly what you mean by 'normal' and 'pathology' in the context of the research question. The method should be a fully crossed design. This means that the same cases must be used across modalities so that the same cases are read, modality A versus modality B. The same readers should be used in the same way so the method then becomes a multiple reader, multiple case (MRMC) paradigm; the most robust possible.

Specific Observer Test Procedures

The Receiver Operating Characteristics (ROC) Method

The ROC method uses a technique taken from Signal Detection Theory (SDT) and has been applied to medical imaging since the 1970s. It works like this. When an observer makes a decision whether an image contains a lesion or if it is normal there are only four possible outcomes to that decision:

True Positive – TP ('yes, pathology is present' when it is)

True Negative – TN ('no, pathology is not present,' when it is not)

False Positive – FP ('yes, pathology is present' when it is not)

False Negative – FN ('no, pathology is not present' when it is)

For each decision the observer is asked to indicate on a rating scale, the level of certainty of that decision. The scale can be a continuous sliding scale but is often a choice on a discrete scale. This may be made between say, 1 (pathology is not present) to 5 (pathology is present). The intervals on the scale from 1 to 5 then indicate the observer's level of confidence in the presence or otherwise of pathology in the image. The actual number of intervals used is a matter of choice but scales of less than 5 are not very precise for curve fitting and 10 is better.

Example: A worked example illustrates how observer decisions are converted to data points on a curve. We will use a 5-point scale to make it simple.

Suppose a test is set up where an observer is shown 200 images in random order; 100 contain a lesion (positives) and 100 have no lesion (negatives). The observer is asked to score each image according to where his decision lies on the scale. So if he is 100 % sure a lesion is present he scores that image as a tick in box 5, but if he is equally sure the image has no lesion he scores it with a tick in box 1. The boxes 2–4 are chosen for different levels of certainty. When all 200 decisions are completed a scale is drawn up by the experimenter using prior knowledge of the ground truth in the test bank:

	1	2	3	4	5	Total
	Lesion not present (normal)	Probably not present (normal)	Unsure	Probably present (positive)	Lesion present (positive)	
Number of lesion images placed in this category	5	10	10	25	50	100
Number of non-lesion images placed in this category	20	40	20	15	5	100

These score categories are then summed from right to left as shown and presented as a percentage of the total of the positive or negative images:

(1+2+3+4+5)	(2+3+4+5)	(3+4+5)	(4+5)	(5)
100 %	95 %	85 %	75 %	50 %
100 %	80 %	40 %	20 %	5 %

The percentage values are then converted to a probability scale (from 0 to 1), and plotted on graph axes as shown in Fig. 36.3 to produce a Receiver Operating Characteristic (ROC)curve.

(1+2+3+4+5)	(2+3+4+5)	(3+4+5)	(4+5)	(5)
1	0.95	0.85	0.75	0.5
1	0.8	0.4	0.2	0.5

The ROC curve is a measure of diagnostic performance that demonstrates the observer's decision thresholds for rating image features as normal or abnormal over a range of true and false positive rates. There are two simple metrics that are commonly extracted from this: the total area under the curve (AUC or Az), or the factor, d-prime (d') as shown in Fig. 36.3. In either case the further the curve extends to the top left hand corner of the graph-space the greater is the performance value; and by producing ROC curves for different conditions it is possible to compare diagnostic efficacy of individuals, groups, equipment or techniques depending on which variables are under fixed control.

The Two-Alternative Forced Choice (2AFC) Method

This method is a close relative of ROC and requires that an observer compares one image with another and makes a decision on whether the images are the same or different. The nature of the difference must be well specified beforehand. The technique has its origins in psychometric efforts to determine a sensory threshold or 'just noticeable difference' (JND) and for vision tasks this was measured as the smallest detectable change in the intensity of a visual signal. It can be used to good effect in medical imaging with a number of variants. Figure 36.4 illustrates a 2AFC task which does not try to reproduce a diagnostic problem but shows an observer exactly where the signal will appear if it is present. In so doing it tests exclusively the observer's ability to detect a signal of known intensity in a noisy background [23].

Adapting the 2AFC principle to mammography images is illustrated if an observer is given a

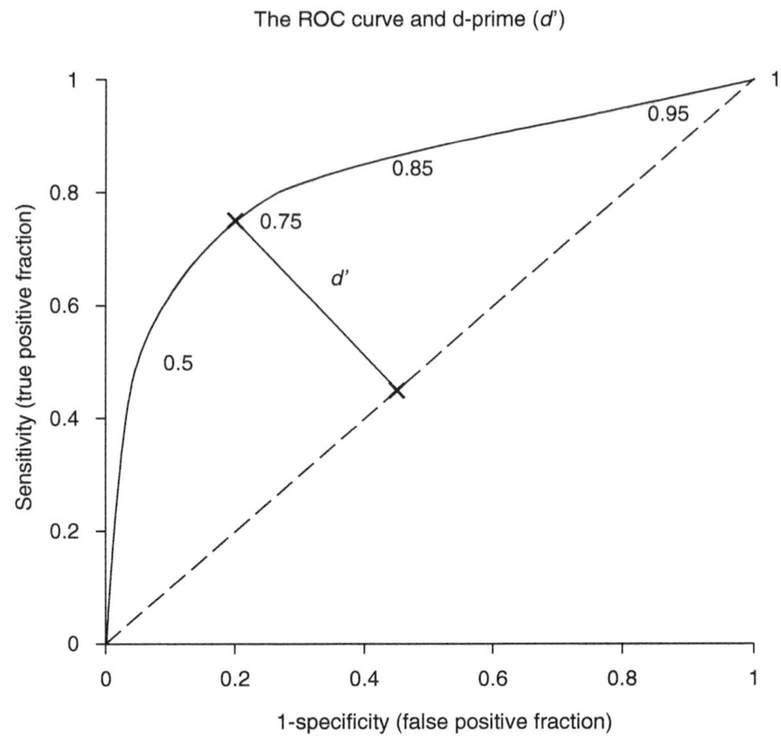

Fig. 36.3 The True Positive Fraction is known as the Sensitivity of the test and is plotted against the False Positive Fraction. The values for the 'lesion present' decisions in the example are shown on the curve. The value *d'* (d-Prime) can be used as a figure of merit to compare one ROC curve with another. More commonly the total area under the curve (*Az or* AUC) is calculated for this comparison

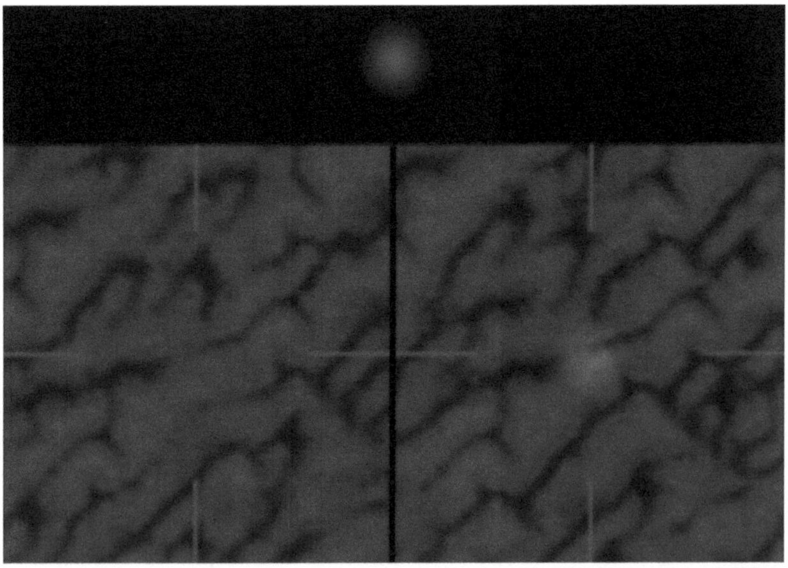

Fig. 36.4 A typical presentation for a 2AFC study. In this case the experiment is a 'Signal Known Exactly' (SKE) design where the observer is guided to the position of the signal by cross-hairs. This isolates the task to one of pure signal detection without search. The signal (*top, centre*) is present in the right hand image in this example and absent from the left hand image Brettle et al [23]

standard, baseline image against which he or she is asked to compare a succession of similar images and to decide for each one if it the same or different. The task usually has a search component because the position of the signal or target for change is not disclosed. This basic model can be made more sophisticated by requiring the observer to score the difference on a pre-defined scale. Such scales can have positive and negative dimensions to accommodate conditions such as 'better' or 'worse' or lesion 'present' or 'absent'. If this is repeated many times the scores can be summed to measure the performance against different imaging conditions or known truth.

It is easy to see that mammography screening uses this principle when the most recent image is compared with that from the last visit. A just noticeable difference is an important threshold in the case management of mammography patients and is implicit in both ROC and 2AFC observer studies.

Summary

Observer studies are well established in medical imaging as a means of measuring diagnostic performance and image quality. By considering the observer as an integral part of the image-diagnosis chain it offers a real world approach to assessing the performance of an imaging method. In some cases it allows analysis of the decision component of the process in the context of the image information presented by the acquisition process. The choice of observer study is an important factor and should be considered as a match for the aim of the investigation. The most rigorous of the observer methods are undoubtedly those using receiver operating characteristic (ROC) techniques or its variants.

References

1. Pushpa T, Vijayalakshmi K, Sulaiman T, Kanaga K. Comparison of image quality criteria between digital storage phosphor plate in mammography and full-field digital mammography in the detection of breast cancer. Malays J Med Sci. 2012;19(1):52–9.
2. Zanca F, Ongeval C, Claus F, Jacobs J, Oyen R, Bosmans H. Comparison of visual grading and free-response ROC analyses for assessment of image-processing algorithms in digital mammography. Br J Radiol. 2012;85(1020):e1233–41.
3. Taplin S, Ichikawa T, Kerlikowske K, Ernster V, Rosenberg R, Yankaskas B, Carney P, Geller G, Urban N, Dignan M, Barlow W, Ballard-Barbash R, Sickles E. Concordance of breast imaging reporting and data system assessments and management recommendations in screening mammography. Radiology. 2002;222:2.
4. Quality assurance guidelines for mammography including radiographic quality control, National Quality Assurance Coordinating Group for Radiography, published by: NHS Cancer Screening Programmes Sheffield. NHS Cancer Screening Programmes. Report 63. 2006. ISBN 1 84463 028 5.
5. Miller J, Diffey J. Audit of Radiography Services Breast Screen South Australia (BSSA), BSSA Review Steering Committee, published by: Department of Health Australia. Digital Mammography System Wide Review. Final Report. 2013.
6. Taplin S, Rutter C, Finder C, Mandelson M, Houn F, White E. Screening mammography: clinical image quality and the risk of interval breast cancer. AJR Am J Roentgenol. 2002;178:797–803.
7. Smith AP. Fundamentals of digital mammography: technology and practical considerations. Hologic, Inc. Bedford U.S.A. 2005. https://www.mmhospital.org/upload/docs/pdf/Fundamentals%20of%20DM.pdf. Accessed 4 June 2014.
8. Samei E. Performance of digital radiographic detectors: quantification and assessment methods. Advances in digital radiography: RSNA categorical course in diagnostic radiology physics. Radiographics. p. 37–47. 25 Feb 2005. http://dx.doi.org/10.1148/rg.252045185. Accessed 5 Jun 2014.
9. Pacifici S. PGMI evaluation system. http://radiopaedia.org/articles/pgmi-evaluation-system. Accessed 3 May 2014.
10. O'Leary D, Teape A, Hammond J, Rainford L. Objective critical appraisal of mammography images in clinical audit: can we achieve this? Breast Cancer Res. 2011;13 Suppl 1:P3.
11. Boyce M, Gullen R, Parashar D, Taylor K. Comparing the use of PGMI scoring systems used in the UK and Norway to assess the technical quality of screening mammograms: a pilot study. Breast Cancer Res. 2012;14(Supplement 1):P41.
12. Moreira C, Svoboda K, Poulos A, Taylor R, Page A, Rickard M. Comparison of the validity and reliability of two image classification systems for the assessment of mammogram quality. J Med Screen. 2005;12:38–42.
13. Commissioning and Routine Testing of Full Field Digital Mammography Systems. NHS Cancer Screening Programmes. Sheffield, NHSBSP Equipment Report 0604. 2009. http://www.screening.org.uk/breastscreen/publications/nhsbsp-equipment-report-0604.html. Accessed 3 May 2014.

14. Bandura A. Social foundations of thought and action: a social cognitive theory. Englewood Cliffs: Prentice Hall; 1986. ISBN 13: 978-0138156145.
15. Mriaty H, England A, Hogg P. Developing and validating a psychometric scale for image quality assessment. Radiography. 2014. doi:10.1016/j.radi.2014.04.002.
16. Mraity H, England A, Akhtar I, Aslam A, De Lange, R, Momoniat H, Nicoulaz S, Ribeiro A, Mazhir S, Hogg P. Development and validation of a psychometric scale for assessing PA chest image quality: a pilot study. Radiography. 2014. http://dx.doi.org/10.1016/j.radi.2014.03.007.
17. RSNA. RadLex: a lexicon for uniform indexing and retrieval of radiology information resources. 2010 [cited 2013 Jan 10]. Available from: http://www.rsna.org/radlex/.
18. Spector P. Summated rating scale construction – an introduction. Newbury Park: Sage Publications; 1992. ISBN 13: 978-0803943414.
19. Abell N, Springer DW, Kamata A. In: Tripodi T, Dattalo P, Thyer BA, Danto EA, Harrington A, Webster JM, et al., editors. Developing and validating rapid assessment instruments. Oxford: Oxford university press; 2009.
20. Bath M, Månsson LG. Visual grading characteristics (VGC) analysis: a non-parametric rank-invariant statistical method for image quality evaluation, 2006. Br J Radiol. 2007;80:169–76.
21. Gale AG. "Maintaining quality in the UK breast screening program", In Manning DJ & Abbey C (Eds.) Proc. SPIE Medical Imaging 2010: Image Perception, Observer Performance, and Technology Assessment. 2010, 7627, 1–11. Pub. SPIE Bellingham Wa. USA.
22. Obuchowski N. Sample size table for receiver operating characteristic studies. AJR Am J Roentgenol. 2000;175:603–8.
23. Brettle DS, Berry E, Smith MA. The effect of experience on detectability in local area anatomical noise. Br J Radiol. 2007;80:186–93.

Bibliography and Further Reading

Berlin L. Errors of omission. AJR Am J Roentgenol. 2005;185:1416–21.

Berlin L. Accuracy of diagnostic procedures: has it improved over the last five decades? AJR Am J Roentgenol. 2007;188:1173–8.

Eddy D. Probabilistic reasoning in clinical medicine. In: Kahnman D, Slovic P, Tversky A, editors. Judgement under uncertainty. Cambridge: Cambridge University Press; 1993.

Gale AG, Scott H. Measuring radiology performance in breast screening. In: Michell M, editor. Contemporary issues in cancer imaging – breast cancer. Cambridge: Cambridge UP; 2010.

Hanley JA, Mcneil BJ. The meaning and use of the area under a receiver operating characteristic(ROC) curve. Radiology. 1982;143:29–36.

Hendee WR, Wells PNT. The perception of visual information. New York: Springer; 1993.

Metz CE. Basic principles of ROC analysis. Semin Nucl Med. 1978;8:283–98.

PERFORMS: personal performance in mammographic screening. Performs AVRC Loughborough University UK. https://performs.lboro.ac.uk/.

Samei E, Krupinski EA. The handbook of medical image perception and techniques. Cambridge: Cambridge University Press; 2010.

Index

A

Absorbed dose, 153–154
AEC. *See* Automatic exposure control (AEC) system
ALARA principle, 153
Amyloid tumour, 34, 36
Asymmetrical density imaging, 215–216
ATEC® VAB systems, 258, 259
Atypical ductal hyperplasia (ADH), 44–45
Atypical lobular hyperplasia (ALH), 44–45
Automatic exposure control (AEC) system, 134, 146–147

B

Bariatric surgery
  CC view, 231, 232
  client care, 231
  for larger breasts, 232
  MLO view, 231, 232
Bilateral dual-energy technique
  CC view, 265, 266
  CESM dose, 265
  MLO view, 266
BI-RADS. *See* Breast imaging reporting and data system (BI-RADS)
Body mass index (BMI), 14
Breast anatomy
  embryology and development, 3–4
  external and internal structures, 4, 5
  innervation, 7
  involuted breast, 9
  lymphatic drainage, 7–8
  macroscopic anatomy
    axillary tail, 5
    fibrous septae and connective tissue stroma, 5
    glandular component, 5
    internal components, 5, 6
    intralobular and interlobular ducts, 5
    superficial and deep layer, 5
    Tail of Spence, 5
  microscopic anatomy, 6–7
  modification, 3
  physiological changes, 3
  pregnancy and lactation, 8
  vascular supply, 7
Breast augmentation
  client expectations, 228–229
  complications, 228
  Eklund technique, 225, 228
  imaging protocols, 224
  implant rupture, 223
  injectable fillers, 229
  radiographer, 223–224
  subglandular placement
    CC view, 225, 226
    MLO view, 225
  subpectoral placement, 224, 225, 227
Breast cancer
  alcohol consumption, 21
  breast density, 19
  clinical examination and patient medical history, 50
  clinical signs and symptoms, 49
  exogenous hormones
    benign breast conditions, 20
    ionising radiation exposure, 20–21
    oral contraceptives/HRT, 20
  genetic risk factors, 18–19
  history, 19
  imaging/radiological assessment, 50
  incidence rates, 17, 18
  lifetime risk (females), 17
  location, 50
  menstrual periods, 20
  mortality rates, 17
  multidisciplinary team, 51
  parity, 20
  pathology assessment, 50
  patient's experience
    chemotherapy, 78, 81, 82
    clinical visit, 78, 79
    diagnosis, 77–78
    infections, 81
    lump, discovery of, 77
    lumpectomy, 79–80
    mastectomy, 80
    radiotherapy, 79, 80, 82
    reconstruction, 80
  physical activity, 21
  referrals, 50

P. Hogg et al. (eds.), *Digital Mammography: A Holistic Approach*,
DOI 10.1007/978-3-319-04831-4, © Springer International Publishing Switzerland 2015

Breast cancer (*cont.*)
  socio-economic status, 19
  uncertain risk factors
    diet, 21
    medications and medical condition, 21–22
    night/shift work, 21
    smoking and passive smoke, 21
  unchangeable risk factors, 18
Breast conserving surgery (BCS), 232
Breast cysts, 172
Breast density
  age, 11, 14
  BMI, 14
  density classification, 12
  focal abnormality, 11, 15
  focal lesion
    dense breast, 13
    fatty area of breast, 13, 14
    mixed breast, 13
  hormonal status, 14
  lifestyle factors, 14–15
  malignant and benign breast disease, 15
  pregnancy and lactation, 14
  PROCAS study, 13
  structure, 11–12
Breast imaging reporting and data system (BI-RADS), 12, 19, 22, 157, 164
Breast Screening Programme, 275

C
Calcifications
  coarse/popcorn, 42, 43
  ductal calcifications, 42
  lobular, 40, 41
  skin, 42, 43
  vascular calcifications, 42
CC view. *See* Cranio-caudal (CC) view
CEDM. *See* Contrast enhanced digital mammography (CEDM)
Charge-coupled devices (CCD), 133–134
Cleavage projection, 205–206
Client–practitioner interactions
  assessment clients, 97
  breast clinic experience, 100–101
  client engagement, 100
  difficult conversations, 102
  incident screen, 100
  interventional procedures, 102
  interventions, 101–102
  practitioner strategy
    client empowerment, 99
    compression techniques, 100
    quality diagnostic images, 99
    rapid assessment, 99
    'tribal' cultural influences, 100
  prevalent screen, 100
  screening experience, 98–99
  symptomatic/screening clinic, 97
Clinical history
  breast surgery, 172–173
  imaging modality, 172
  initial client contact, 171
Compression force, 295. *See also* Mechanical compression
  balance
    CC view, 177–179
    MLO, 179–188
  pressure, 176
  screening mammography, 176
Compression views. *See* Coned compression views
Computed radiography (CR), 132–133
Coned compression views
  asymmetrical density, 215–216
  focal compression paddle, 213
  mammographic technique
    localising abnormal area, 213–214
    positioning, 214–215
Continuous professional development (CPD)
  good images, 279–282
  inadequate images, 287–289
  moderate images, 283–286
  perfect images, 277–278
Contrast agents. *See* Iodinated contrast agents
Contrast enhanced digital mammography (CEDM)
  bilateral dual-energy technique
    CC view, 265, 266
    CESM dose, 265
    MLO view, 266
  clinical applications, 268
  high and low energy images, 264
  iodinated contrast agents
    allergic reactions, 267–268
    concentrations, 266–267
    contrast medium nephrotoxicity, 267
    extravasation, 268
    interaction with thyroid gland, 267
  iodine uptake, 264
  side effects and reactions, 268
  temporal subtraction technique, 264
Cranio-caudal (CC) view
  breast on image receptor placement, 178
  check list, 184
  compression force application, 177
  extended (cleopatra), 204
  initial client position, 177
  inverted, 207–208
  laterally extended, 203–204
  medially extended, 204
  nipple position, 178
  problem solving, 184
  raising breast, 178
Cysts, 27–28

D
Digital breast tomosynthesis (DBT), 138
  advantages, 249

compression force, 248
dose estimation, 157–158
FFDM platform, 247–249
filtered back projection, 242
future aspects, 245
glandular tissue detection, 241, 242
image acquisition, 138, 139
image interpretation, 139–140
indications
asymmetry, distortions/masses, 244
cancer detection, 242–243
factors, 243–244
microcalcification, 244–245
iterative reconstruction, 242
principle of, 241
radiation dose, 140
reconstruction, 138–139
"step and shoot" method, 241
Digital health
DSN (*see* Digital social network (DSN))
healthcare access, 105
information access, 105
key performance indicators (KPIs), 107
medical apps, 106
mobile devices, 105–106
NHSBSP website, 106
social media, 106
symptomatic service-users, 106
technological developments, 105
Digital social network (DSN)
anxiety reduction, 108
development, 108–110
online appointments, 107–108
post examination, 108
pre-examination, 107
professional social networking, 108
Disabled clients. *See* Limited mobility clients
Disease progression
atypical and in situ disease, 56
cell adhesion, 54
cell communication, 54
cell death, 54
cell reproduction, 54
cell specialization, 54
hallmark features, 54
invasive tumour, 57
local invasion, 55
metastasis, 55–56
metastatic spread, 57
neoplastic cells, 53
oncogenes, 53
regional nodes, 57
tumour establishment, 54–55
tumour suppressor genes, 53
DSN. *See* Digital social network (DSN)
Ductal carcinoma in situ (DCIS), 45, 56, 239
Duct ectasia, 37–38
Dutch breast cancer screening program, 190

E
Eklund technique, 225, 228
Emotional intelligence (EI)
ability model, 90
anxiety
facial expressions, 92–93
recognising anxiety, 93
reducing anxiety, 93–94
controlled experimental design, 92
definition, 89–90
Greater Good site, 92
mixed model, 90
negative emotions/feelings, 89
nursing, 91
physiotherapy, 91
radiography, 91–92
trait model, 90, 91
EnCore Enspire® VAB system, 258, 259
European Federation of Organisations in Medical Physics (EFOMP), 143, 144
European Free Trade Association (EFTA), 72
European Pressure Ulcer Advisory Panel (EPUAP), 119
European Protocol (EP), 143
Excellent, Adequate, Repeat (EAR) grading system, 295

F
Fat necrosis
lucent "bubbles," 39, 40
oil cysts, 38, 40
with/without wall calcifications, 38, 40
FFDM. *See* Full-field digital imaging (FFDM)
Fibroadenoma
juvenile, 27
lactating adenomas, 27
lobulated masses, 27, 28
ovoid, 27, 28
tubular adenomas, 27
typical popcorn-shaped pattern, 27, 29
well-defined round mass, 27, 28
Fibrocystic changes, 44
Focal fibrosis, 42, 44
Full-field digital imaging (FFDM)
DBT, 247–249
MGD estimation
BI-RADS category, 157
c-factor, 156–157
conversion factors, 154–155
g-factor, 155–156
s-factor, 157
typical target-/filter-combinations, 155

G
Galactocele, 33
Greyscale standard display function (GSDF), 135–136
Gynaecomastia
dendritic growth pattern, 30, 31
diffuse pattern, 30

Gynaecomastia (*cont.*)
  endogenous hormonal imbalance, 30
  firm and palpable subareolar mass, 30
  florid phase, 30, 31
  heterogenously dense breast tissue, 30, 32
  hormone producing tumours, 30
  male mammography, 239
  nodular pattern, 30
  obesity, 30
  pseudogynecomastia, 31, 32
  systemic disease, 30

H
Haemangioma, 28, 30
Haematoma, 33, 35
Half value layer (HVL), 155–156
Hamartoma, 31–32, 34
Hormone replacement therapy (HRT), 172–173
HVL. *See* Half value layer (HVL)

I
Image quality assessment
  assessment form, 275–276
  audit procedures, 275–276
  clinical setting
    client positioning, 293
    compression force, 293
    contrast, 294
    exposure factors, 293
    NHSBSP criteria, 292–294
    noise, 294
    sharpness, 294
  CPD application
    good images, 279–282
    inadequate images, 287–289
    moderate images, 283–286
    perfect images, 277–278
  grading system, 273–274
  monitor quality, 296
  observer test
    2AFC principle, 299–301
    ROC method, 298–300
  peer review, 274
  PERFORMS system, 297
  using phantoms, 149–150
  QA visits, 275
  quality standards, 273
  repeat images, 274
  technical recall, 274
  technical repeat, 274
  VGA tool (*see* Visual grading analysis)
Implants. *See* Breast augmentation
Institute of Physics and Engineering in Medicine (IPEM), 143
International Atomic Energy Agency (IAEA), 143, 144
Interventional procedures. *See also* Stereotactic image guided interventional techniques
  biopsy diagnosis, 251
  calcification, 252
  contraindications, 253
  localisation procedures, 252, 254
  methods, 251
  stereotaxis, 251, 253
  3D perception, 252
Invasive ductal carcinoma, 239–240
Invasive lobular carcinoma, 239–240
Iodinated contrast agents
  concentrations, 266–267
  side effects
    allergic reactions, 267–268
    contrast medium nephrotoxicity, 267
    extravasation, 268
    interaction with thyroid gland, 267

K
Key performance indicators (KPIs), 107
Kinetic energy released per unit mass (kerma), 153–154

L
Lateromedial projection, 205
Likert scale, 297
Limited mobility clients
  disability, defined, 234
  patient care, 236–237
  risk factors, 235
  technical points, 235–236
Lipoma, 32, 35
Lobular carcinoma in situ (LCIS), 45, 56
Lymphoma, 37

M
Magnification views
  magnification table, 211
  mammographic technique
    localising abnormal area, 213–214
    positioning, 214–215
  microcalcification, 211
  paddle selection, 212
  pleomorphic microcalcification, 216–218
Male breast cancer
  ductal carcinoma in situ (DCIS), 239
  vs. female breast cancer, 239
  gynaecomastia, 239
  mammography, 240
  risk factors, 239–240
Mammographic breast screening
  acceptable and desirable quality levels, 67
  accreditation and certification, 72, 74
  assessment, 60
  communication, 71
  examination, 70
  implementation, 68

lead time bias, 59–60
meta-analysis, 60
mortality, 60
organization models
centralised/decentralized organisation, 69
disadvantages, 68
geographically spread units, 69
grey screening, 70
image reading, 69
intervals, 68
mobile and stationary units, 69
participation rates, 69
screening test, 68
target population, 68
overdiagnosis
definition, 63
estimation, 64
hypothetical cumulative incidence, 63, 64
statistical methods, 65
valid method, 64
quality assurance, 70–71
radiographers training programs, 71–74
recall rate, 62–63
risk of dying, 59, 61
Mammographic density (MD)
cancerous tissue, 163
fully automated method, 165–166
risk estimation, 163–164
semi-automated methods, 164–165
subjective classification, 164
Mammographic technique
cleavage projection, 205–206
extended CC (cleopatra) projection, 204
inverted CC projection, 207–208
laterally extended CC projection, 203–204
lateromedial projection, 205
medially extended CC projection, 204
mediolateral axillary tail projection, 206
mediolateral projection, 204–205
nipple, profile projection, 206–207
rolled projection, 208–209
skin lesions, 208
Mammography equipment
AEC system, 134
amorphous selenium, 131
CCD, 133–134
compression paddle
advantage, 128
biopsy compression plate, 129, 130
compression force, 130
disadvantage, 128
flat rigid paddle, 129
magnification compression plate, 129
pressure reduction, 130
sliding compression plate, 129
S.O.F.T, 129–130
spot compression plate, 129
tilting flat paddle, 129
computed radiography, 132–133
digital breast tomosynthesis (DBT)
image acquisition, 138, 139
image interpretation, 139–140
radiation dose, 140
reconstruction, 138–139
digital image, 130–131
goal, 125
greyscale standard display function (GSDF), 135–136
medical-grade display monitors, 135
optimisation, 134–135
quality control (*see* Quality control (QC))
scanned slit linear detectors, 133
scintillator and amorphous silicon, 132
spatial frequency filtering, 136–137
windowing, 136
X-ray photons, 125
X-ray spectrum, 127–128
X-ray unit, 126–127
Mammography Quality and Standards Act (MQSA), 189
Mastitis/abscess, 36
Mayer, Salovey and Caruso Emotional intelligence test (MSCEIT), 90
Mean glandular dose (MGD)
definition, 154
mammography unit, 158
SFM and FFDM estimation
BI-RADS category, 157
c-factor, 156–157
conversion factors, 154–155
g-factor, 155–156
s-factor, 157
target-/filter-combinations, 155
Mechanical compression
absorbed glandular dose *vs.* contact area, 192
benefits, 189
breast thickness *vs.* contact area, 192
breast volume and density, 190, 191
compression force, 191
contact pressure, 190, 191
mammographic monitoring software, 190
Mammography Quality and Standards Act (MQSA), 189
modeled compressions, 192, 193
pressure-standardized compression approach, 190
Mediolateral axillary tail projection, 206
Medio-lateral oblique (MLO) view
check list, 184
IR angle selection, 179–184
problem solving, 186–187
risk of pain, 116
step by step guide, 179
Metastases, 37
MGD. *See* Mean glandular dose (MGD)
Microcalcification analysis, 211
MLO view. *See* Medio-lateral oblique (MLO) view
Monte Carlo techniques, 154
Musculoskeletal disorders (MSKD). *See* Repetitive strain injury (RSI)

N
National Health Service (NHS), 106
National Health Service Breast Screening Program (NHSBSP), 97, 106, 143, 196, 273, 275, 292
National Pressure Ulcer Advisory Panel (NPUAP), 119
Needle localisation (NL), 260–261
Nipple, profile projection, 206–207
Numerical rating scale (NRS), 113, 114

O
Obesity. *See* Bariatric surgery
Oslo Tomosynthesis Screening Trial (OTST)
compression force, 248
digital breast tomosynthesis (DBT), 248–250
Norwegian Breast Cancer Screening Program (NBCSP), 247
PGMI classification system, 248
positioning errors, 248
training process, 249

P
Paddle views. *See* Coned compression views
Pagets disease, 45
Pain
behavioural indicators, 113
cranio-caudal projection, 116
definition, 113
vs. discomfort, 113
importance of, 114
level of compression, 113
McGill Pain Questionnaire, 114
MLO projection, 116
NRS, 113, 114
premedication trail, 115–116
randomised controlled trials, 115, 116
reliable scale, 113
self-report method, 113
valid scale, 113
VAS, 113, 114
VRS, 113, 114
women, risk of, 114–115
Papilloma, 33–35
Peer review, 274
Perfect, Good, Moderate, Inadequate (PGMI) system, 273, 295
Phyllodes tumours, 28, 29
Pleomorphic microcalcification, 216–218
Post-surgical imaging
BCS, 232
client care, 234
distortion, 233, 236
fat necrosis, 233, 235
oedema and skin thickening, 233, 234
technical points, 233–234
UK NICE Guidance (CG80), 232
Pressure ulcers
classification systems, 121
definition, 119
mammography, risk of, 119
management considerations, 121–122
occurrence, 120
predisposing risk factors, 120
prevention, 120–121
Pseudoangiomatous stromal hyperplasia (PASH), 32–33
Psychological considerations
Health Beliefs Model
cause of illness, 83
cost benefit analysis, 84
culturally distinct factors, 85
fewer ethnic-group differences, 85
risk assessment, 84–85
self-examination and clinical consultation, 85
social support, 85
Theory of Planned Behaviour, 85
negative psychological factors
depression levels, 86
emotional impact, 86
false-positives result, 87
fear and anxiety, 86
practical solutions, 86
sense of helplessness, 86
UK-wide evaluation, 86
perception of risk and pain, 83, 84
practitioner's efforts, 83

Q
Quality control (QC)
AAPM TG-18 pattern, 137
acquisition systems, 144
AEC, 146–147
compression force and thickness accuracy, 145
detection systems, 144–145
detector uniformity and artifacts, 147–148
EFOMP guidelines, 143, 144
EP guidelines, 143
IAEA guidelines, 143, 144
image retention evaluation test, 148–149
IPEM guidelines, 143
IQ assessment, 149–150
luminance measurement, 138
NHSBSP guidelines, 143
STP, 145–146
Quantra™ method, 165

R
Radial scars and complex sclerosing lesions, 38, 39
Radiation dose
absorbed dose, 153
ALARA principle, 153
digital breast tomosynthesis (DBT) units, 157–158
entrance dose, 158
kerma, 153–154
measuring purposes, 153
MGD (*see* Mean glandular dose (MGD))
national surveys, 158–159
tube output, 154

Radio-guided occult lesion localisation (ROLL), 261
Receiver operating characteristics (ROC), 298–299
Repetitive strain injury (RSI)
  acquisition workstation
    patient positioning, 198–201
    room design, 198
  column/gantry equipment, 196, 197
  height adjustment equipment, 196, 197
  occupational, causal/contributory factors, 196
  smooth breast compression technology, 198
  symptoms, 196
ROLL. *See* Radio-guided occult lesion localisation (ROLL)
Rolled projection, 208–209
RSI. *See* Repetitive strain injury (RSI)

S
Sarcoma, 37
SCB. *See* Stereotactic core biopsy (SCB)
Schwannoma, 31, 33
Sclerosing adenosis, 44
Screen film mammography (SFM)
  BI-RADS category, 157
  c-factor, 156–157
  conversion factors, 154–155
  g-factor, 155–156
  s-factor, 157
  target-/filter-combinations, 155
Sentinel node biopsy (SNB), 261
SFM. *See* Screen film mammography (SFM)
Signal difference to Noise Ratio (SdNR) method, 146–147
Signal transfer property (STP), 145–146
Skin Tear Audit Research (STAR) Classification System, 121
Skin tears
  classification systems, 121
  definition, 120
  mammography, risk of, 119
  management considerations, 121–122
  occurrence, 120
  predisposing risk factors, 120
  prevention, 120–121
Society of Radiographers (SoR), 196
Specimen imaging
  cabinet houses, 219, 220
  core biopsy calcification, 219–220
  core biopsy report, 219–220
  fixed pathology, 221–222
  surgical excision, 220–221
  types, 219
Stereotactic core biopsy (SCB)
  biopsy needle, 257
  client and breast positioning, 256–257
  informed consent, 256
  prone biopsy system, 256
  sampling, 258
  upright stereotactic system, 256
Stereotactic image guided interventional techniques
  pre-operative needle localisation, 260–261
  ROLL, 261
  SCB (*see* Stereotactic core biopsy (SCB))
  VAB (*see* Vacuum assisted biopsy (VAB))
Stereotactic mammography biopsy system, 251
Stereotaxis, 251, 253
STP. *See* Signal transfer property (STP)
Subglandular implant placement
  CC view, 226
  MLO view, 225
Subpectoral implant placement, 224, 225, 227
Surgical scar, 39–41
Surveillance mammography, 234

T
Temporal subtraction technique, 264
Tomosynthesis. *See* Digital breast tomosynthesis (DBT)
TORMAM phantoms, 149–150
Trait Emotional Intelligence Questionnaire (TEIQue), 90
Two-alternative forced choice (2AFC), 299–301

U
UK Breast Screening programme, 158, 159
UK NICE Guidance (CG80), 232

V
Vacuum assisted biopsy (VAB)
  biopsy sample, 259, 260
  indications, 258
  lateral arm, 259
  types, 258–259
Verbal rating scale (VRS), 113, 114
Visual analogue scales (VAS), 113, 114, 164
Visual grading analysis
  Bandura's theory, 296
  EAR tool, 295
  European quality criteria, 296
  Likert scale, 297
  PGMI system, 295
  ROC analysis, 297
Volpara™ method, 165

FSC
www.fsc.org
MIX
Papier | Fördert
gute Waldnutzung
FSC® C083411

Kolibri 360 GmbH
Ferdinand-Jühlke-Straße 7
99095 Erfurt, Deutschland
produktsicherheit@kolibri360.de